# Objective Measures in Cochlear Implants

**Core Clinical Concepts in Audiology**

*Series Editor*
Brad Stach, PhD

**Basic Audiometry**
*Editors*
James W. Hall III & Virginia Ramachandran

*Pure-Tone Audiometry and Masking* by Maureen Valente, PhD
*Basic Audiometry Learning Manual* by Mark DeRuiter, PhD, and Virginia Ramachandran, AuD
*Speech Audiometry* by Gary D. Lawson, PhD, and Mary E. Peterson, PhD

**Electrodiagnostic Audiology**
*Editors*
James W. Hall III & Virginia Ramachandran

*Objective Assessment of Hearing* by James W. Hall III, PhD, and De Wet Swanepoel, PhD
*Otoacoustic Emissions: Principles, Procedures, and Protocols* by Sumitrajit Dhar and James W. Hall III

**Cochlear Implants**
*Editors*
Terry Zwolan & Jace Wolfe

*Programming Cochlear Implants* by Jace Wolfe, PhD, and Erin C. Schafer, PhD
*Objective Measures in Cochlear Implants* by Michelle L. Hughes, PhD, CCC-A

**Vestibular Assessment**
*Editors*
Ken Bouchard & Virginia Ramachandran

*Vestibular Learning Manual* by Bre L. Myers, AuD

# Objective Measures in Cochlear Implants

Michelle L. Hughes, PhD, CCC-A

Plural Publishing
Inc.
San Diego
Oxford
Melbourne

PLURAL PUBLISHING INC.

5521 Ruffin Road
San Diego, CA 92123

e-mail: info@pluralpublishing.com
Web site: http://www.pluralpublishing.com

49 Bath Street
Abingdon, Oxfordshire OX14 1EA
United Kingdom

FSC
www.fsc.org
MIX
Paper from responsible sources
FSC® C011935



Typeset in 11/13 Palatino by Flanagan's Publishing Services, Inc.
Printed in the United States of America by McNaughton & Gunn



Library of Congress Cataloging-in-Publication Data

Hughes, Michelle L.
Objective measures in cochlear implants / Michelle L. Hughes.
p. ; cm. — (Core clinical concepts in audiology)
Includes bibliographical references and index.
ISBN-13: 978-1-59756-435-9 (alk. paper)
ISBN-10: 1-59756-435-4 (alk. paper)
I. Title. II. Series: Core clinical concepts in audiology.
[DNLM: 1. Cochlear Implants. 2. Evoked Potentials, Auditory. 3. Treatment Outcome. WV 274]
LC Classification not assigned
617.8'8220592—dc23

2012021004

# Contents

# Foreword

*Objective Measures in Cochlear Implants* by Michelle Hughes is the latest addition to the Cochlear Implant component of the Core Clinical Concepts in Audiology series. Dr. Hughes begins by providing us with a thorough historical overview of commercially available cochlear implant systems (Chapter 1), followed by a detailed description of signal delivery with cochlear implants (Chapter 2). These two chapters lay important groundwork for information provided in the following chapters, where she describes both nonphysiological and physiological objective measures. The chapter on nonphysiological measures is a "must read" for all clinicians who work with implant recipients, as it provides an overview of the basic principles of impedance testing, where Dr. Hughes reviews important clinical issues such as short circuits, open circuits, and changes over time. Chapters 4 and 5 provide a brief overview of electrical field potentials and averaged electrode voltages, respectively. In the final five chapters (Chapters 6–10), Dr. Hughes describes physiological measures from different levels of the auditory system in response to electrical stimulation through a cochlear implant, including electrically evoked stapedial reflexes, electrically evoked compound action potentials, electrically evoked auditory brainstem response, electrically evoked auditory middle latency response, and electrically evoked auditory cortical potentials.

We appreciate that Dr. Hughes has taken the time to share her expertise with us, and we are pleased to provide you with this book, which helps us understand the important and complex topic of objective measures with cochlear implants.

Terry Zwolan, PhD
Jace Wolfe, PhD
*Series Editors*

# Preface

This text represents one of the few books ever published dedicated solely to objective measures in cochlear implants. It is designed to provide a strong foundation for many of the basic concepts that underlie physiological and nonphysiological objective measures, and to do so in a clear, straightforward way. When I teach, I rely heavily on that old adage, "A picture is worth a thousand words." So, I have packed this book with as many schematics, pictures, and graphs as possible to clearly demonstrate the concepts described within. Furthermore, each chapter ends with a brief summary of the key points presented. My hope is that I have created a clear, concise tutorial that is useful for students, clinicians, and practicing scientists. This book is by no means exhaustive in its coverage of the topic (after all, I had a page limit). But, I hope that you will find it provides a good foundation for understanding objective measures in cochlear implants, and that you will learn a thing or two along the way.

# Acknowledgments

My friend and mentor, Carolyn Brown, once told me that I should write a book like this. At the time, I laughed and said something like, "Are you crazy? Can you even imagine how hard that would be?" But, it was something that remained in the back of my mind, and I guess I put it on my professional bucket list at that point. Years later when Jace Wolfe called to ask if I'd be interested in writing a book on objective measures in cochlear implants as part of Plural Publishing's Core Clinical Concepts in Audiology series, I thought, Hey, here's an opportunity to make it happen. (I had no idea what I was getting myself into.) But, the process was a beautiful learning experience and one that I truly value. So, thank you Carolyn for believing long ago that I could do something like this, and thank you Jace for asking. I'd also like to thank Mandy Licata at Plural Publishing for being gentle, supportive, and positive throughout this process.

I am deeply indebted to many people who assisted me with this undertaking. For Chapter 1, the following people helped secure photos of old and new internal and external devices, checked facts regarding the history of each manufacturer's devices, and provided permissions to reproduce photos: Mike Brownen, Tracey Kruger, Arlie Adam, Cheryl Garma, Mark Downing, Sharon Smith, and Darci Teobaldi from Advanced Bionics LLC; Susan Trouba and Darla Franz from MED-EL; and Peter Arkis, Barbara Buck, and Mike Leman from Cochlear Americas. Bas Van Dijk (Cochlear Europe) and Prasanna Aryal (Boys Town National Research Hospital) provided feedback on an earlier version of Chapter 3. Filiep Vanpoucke (formerly with Advanced Bionics Europe) provided figures and feedback for an earlier version of Chapter 4. Paul Abbas, Carolyn Brown, and Christine Etler (University of Iowa) provided EABR waveforms for Chapter 8. Shuman He (University of North Carolina-Chapel Hill) provided BIC waveforms from her dissertation work at the University of Iowa for Chapter 8. Karen Gordon and Salima Jiwani (Hospital for Sick Children, Toronto) provided EMLR and cortical waveforms for Chapters 9 and 10. Kelly Tremblay (University of Washington) provided valuable feedback for Chapter 10, and was willing to do so with a *very* short time line. Thank you all so very much.

As for the local crowd: I would like to thank Skip Kennedy from Boys Town National Research Hospital, who always made time for me (also usually on short notice), and Gina Diaz, who helped with literature searches and securing articles. I would also like to extend a special thanks to Jenny Goehring and Jacquelyn Baudhuin of Boys Town National Research Hospital, who generously agreed to read every chapter, and kindly provided feedback on many earlier drafts of the chapters that follow. I appreciate you more than you know. Finally, I would like most to thank my husband Troy, who did more than his fair share of the domestic duties and was always willing to be flexible so that I could finish this project. And, of course, I want to thank our two beautiful children, Owen and Joslyn, for allowing me to take some of "their time" to work on this book. I know it wasn't easy for you. I couldn't have done it without you. Thank you all!

# About the Author

**Michelle Hughes, PhD, CCC-A,** is the Coordinator of the Cochlear Implant Program and Director of the Cochlear Implant Research Laboratory at Boys Town National Research Hospital in Omaha, Nebraska. She is also an adjunct associate professor in the Department of Special Education and Communication Disorders at the University of Nebraska-Lincoln. Her NIH-funded research program is aimed at investigating the relationships between physiological and perceptual measures in cochlear implant recipients. She has published numerous peer-reviewed journal articles on evoked potentials in cochlear implants, and has presented her work nationally and internationally.

Dr. Hughes received her bachelor's degree from the University of Nebraska-Lincoln, and her MA and PhD degrees from the University of Iowa. She has served as a Contributing Editor in cochlear implants for *Audiology Online*, an ad-hoc reviewer for national and international grant institutes, and an ad-hoc reviewer for a number of highly ranked journals. Dr. Hughes currently serves on the editorial board for *Ear and Hearing*, and is a member of the American Academy of Audiology Clinical Practice Guidelines Task Force for Cochlear Implants.

*This book is dedicated to my children,*
*Owen and Josie,*
*who inspire me every day.*

# Part I

## Laying the Foundation

# 1

# The Basics of a Cochlear Implant

## INTRODUCTION

As children receive cochlear implants at increasingly younger ages, the use of objective measures for clinical management becomes ever more important. For the purposes of this book, "objective measures" encompass two general areas: (1) nonphysiological measures (i.e., device function and current fields), and (2) physiological (neural) measures. Objective measures are used to serve a number of purposes:

1. To verify device function,
2. To identify malfunctioning electrodes,
3. To verify the integrity and function of the auditory pathway,
4. To obtain a baseline of neural function for tracking potential changes over time,
5. To assist in programming the cochlear implant sound processor,
6. To measure discrimination of different stimuli, and
7. To measure the plasticity of the auditory system.

The first step in learning about evoked potentials with cochlear implants is to gain a solid understanding of: (1) the limitations of the impaired auditory system, (2) how responses to electrical stimulation differ from those to acoustic stimulation, and (3) the device that delivers stimulation to the auditory system. A cochlear implant is an electronic device that is surgically implanted into the cochlea to provide electrical stimulation to the auditory nerve. The implant bypasses damaged or malformed cochlear structures that would normally convert the mechanical motion of the traveling wave into neural impulses. The cochlear implant is therefore indicated for severe to profound hearing loss secondary to cochlear damage, not neural loss. A critical component for successful cochlear implant use is that there must be a functioning auditory nerve.

This chapter begins with some basic concepts regarding the anatomical changes that follow severe to profound hearing loss. Next, the basic principles of electrical stimulation of the auditory system are discussed, focusing on the primary differences in physiology between acoustic and electrical stimulation. The basic parts and functions of a cochlear implant are described, and more in-depth information about past and current devices for each manufacturer is provided. Finally, although not the focus of this textbook, a brief description of present candidacy criteria is included.

## ANATOMY OF SEVERE TO PROFOUND HEARING LOSS

### The Normal Auditory System

In the normal auditory system, sound waves enter the ear canal (Figure 1–1A), causing the tympanic membrane to vibrate (Figure 1–1B), which in turn sets the ossicles (malleus, incus, stapes) into motion (Figure 1–1C). The stapes footplate is connected to the cochlea via the oval window (Figure 1–1D). As the stapes pushes inward, fluid in the cochlea is displaced, generating a traveling wave. The cochlea is divided into three sections: scala tympani, scala media, and scala vestibuli (Figure 1–1E).

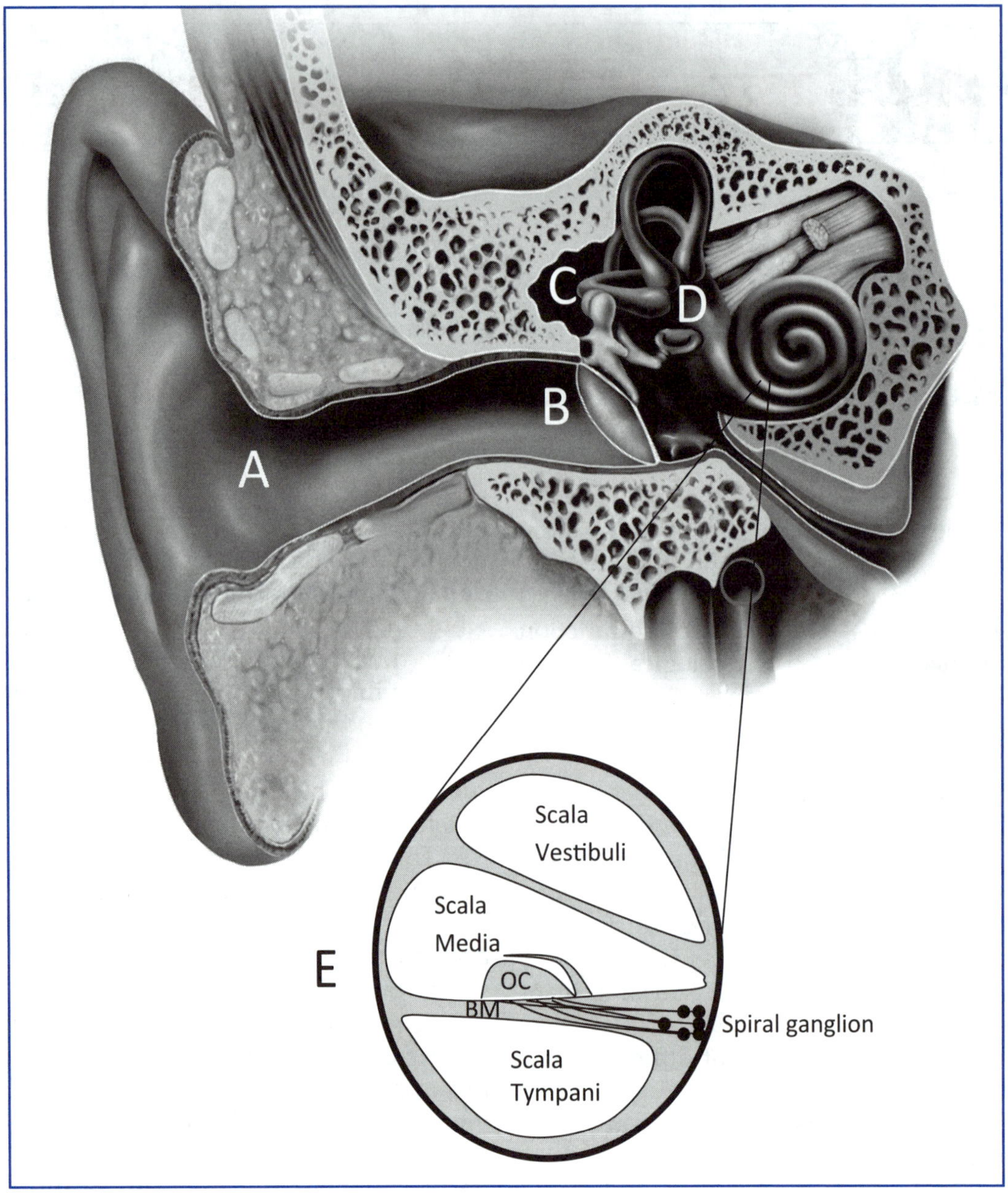


**FIGURE 1–1.** Schematic illustrating the normal auditory pathway. **A.** External auditory canal. **B.** Tympanic membrane. **C.** Ossicular chain (malleus, incus, stapes). **D.** Stapes footplate and oval window, leading to the cochlea. Inset **E.** Cross-section of one cochlear turn. OC: Organ of Corti. BM: Basilar membrane. Illustration of the cross-section of the ear courtesy of MED-EL.

The basilar membrane separates the scala tympani from the scala media. The organ of Corti, which contains inner and outer hair cells, sits atop the basilar membrane (Figure 1–2). As the traveling wave pushes up on the basilar membrane, stereocilia on the tips of the inner and outer hair cells bend open to allow potassium ions to enter the cell, resulting in cell depolarization (Pickles, 1988). Outer hair cells provide active mechanical feedback (via efferent neurons) to amplify the motion of the basilar membrane, resulting in fine frequency tuning. Depolarization of the inner hair cells results in release of neural transmitter, which causes auditory nerve fibers to produce action potentials. These action potentials propagate along the brainstem to the auditory cortex, where the acoustic sound wave is perceived as meaningful sound. In brief, the organ of Corti serves as a transducer that converts the mechanical energy from the traveling wave into electrical neural impulses.

## The Impaired Auditory System

When substantial inner and outer hair cell loss, damage, or dysfunction occurs, as is often the case with severe or profound sensorineural hearing loss, the cochlea loses its ability to convert the mechanical energy from sound waves into neural impulses. The cochlear implant provides a means to generate neural action potentials in lieu

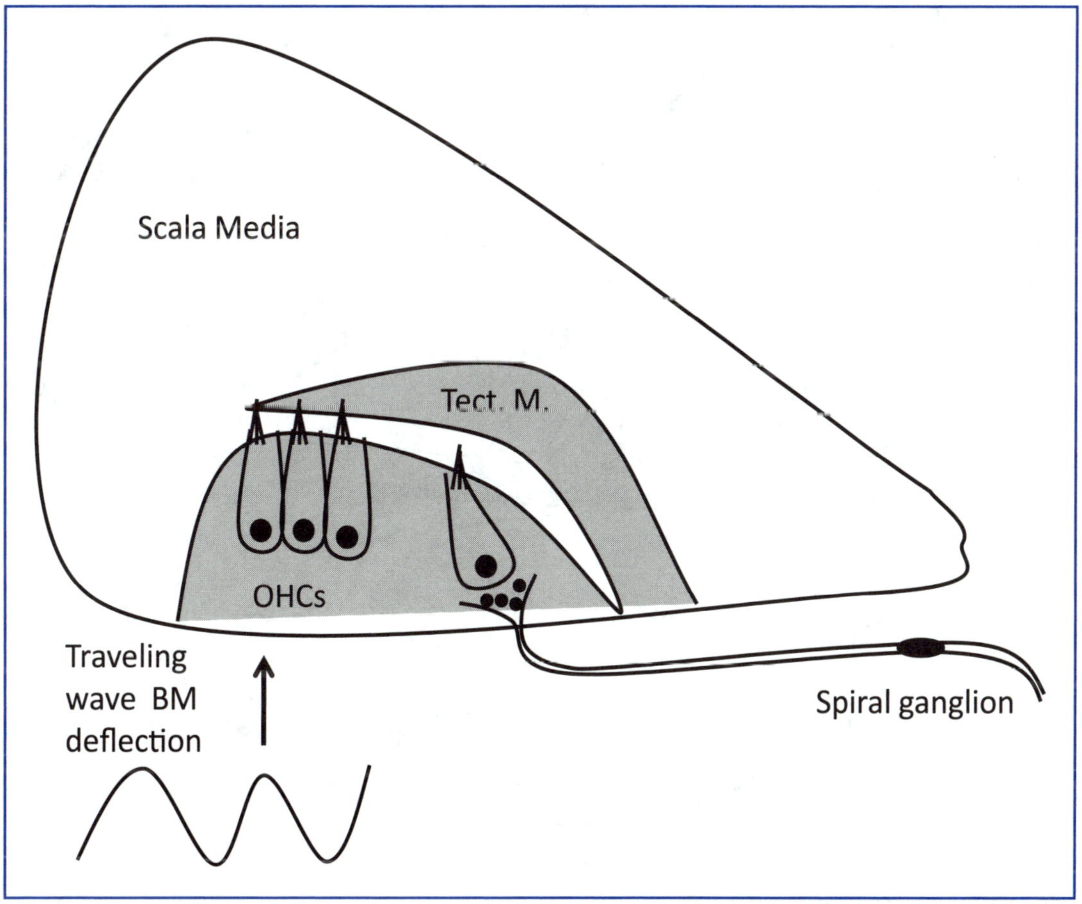


**FIGURE 1–2.** Schematic illustrating normal cochlear function. As the traveling wave pushes up on the basilar membrane, stereocilia on the tips of the inner and outer hair cells bend open to allow potassium ions to enter the cell. This results in the release of neural transmitter, which causes afferent auditory nerve fibers to produce action potentials. (Efferent and afferent fibers for the OHCs are not shown.) OHCs: Outer hair cells. Tect. M.: Tectorial membrane.

of functioning hair cells by depolarizing the auditory neurons directly via electrical current instead of neural transmitter. This process is illustrated in Figure 1–3.

Sensorineural hearing loss is typically associated with a number of peripheral and central anatomical changes. The loss of cochlear hair cells results in the loss of compression and spontaneous activity of auditory neurons. Hair cell loss can also lead to degeneration of the peripheral portion of auditory neurons (Figure 1–4B), reduction in spiral ganglion cell volume (Figure 1–4C), demyelination of the cell body and/or axon (Figure 1–4D), and axonal degeneration (Figure 1–4E) (e.g., Otte, Schuknecht, & Kerr, 1978; Spoendlin, 1975). These degenerative processes can progress over the course of months to several years (Leake & Hradek, 1988). Similar changes have been noted in the central auditory pathway, including cortical reorganization (see Hartmann & Kral, 2004, for a

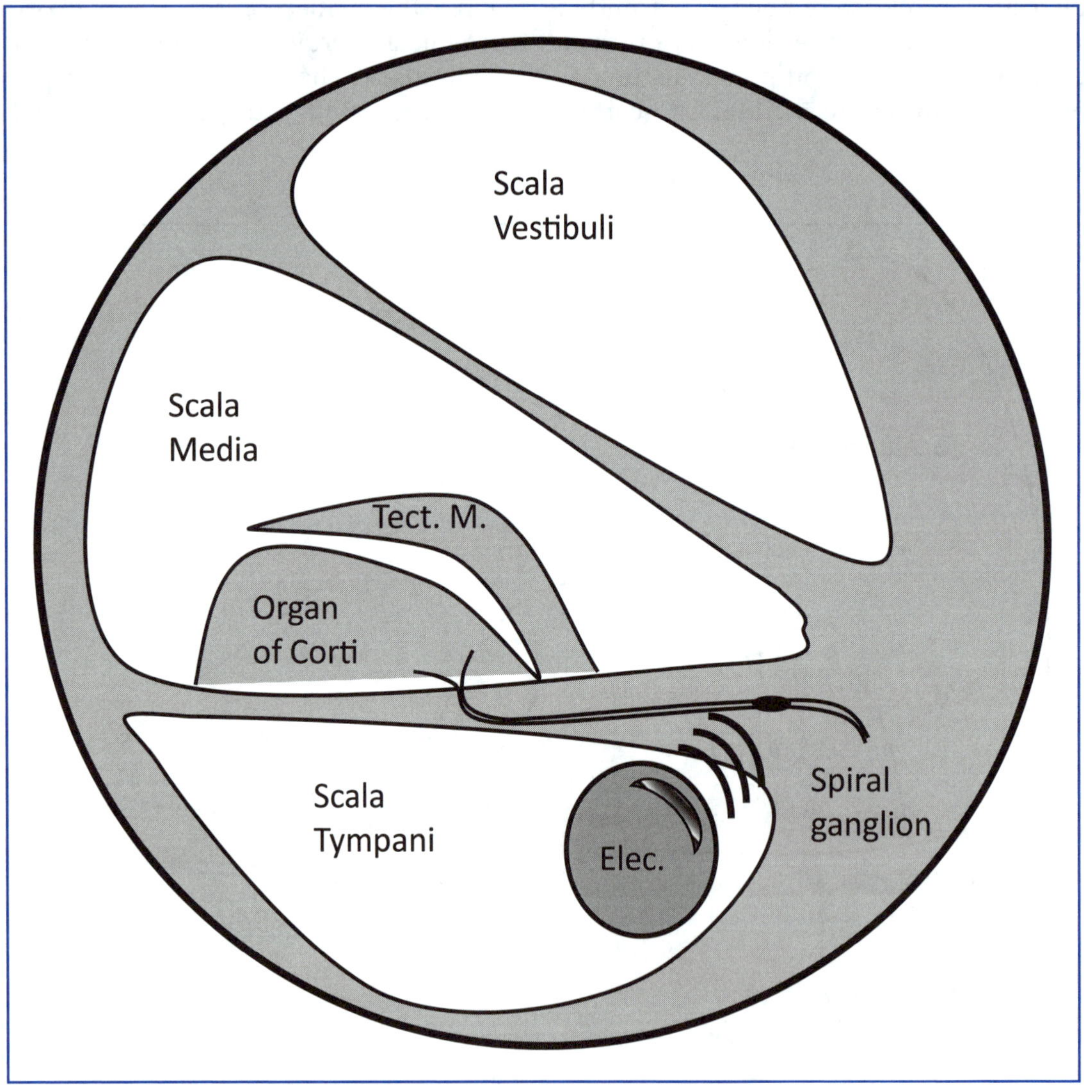


**FIGURE 1–3.** Schematic illustrating a cross-section of the impaired cochlea with a cochlear implant electrode array (Elec.) in the scala tympani. Note the loss of cochlear hair cells within the organ of Corti. Electrical current from the implanted electrode array compensates for hair cell loss (or other forms of cochlear dysfunction) by directly depolarizing the auditory neurons, and bypassing the normal mechanism of neural transmitter release. Tect. M.: Tectorial membrane.

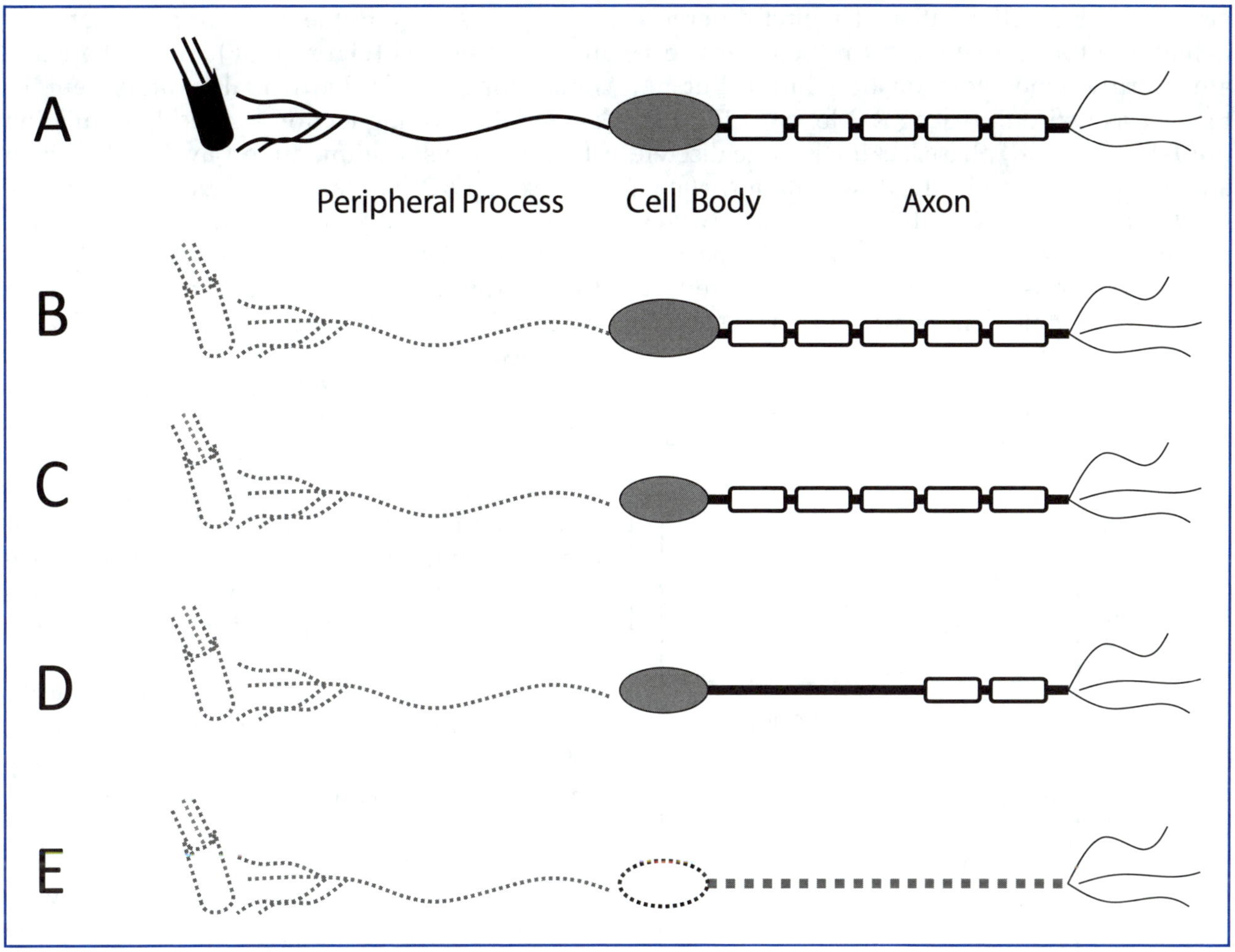


**FIGURE 1–4.** Schematic illustrating the course of retrograde degeneration. **A.** Healthy ear. **B.** Hair cell loss leading to degeneration of the peripheral axon. **C.** Further degeneration involving reduced volume of the cell body. **D.** Demyelination of the central axon. **E.** Degeneration of the central axon.

review). Research has shown, however, that the presence of supporting cells in the organ of Corti can delay degeneration of auditory neurons (Sugawara, Corfas, & Liberman, 2005). Interestingly, there does not appear to be a clear association between the number of surviving spiral ganglion cells and speech perception with a cochlear implant (Fayad, Linthicum, Otto, Galey, & House, 1991; Linthicum, Fayad, Otto, Galey, & House, 1991).

When hearing loss occurs, hearing aids are typically recommended for amplifying sound to a level that is audible. However, hearing aid benefit is often limited for greater degrees of hearing loss. Hair cell loss results in broader tuning curves (due to the loss of active mechanical feedback of the outer hair cells), which effectively degrades the fine spectral resolution of the normal cochlea (Liberman & Dodds, 1984). Functionally, this translates into poorer speech understanding, despite adequate amplification of sound with a hearing aid.

## BASIC PRINCIPLES OF ELECTRICAL STIMULATION OF THE AUDITORY SYSTEM

In the context of auditory evoked potentials, it is important to understand the basic differences between neural responses obtained with acoustic versus electrical stimulation. The first difference is that auditory nerve fibers (in the normal ear) are sharply tuned to acoustic stimuli, but not to electrical stimuli (Kiang & Moxon, 1972; Figure 1–5A). Second, phase locking is more discrete and focused with electrical stimulation (Javel, 1989; Kiang & Moxon, 1972). For sine waves, phase locking occurs in response to the positive phase for acoustic stimulation (which reflects basilar membrane deflection), whereas responses occur in response to the negative phase for electrical stimulation (Figure 1–5B). Third, the maximum firing rate for individual auditory neurons is significantly higher for electrical stimulation than for acoustic stimulation (Javel, 1989; Kiang & Moxon, 1972; Figure 1–5C). Fourth, the dynamic range for fiber rate-level functions is much narrower for electrical stimulation (typically less than 10 dB) than for acoustic stimulation (on the order of 20–50 dB) (Kiang & Moxon, 1972; Pickles, 1988; see Figure 1–5C). Fifth, rate-level functions for acoustic stimulation tend to plateau, whereas functions for electrical stimulation typically do not (Kiang & Moxon, 1972; see Figure 1–5C).

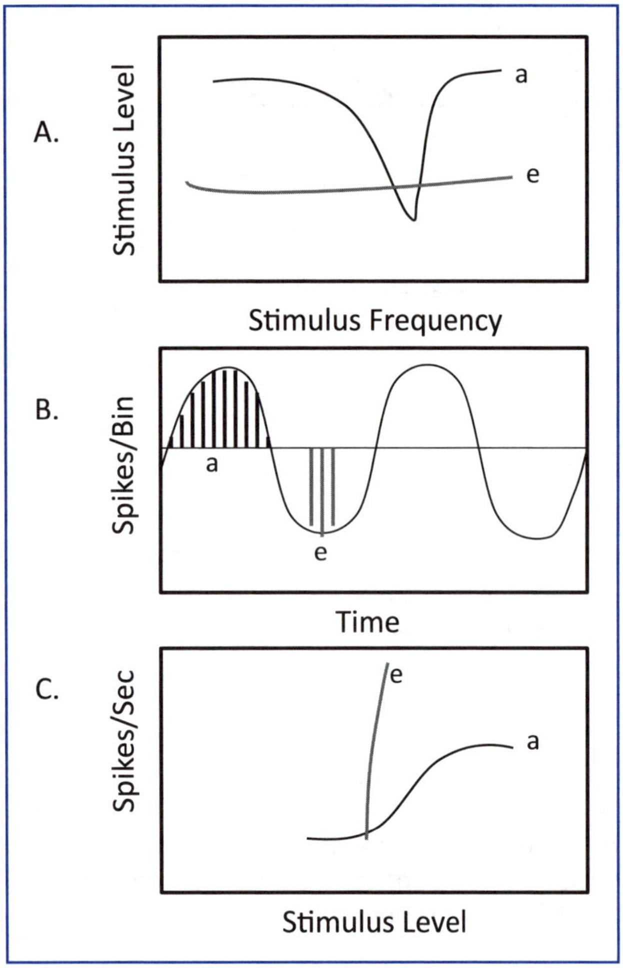


**FIGURE 1–5.** Examples of differences in neural response properties for acoustic (a) versus electrical (e) stimulation. **A.** Frequency tuning curves. **B.** Poststimulus time histograms for a sine wave. Neural responses encompass the entire positive phase for acoustic stimulation. For electrical stimulation, responses are highly synchronized to the peak of the negative phase. **C.** Rate-level functions for acoustic versus electric stimulation. Adapted from Kiang and Moxon, 1972.

In general, electrical stimulation yields highly synchronous neural responses, compared with acoustic stimulation. This is because electrical stimulation does not typically involve synaptic activity between the inner hair cells and afferent auditory neurons in the deafened ear. Synaptic processes introduce small time variations, or jitter, in fiber response probability functions (Javel, 1989). Secondary outcomes of greater synchrony with electrical stimulation are that: (1) input/output (or amplitude growth) functions are steeper for electrical stimulation, and (2) amplitudes are typically larger than responses obtained with acoustic stimulation. The third difference between acoustically evoked and electrically evoked potentials is that electrically evoked neural responses have shorter latencies. With acoustic stimulation, latencies are longer because of the time it takes for sound to travel down the ear canal, through the middle ear structures, and to activate the traveling wave. Because these structures and mechanisms are bypassed with the cochlear implant (i.e., neurons are stimulated directly), the resulting latencies are shorter for electrical stimulation.

## BASIC PARTS AND FUNCTIONS OF A COCHLEAR IMPLANT

Although cochlear implants differ slightly in appearance across manufacturers and generations of technology, all cochlear implants share the same basic design and function. Figures 1–6 through 1–8 illustrate the basic parts and function of a cochlear

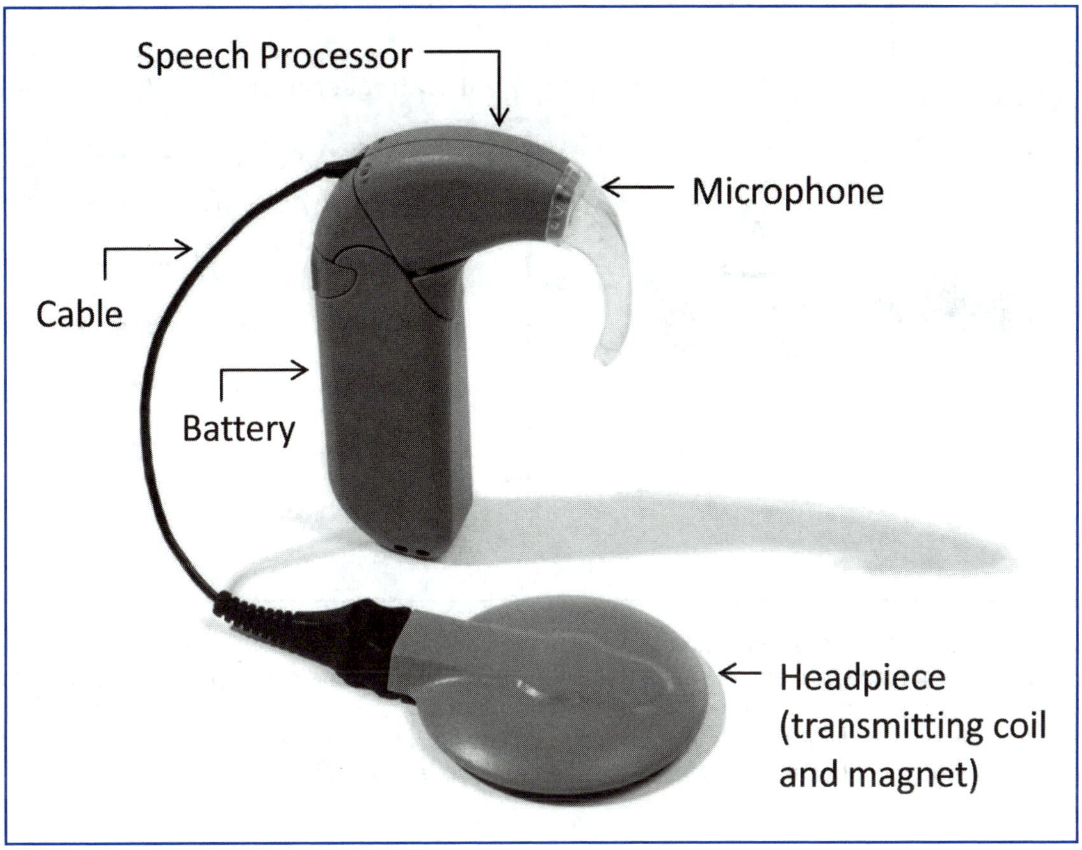


**FIGURE 1–6.** Parts of the externally worn sound processor. This example is a MED-EL OPUS 2 behind-the-ear processor. Photo courtesy of MED-EL.

implant. The cochlear implant is composed of two basic components: (1) the external sound processor (see Figure 1–6), and (2) the surgically implanted internal device (see Figure 1–8).

## External Sound Processor

The sound processor is worn externally, either as a body-worn processor or an ear-level processor, much like a behind-the-ear hearing aid (see Figure 1–6 for an example of the latter). Figure 1–7 illustrates how a cochlear implant processor works.

The sound processor consists of the following:

1. Microphone—Captures sound and converts it to an electrical signal (see Figures 1–6 and 1–7A).
2. Sound processor—Breaks down the incoming signal into different band-pass filters (see Figure 1–7B) and then compresses the signal into the recipient's electrical dynamic range. The output of each filter corresponds to an electrode in the recipient's sound processor program, or map (see Figure 1–7C). The number of filters may be equal to, less than (e.g., because of malfunctioning electrodes that are disabled), or greater than (in the case of virtual channels) the number of physical electrodes in the implanted array.
3. Battery—Sound processors may be powered by disposable or rechargeable batteries (see Figure 1–6). Most newer models have both options. Some processors have off-the-ear power options, to reduce the size and weight of the portion that sits on the pinna.
4. Headpiece—The processed information is sent down a cable to the headpiece (see Figure 1–6), which contains a radio frequency (RF) transmitting coil. The RF transmission link

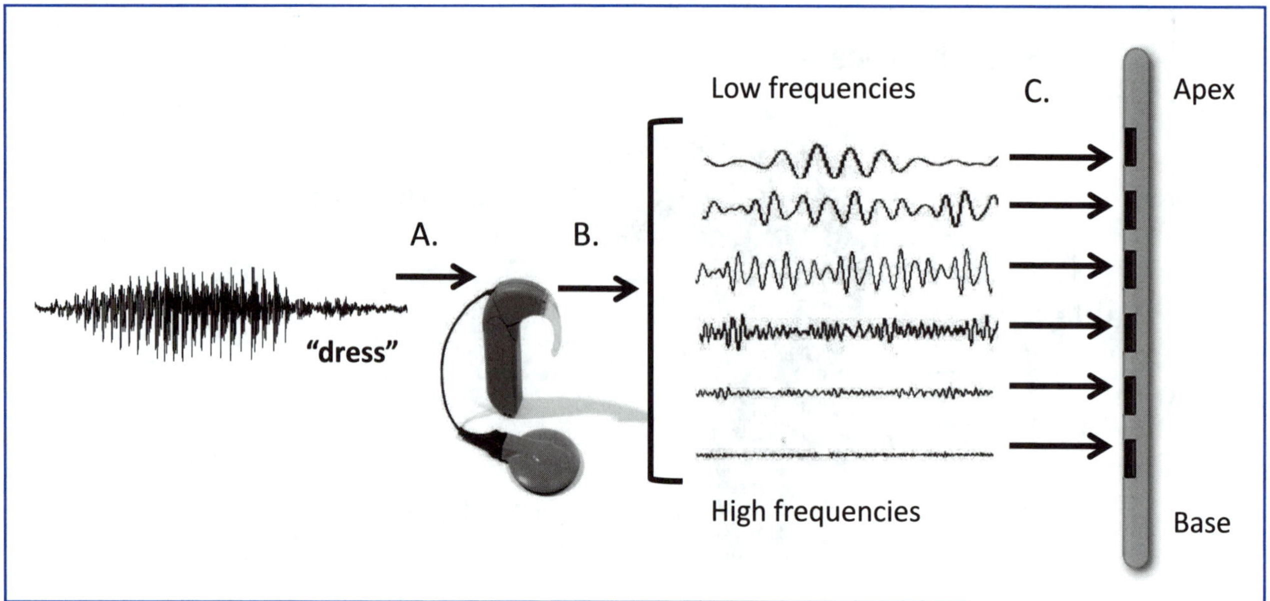


**FIGURE 1–7.** Schematic illustration of how a cochlear implant works. **A.** Sound enters the microphone, where it is converted to an electrical signal and sent to the sound processor. **B.** The sound processor breaks the signal into band-pass filters and compresses the signals. **C.** The output of each filter is mapped to a different electrode, where the lowest-frequency filter band is mapped to the most apical electrode, and the highest-frequency filter band is mapped to the most basal electrode. Processor photo courtesy of MED-EL.

allows for information transfer across the skin (transcutaneous connection), which obviates the need for a direct connection between the external and internal portions of the device, thereby reducing the risk of infection. The transmitting coil sends the processed information across the skin to the internal receiver/stimulator. The transmitting coil connects to the internal portion of the device via a magnet in the center, which holds the coil against the head directly over the magnet contained in the internal portion of the device.

## Internal Device

The internal receiver/stimulator (see Figure 1–8) is surgically placed into a small bed drilled in the skull, just behind the pinna. (Some newer devices do not require a bed to be drilled.) A template of the behind-the-ear portion of the external processor is typically used to guide the placement of the internal receiver/stimulator so that the external processor will not overlay the internal portion of the device (which could cause skin breakdown). The electrode array is inserted into the cochlea either through a small hole drilled into the cochlea (cochleostomy), or directly through the round window (not as common of an approach).

The internal device (see Figure 1–8) consists of the following:

1. Antenna/receiver coil—Receives the RF signal from the external transmitting coil.
2. Magnet—Holds the external coil against the head so that the external and internal coils align.
3. Electronics package—Decodes the RF signal, which contains information about the amount of current to be delivered, the speed at which it is delivered, and which electrodes will be stimulated in what order.
4. Electrode lead—Contains the lead wires that carry current from the internal electronics package to the individual electrode contacts implanted in the cochlea.

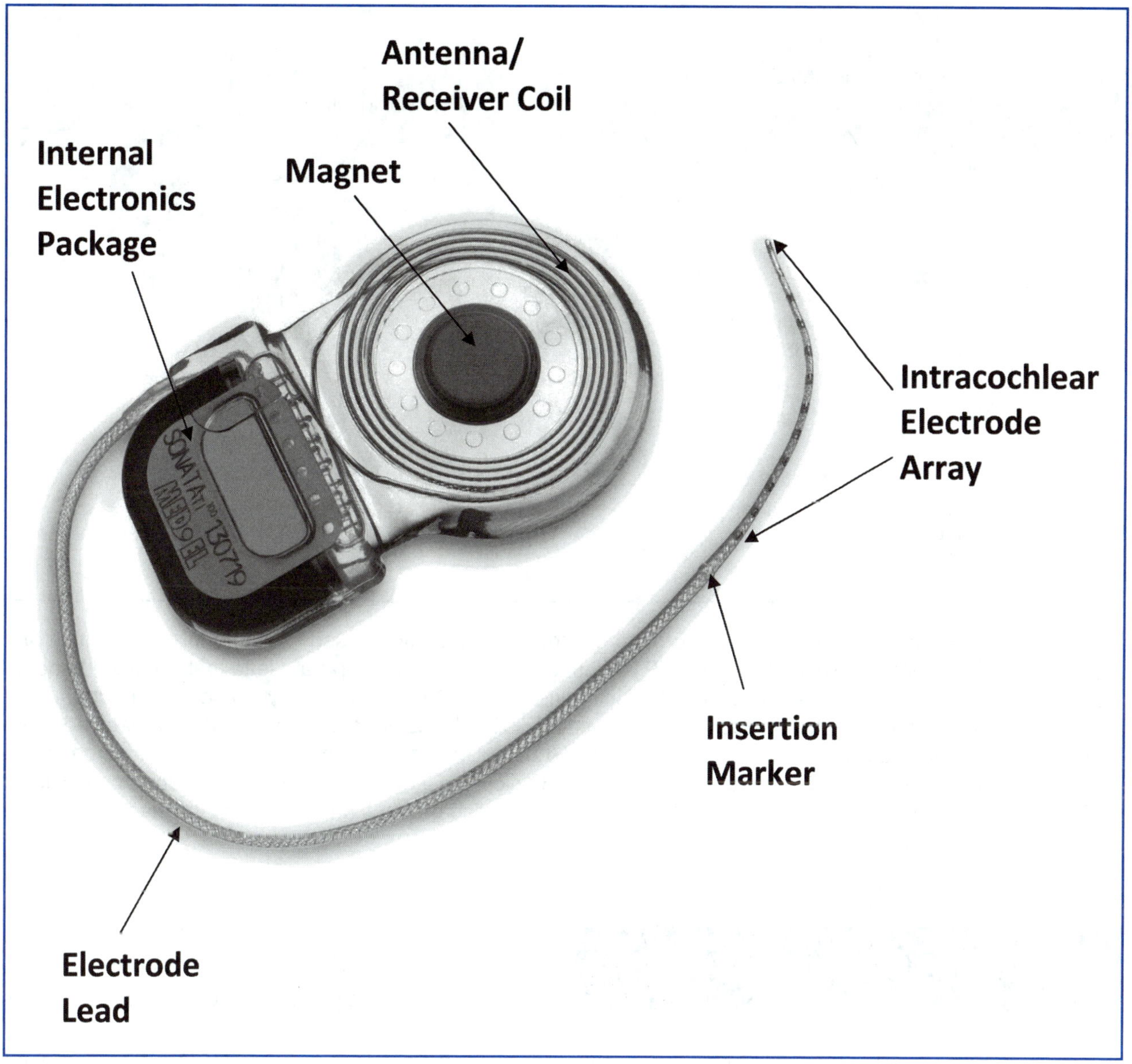


**FIGURE 1–8.** Parts of the surgically implanted internal device. This example is a MED-EL SONATATI$^{100}$ device. Photo courtesy of MED-EL.

5. Intracochlear electrode array—Contains tonotopically arranged electrode contacts, which provide the point of current injection into the tissue. The electrode array may have a marker that indicates the point at which a full insertion is achieved (see Figure 1–8).
6. Extracochlear electrodes—All of the newer-generation devices have one or two extracochlear electrodes that are used for monopolar stimulation. These are typically located on the case/housing of the internal electronics package, on the electrode lead bundle near the electronics package, or on a separate electrode lead. Figure 1–9 shows several examples of different locations for the extracochlear electrodes.

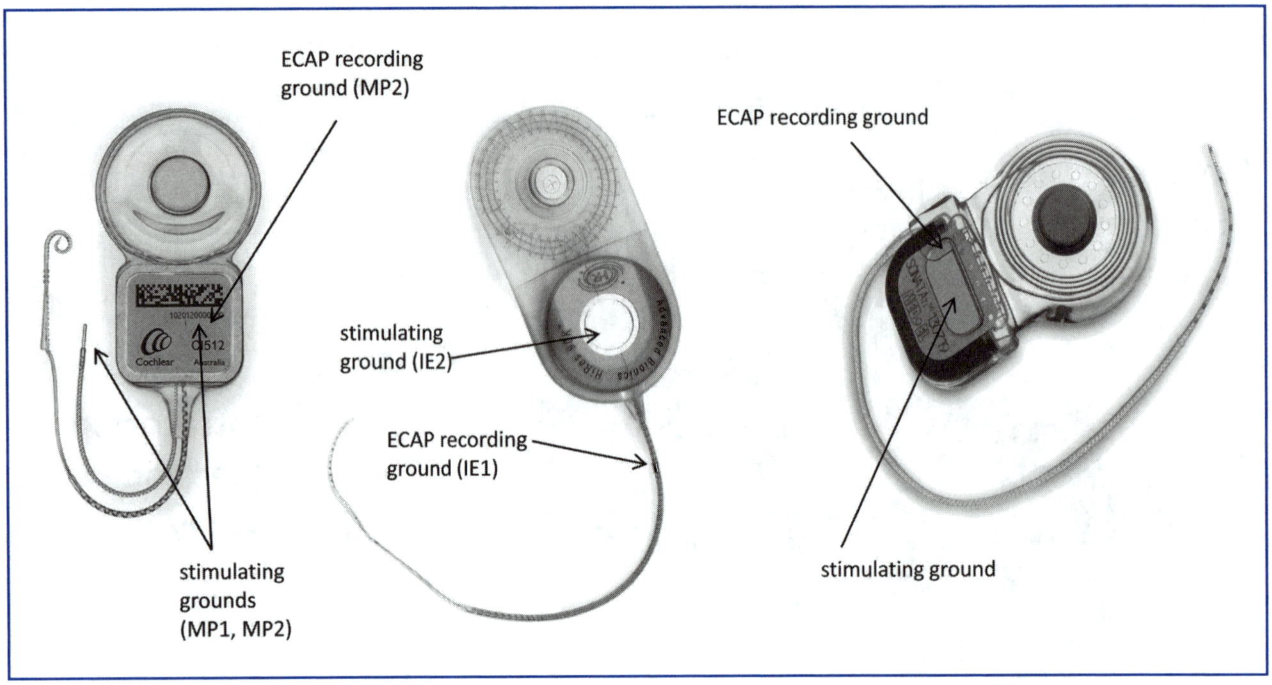


**FIGURE 1–9.** Examples of extracochlear ground electrode configurations used for monopolar stimulation and recording. **Left:** Cochlear Ltd. CI512 device. MP1 is located at the end of a separate lead that is placed beneath the temporalis muscle. MP2 is located on the electronics case. ECAP = electrically evoked compound action potential. Photo provided courtesy of Cochlear™ Americas, ©2011 Cochlear Americas. Middle: Advanced Bionics HiRes 90K device. IE1 is a ring ground at the base of the lead for the intracochlear array. IE2 is located on the electronics case. Image provided courtesy of Advanced Bionics, LLC, http://www.AdvancedBionics.com. **Right:** MED-EL SONATATI[100] device. Both stimulating and ECAP recording grounds are located on the electronics case. Photo courtesy of MED-EL.

## PAST AND PRESENT DEVICES

Because cochlear implants have been designed to last a lifetime, it is useful to have a brief summary of all past and present devices. After all, recipients with any of the devices discussed below may show up in the clinic for programming or troubleshooting needs, which may involve the use of objective measures. So, it is worthwhile to know whether the recipient's device is one that you can connect to the clinical software and measure ECAPs, impedance, electric field potentials, or none of these. For practical purposes, the following section focuses on multichannel devices (i.e., it excludes single-channel devices) because most can be evaluated with objective measures that utilize clinical software. The purpose of this section is to provide the reader with the necessary background to understand how present technology has evolved. Specifically, this section outlines the primary differences between generations of each manufacturer's devices, as well as a brief summary of what processors work with what internals.

### Advanced Bionics

Advanced Bionics, LLC, is based in Sylmar and Valencia, California in the United States. The company was acquired in 2009 by Sonova Holding, AG (Switzerland), which is also the parent company for the hearing aid manufacturer, Phonak. Advanced Bionics has produced four generations of cochlear implants, each outlined in the following sections, and summarized in Table 1–1.

**Table 1–1.** Summary of Advanced Bionics Devices

| *Internal Device* | *Electrode Array* | *Sound Processors (Strategies)* | *Impedance/ ECAP* |
|---|---|---|---|
| **Clarion 1.0** (1991)<br>• Ceramic case<br>• Nonremovable magnet<br>• Left- and right-side devices | **Radial bipolar**<br>• 8 medial/lateral electrode pairs<br>• Precoiled array | ***1.0** (*CA, CIS)<br>*1.2 (*CA, CIS, SAS, MPS)<br>S-Series (*CA, CIS, SAS, MPS)<br>PSP (*CA, CIS, SAS, MPS)<br>*Platinum BTE (CIS, SAS, MPS)<br>Harmony BTE (CIS, SAS, MPS) | Impedance telemetry;<br>EFI;<br>No ECAP capability |
| **Clarion 1.2** (1996)<br>• Ceramic case<br>• Nonremovable magnet<br>• Left- and right-side devices | **Radial bipolar**<br>• 8 medial/lateral electrode pairs<br>• Precoiled array | ***1.2** (*CA, CIS, SAS, MPS)<br>S-Series (*CA, CIS, SAS, MPS)<br>PSP (*CA, CIS, SAS, MPS)<br>*Platinum BTE (CIS, SAS, MPS)<br>Harmony BTE (CIS, SAS, MPS) | Impedance telemetry;<br>EFI;<br>No ECAP capability |
| | **Enhanced bipolar**<br>• 8 medial/lateral electrode pairs (for monopolar CIS/ MPS)<br>• 7 medial/lateral electrode pairs (for bipolar SAS)<br>• Precoiled array<br>• Separate positioner | *1.2 (*CA, CIS, SAS, MPS)<br>**S-Series** ( *CA, CIS, SAS, MPS)<br>PSP (*CA, CIS, SAS, MPS)<br>*Platinum BTE (CIS, SAS, MPS)<br>Harmony (CIS, SAS, MPS) | |
| | **HiFocus I & II**<br>• 8 medial/lateral electrode pairs<br>• Separate positioner (HF I)<br>• Attached positioner (HF II) | S-Series (*CA, CIS, SAS, MPS)<br>**PSP** (CIS, SAS, MPS)<br>*Platinum BTE (CIS, SAS, MPS)<br>Harmony BTE (CIS, SAS, MPS) | |
| **CII** (2001)<br>• Ceramic case<br>• Nonremovable magnet | **HiFocus I & II**<br>• 16 electrodes<br>• Separate positioner (HF I)<br>• Attached positioner (HF II)<br>**HiFocus IJ**<br>• 16 electrodes | PSP (CIS, SAS, MPS, HiRes, HR120)<br>***CII BTE** (CIS, SAS, MPS, HiRes)<br>***Platinum BTE** (CIS, SAS, MPS, HiRes)<br>**Auria** (CIS, SAS, MPS, HiRes)<br>Harmony (CIS, MPS, HiRes, HR120, CV)<br>Neptune (CIS, MPS, HiRes, HR120, CV) | Impedance telemetry;<br>EFI; BEIT;<br>ECAP capability |

*continues*

**Table 1–1.** *continued*

| *Internal Device* | *Electrode Array* | *Sound Processors (Strategies)* | *Impedance/ ECAP* |
|---|---|---|---|
| **HiRes 90K** (2003)<br>• Titanium case<br>• Removable magnet | **HiFocus IJ**<br>• 16 electrodes<br>**HiFocus Helix**<br>• 16 electrodes<br>• Pre-coiled | PSP (CIS, SAS, MPS, HiRes, HR120)<br>*CII BTE (CIS, SAS, MPS, HiRes)<br>*Platinum BTE (CIS, SAS, MPS, HiRes)<br>Auria (CIS, SAS, MPS, HiRes)<br>**Harmony** (CIS, MPS, HiRes, HR120, CV)<br>**Neptune** (CIS, MPS, HiRes, HR120, CV) | Impedance telemetry;<br>EFI; BEIT;<br>ECAP capability |

*Note:* All devices listed are capable of monopolar or bipolar stimulation, sequential or simultaneous stimulation, and analog or pulsatile stimulation. All intracochlear arrays are numbered such that electrode 1 is most apical. All sound processors are listed in the order in which they were released/available for a given internal device. Boldface indicates processors that were developed with or shortly after the associated internal device (but before the next-generation internal was released). Asterisks indicate processors/strategies that are now obsolete. ECAP = electrically evoked compound action potential. EFI = electric field imaging. BEIT = Bionic Ear integrity test. CA = compressed analog. CIS = continuous interleaved sampling. SAS = simultaneous analog stimulation. MPS = multiple pulsatile sampler. HiRes = high resolution, which includes HiRes-P (paired) and HiRes-S (sequential). HR120 = HiRes 120. CV = ClearVoice. PSP = Platinum Series Processor. BTE = behind the ear. HF = HiFocus.

All Advanced Bionics devices are capable of monopolar or bipolar electrode coupling, sequential or simultaneous stimulus delivery, and analog or pulsatile stimulation (all described further in Chapter 2); however, not all of these options are utilized for all devices within the commercial software. All of the devices' electrodes (or electrode pairs, in the case of the Clarion 1.0 and 1.2) have independent current sources, which allow for simultaneous stimulation. All electrodes are numbered such that electrode 1 is most apical.

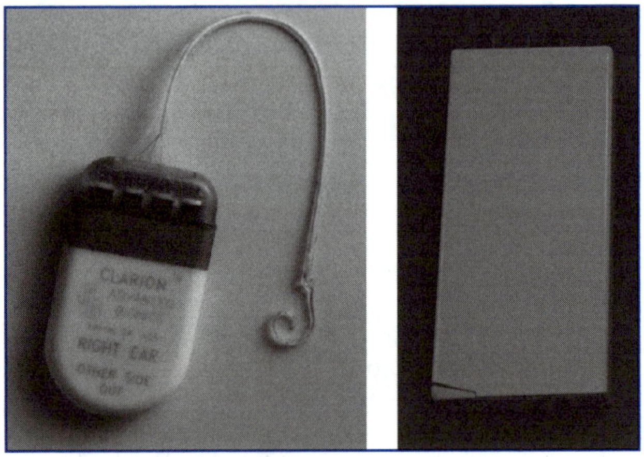


**FIGURE 1–10.** Clarion 1.0 internal device (*left*) and 1.0 sound processor (*right*). Photo of 1.0 internal provided courtesy of Advanced Bionics, LLC, http://www.AdvancedBionics.com.

### *Clarion 1.0*

The original Advanced Bionics internal receiver/stimulator was called the Clarion 1.0 (Figure 1–10, left photo). This device was only trialed with adults. The Clarion 1.0 was introduced in 1991 and was never FDA approved due to efforts dedicated to developing the second-generation device (Clarion 1.2) for use with children.

The body of the implant is ceramic, and therefore has a nonremovable magnet. The device also has impedance telemetry (see Chapter 3) and electric field imaging (EFI; see Chapter 4) capabilities. The intracochlear electrode array is a spiral precoiled array, so left-side and right-side devices were manufactured. The intracochlear array consists of a radial bipolar design, where medial and lateral pairs of ball electrodes serve as a bipolar stimulating pair (see circled electrode pairs, left panel, Figure 1–11). The extracochlear electrode (used for monopolar stimulation) is a metal band on the ceramic case.

The Clarion 1.0 was introduced with the 1.0 sound processor (see Figure 1–10, right photo), which was a rather large body-worn processor that ran the compressed analog (CA; now obsolete) and continuous interleaved sampling (CIS) processing strategies. This processor has since become obsolescent. Subsequent generations of internal devices were each released with one or more new processors, which were typically backward compatible with older-generation internal devices. Compatible processors (and processing strategies, in parentheses) are listed in Table 1–1. The sound processor listed in boldface is the processor that was introduced with (or shortly after) the corresponding internal device.

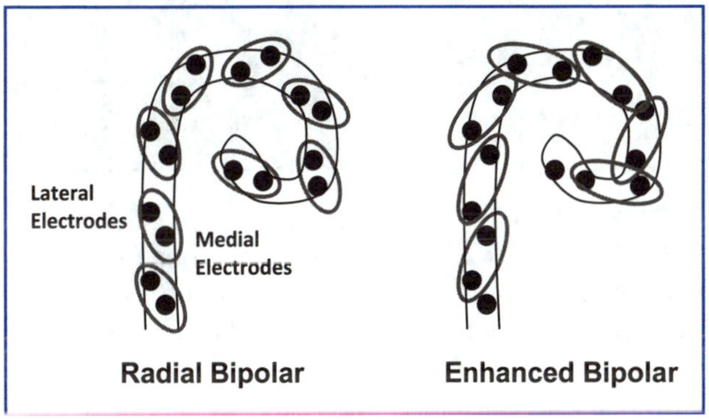


**FIGURE 1–11. Left:** Radial bipolar stimulation mode, where medial and lateral electrodes are paired for stimulation. **Right:** Enhanced bipolar stimulation mode, where the lateral electrode of the more basal pair is linked to the medial electrode of the more apical pair.

### *Clarion 1.2*

The second-generation Advanced Bionics device is called the Clarion 1.2 (Figure 1–12, left photo). The internal electronics package was redesigned to be significantly smaller than the Clarion 1.0 so it could be implanted in children. The 1.0 and 1.2 internal devices are collectively referred to as C-1 devices. The Clarion 1.2 received FDA approval in 1996 for adults and in 1997 for children ages 2 years and older.

Like the 1.0, the body of the 1.2 is ceramic. The 1.2 also has an extracochlear electrode on the ceramic case, and it has impedance telemetry and EFI capabilities. The 1.2 has four different iterations for the intracochlear electrode array. The first version of the array is the same as in the 1.0 (radial bipolar), but the narrow spacing between the electrodes in the pair resulted in problems achieving adequate loudness growth. The second version of the array is modified so that the lateral electrode of one pair and the medial electrode of the next apical pair create a bipolar pair (for the simultaneous analog stimulation, or SAS, strategy). This configuration is shown in Figure 1–11 (right panel) and

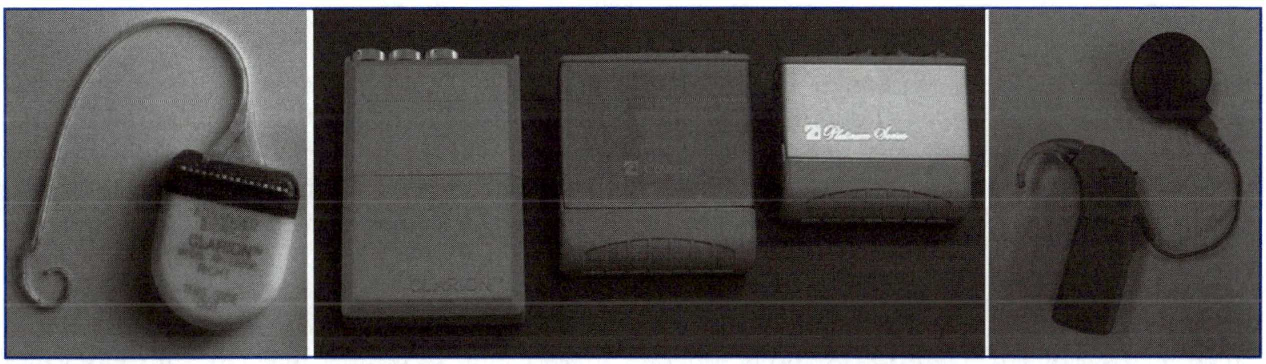

**FIGURE 1–12.** Clarion 1.2 internal device (*left*), 1.2 sound processor (*second from left*), S-Series sound processor (*middle*), Platinum Series Processor (*second from right*), and Platinum series behind-the-ear processor (*right*). Left and middle photos provided courtesy of Advanced Bionics, LLC, http://www.AdvancedBionics.com.

is termed enhanced bipolar, or more commonly, the S-Series device. Because the electronics package is designed for 16 electrodes (8 pairs, used for monopolar CIS and multiple pulsatile sampler, or MPS strategies), this change results in only 7 bipolar pairs. The medial electrode of the most basal pair, 8M, and the lateral electrode of the most apical pair, 1L, are not linked to any other electrode. The enhanced bipolar array was available with a separate positioner, which was inserted lateral to the electrode array for the purpose of holding the array in a perimodiolar position. The last two versions of the electrode array, the HiFocus I and II, consist of 16 equally spaced, individual electrodes (1.1 mm apart for HF I; 0.9 mm for HF II). With the 1.2 internal device, these 16 electrodes were coupled as 8 pairs. Because the electrodes in the HiFocus are spaced longitudinally along a slightly precurved array, these were the first Advanced Bionics arrays that could be used for either a left- or right-side implant (i.e., the arrays were not ear specific). The HiFocus I was available with a separate positioner; the HiFocus II had the positioner attached to the electrode array.

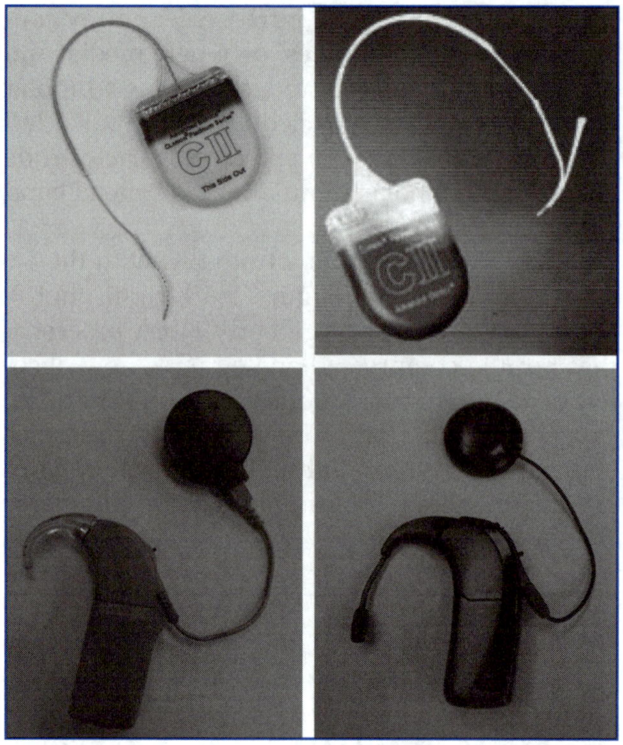


**FIGURE 1–13.** Clarion CII without positioner (*top left*), Clarion CII with attached positioner (*top right*), CII behind-the-ear processor (*bottom left*), and Auria behind-the-ear processor (*bottom right*). CII photos provided courtesy of Advanced Bionics, LLC, http://www.AdvancedBionics.com.

The Clarion 1.2 (with the radial bipolar array) was introduced with the 1.2 body-worn sound processor (see Figure 1–12, left processor), which was several inches shorter than the 1.0 processor. Shortly after the enhanced bipolar array was introduced with the 1.2 internal, the S-Series body-worn processor was introduced (see Figure 1–12, middle photo, middle processor). Finally, the body-worn Platinum Series Processor (PSP) was introduced in 2000 after the HiFocus arrays were released (see Figure 1–12, middle photo, right processor). Later-generation processors that are backward compatible with the Clarion 1.2 internal device, including Advanced Bionics' first behind-the-ear (BTE) processor for C-1 devices, the Platinum BTE (see Figure 1–12, far right), are listed in Table 1–1.

### *Clarion CII*

The third-generation Advanced Bionics device is called the Clarion CII (Figure 1–13, top two photos). The internal receiver/stimulator contains added electronics for measurement of two objective measures (in addition to impedance and EFI): the electrically evoked compound action potential (ECAP; see Chapter 7) and Bionic Ear Integrity Test (BEIT). The CII received FDA approval in 2000 for adults and children ages 18 months and older, and was released to the market in 2001.

Like the 1.0 and 1.2, the body is ceramic, although a slightly different manufacturing process was used to make the ceramic more durable. The CII has three different versions of the intracochlear electrode array: the HiFocus I, HiFocus II (which are described above for the 1.2 device), and HiFocus Ij. The HiFocus Ij is a slightly precurved 16-electrode array that is very similar to the HiFocus I, with evenly spaced electrodes (1.1 mm apart, center to center). The CII with HiFocus I and HiFocus II arrays are shown in Figure 1–13, top left and top right photos, respectively. Following an increased incidence of meningitis in recipients with the positioner, the positioner was removed from the market. The HiFocus II never received FDA approval because it was designed to be used with the positioner.

The CII was introduced with the CII and Platinum BTEs in 2001 (Figure 1–13, bottom left photo), which look virtually identical. The only way to tell the processors apart is to examine the color on the underside of the processor (after removing the battery pack): a Platinum BTE is black and a CII BTE is blue. The primary difference between the two processors was that the Platinum BTE could power the C-1 internals (1.0, 1.2); the CII BTE was designed for power efficiency and did not have enough power to operate the earlier-generation internal devices. Finally, the Auria BTE (Figure 1–13, bottom right photo) was introduced for the CII in 2002. Later-generation processors that are backward compatible with the CII internal device are listed in Table 1–1 along with the respective processing strategies.

### *HiRes 90K*

The fourth-generation, and currently used, Advanced Bionics device is the HiRes 90K (Figure 1–14, left photo). The primary changes from its predecessors are that the HiRes 90K has a titanium case, a removable magnet, and two extracochlear ground electrodes. Like the CII, it is equipped with a back-telemetry system that supports impedance, EFI, BEIT, and ECAP measures. The HiRes 90K received FDA approval in 2003 for adults and children ages 12 months and older.

The HiRes 90K has two different electrode arrays. The first is the HiFocus Ij (described above for the CII). The second is the HiFocus Helix, which is precoiled to achieve a more perimodiolar position within the scala tympani. The Helix also consists of 16 equally spaced electrodes (0.85 mm apart, center to center).

When the HiRes 90K was introduced, it utilized the existing Platinum body processor or Auria BTE. (The CII and Platinum BTEs could technically be fit with the HiRes 90K internal, but they were older processors.) In 2006, the Harmony BTE was released (see Figure 1–14, middle photo). The Harmony had improved front-end processing and was the first BTE processor that could run Advanced Bionics' virtual channels strategy, HiRes 120. The Auria and Harmony are virtually identical in appearance, except that the Harmony has an LED indicator light behind the microphone. Finally, the newest body-worn processor is the Neptune, which is much smaller than the PSP, has numerous wearing options, and is fully submergible and swimmable (see Figure 1–14,

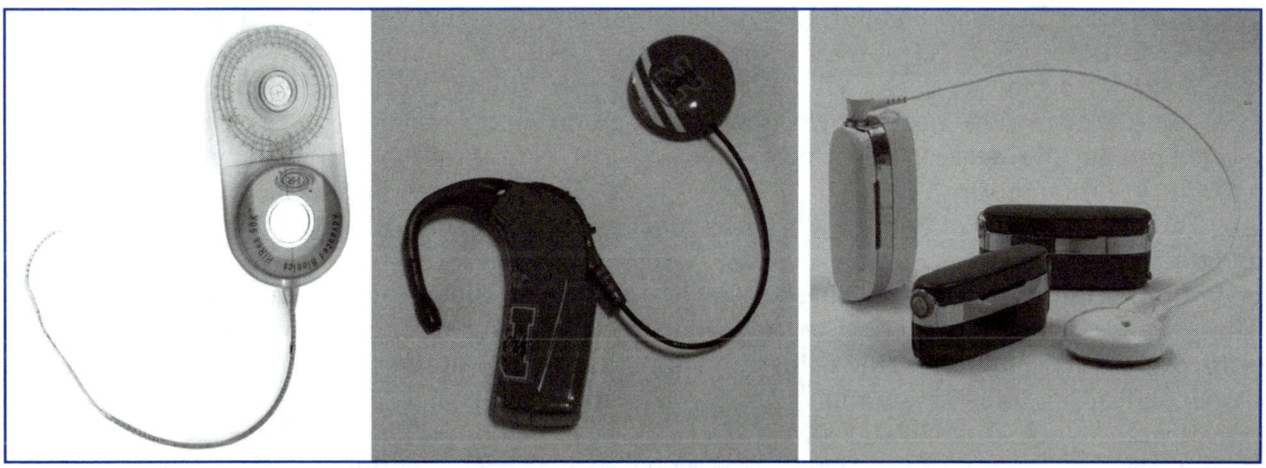

**FIGURE 1–14.** Advanced Bionics HiRes 90K internal device (*left*), Harmony behind-the-ear sound processor (*middle*), and Neptune freestyle body-worn processor (*right*). 90K and Neptune photos provided courtesy of Advanced Bionics, LLC, http://www.AdvancedBionics.com.

right photo). Table 1–1 lists all processors and strategies that are compatible with the HiRes 90K internal device.

## Cochlear

Cochlear Ltd. is based in Macquarie, New South Wales, Australia. Cochlear has produced five generations of cochlear implants, each outlined in the following sections, and summarized in Table 1–2. All of Cochlear's devices have a titanium electronics package and are capable of sequential, pulsatile stimulation. None of the Cochlear devices produce analog signals. All generations of the Cochlear devices have 22 intracochlear electrodes, which are numbered 1 to 22 from base to apex.

### *Nucleus 22*

The Nucleus 22 (Figure 1–15, top left photo) was the first multichannel cochlear implant to receive FDA approval in the United States. It was approved in 1985 for adults and in 1990 for children ages 2 years and older. The body of the Nucleus 22 implant is titanium, with a nonremovable magnet (although some Nucleus 22 devices were manufactured with a removable magnet). The electronics package allows for either bipolar (or various combinations thereof) or common ground stimulation (see Chapter 2). The electrode array consists of 22 equally spaced, full-band (see Chapter 2) intracochlear electrodes spaced 0.45 mm apart (0.75 mm center to center). In addition, ten stiffening rings (inactive electrodes) are located proximal to the most basal electrode to aid with the insertion process.

Three generations of body-worn processors and three generations of ear-level processors have been used with the Nucleus 22 internal device. These are detailed in Table 1–2. The three body-worn processors (shown in Figure 1–15) were each developed after different iterations of speech-processing strategies for the Nucleus 22. The first body-worn processor was the analog Wearable Speech Processor (WSP) (see Figure 1–15, top right photo). The WSP was only used with adults, and ran the F0/F2 (WSP II) and F0/F1/F2 (WSP III) strategies. The second body-worn processor for the Nucleus 22 was the smaller, digital Mini Speech Processor (MSP) (see Figure 1–15, bottom left photo), which was introduced with the Multipeak (MPEAK) processing strategy. The MSP was the first processor used for children implanted with the Nucleus 22 device. The last body-worn processor for the Nucleus 22 was the Spectra 22 (see Figure 1–15, bottom right photo), which was introduced with the SPEAK processing strategy. All three of these body-worn devices are now obsolete. Each of the three ear-level processors (ESPrit 22, ESPrit 3G for 22, and Freedom for 22) were developed later (initially for later-generation internals) and were made back-compatible for the Nucleus 22. Presently, the Freedom for 22 is the only processor that is supported for the Nucleus 22 internal device; the other five are obsolete (see Table 1–2).

### *Nucleus CI24M*

The Nucleus CI24M was the second-generation internal device released by Cochlear (Figure 1–16, left photo). It received FDA approval in 1998 for use in adults and children ages 18 months and older. This device differs from the Nucleus 22 in several important ways. First, the internal receiver/stimulator portion is thinner than that of the N22. Second, the CI24M has two extracochlear electrodes that allow for monopolar stimulation (MP1, a ball electrode at the end of a separate lead; and MP2, a plate electrode on the case of the internal receiver/stimulator). The capability for monopolar stimulation allowed for implementation of a number of new speech-processing strategies (such as CIS and Advanced Combination Encoder, or ACE). Third, the CI24M has a removable magnet for patients with future MRI needs. Last, the CI24M has added circuitry in the receiver/stimulator that allows for impedance and ECAP telemetry measures. The CI24M was the first device (across all manufacturers) that made ECAP telemetry commercially available. The CI24M was also later introduced with a double array for ossified cochleae. This option consists of two electrode leads, each containing 11 full-band electrodes, and a third lead for the MP1 ball electrode. The basal and apical electrode leads have 10 and 9 stiffening rings, respectively.

**Table 1–2.** Summary of Cochlear Corporation Devices

| *Internal Device* | *Electrode Array* | *Sound Processors (Strategies)* | *Impedance/ ECAP* |
|---|---|---|---|
| **Nucleus 22** (1985)<br>• Titanium case<br>• Nonremovable magnet | **Straight**<br>• 22 full-band electrodes<br>• 10 full-band stiffening rings | ***WSP** (*F0/F2)<br>***MSP** (*F0/F1/F2)<br>***Spectra 22** (*MPEAK, SPEAK)<br>*Esprit 22 (SPEAK)<br>*ESPrit 3G for 22 (SPEAK)<br>Freedom for 22 (SPEAK) | No impedance telemetry;<br>No ECAP capability |
| **Nucleus 24M** (1998)<br>• Titanium case<br>• Removable magnet<br>• 2 extracochlear electrodes for monopolar stimulation | **Straight**<br>• 22 full-band electrodes<br>• 10 full-band stiffening rings<br>**Double array**<br>• 2 leads with 11 full-band electrodes each (10 stiffening rings basal lead, 9 for apical) | ***SPrint** (SPEAK, ACE, CIS)<br>***ESPrit** (SPEAK)<br>*ESPrit 3G (SPEAK, ACE, CIS)<br>Freedom (SPEAK, ACE, CIS)<br>CP810 (SPEAK, ACE, CIS) | Impedance telemetry;<br>First device with ECAP capability |
| **Nucleus 24R** (2000)<br>• Titanium case<br>• Removable magnet<br>• Smaller electronics package<br>• 2 extracochlear electrodes for monopolar stimulation | **Contour (CS, CA)**<br>• 22 half-band electrodes<br>• Precoiled array<br>• 3 silicone rings<br>**Straight**<br>• 22 full-band electrodes | *SPrint (SPEAK, ACE, CIS)<br>*ESPrit (SPEAK)<br>***ESPrit 3G** (SPEAK, ACE, CIS)<br>Freedom (SPEAK, ACE, CIS)<br>CP810 (SPEAK, ACE, CIS) | Impedance telemetry;<br>ECAP capability |
| **Nucleus 24RE** (2005)<br>• Titanium case<br>• Removable magnet<br>• 2 extracochlear electrodes for monopolar stimulation | **Contour Advance**<br>• 22 half-band electrodes<br>• Precoiled array<br>**Straight**<br>• 22 full-band electrodes | **Freedom** (SPEAK, ACE, CIS)<br>CP810 (SPEAK, ACE, CIS) | Impedance telemetry;<br>ECAP capability |
| **CI512** (2009)<br>• Titanium case<br>• Removable magnet<br>• 2 extracochlear electrodes for monopolar stimulation | **Contour Advance**<br>• 22 half-band electrodes<br>• Precoiled array | CP810 (SPEAK, ACE, CIS) | Impedance telemetry;<br>ECAP capability |

*Note:* All devices listed are capable of sequential pulsatile stimulation. All standard intracochlear arrays consist of 22 electrodes, numbered 1 to 22 from base to apex. All sound processors are listed in the order in which they were released for a given internal device. Boldface indicates processors that were developed with or shortly after the associated internal device (but before the next-generation internal was released). Asterisks indicate sound processors and strategies that are now obsolete. ECAP = electrically evoked compound action potential. WSP = wearable speech processor. MSP = mini speech processor. MPEAK = multipeak. SPEAK = spectral peak. ACE = advanced combination encoder. CIS = continuous interleaved sampling. CS = contour with stylet. CA = contour advance.

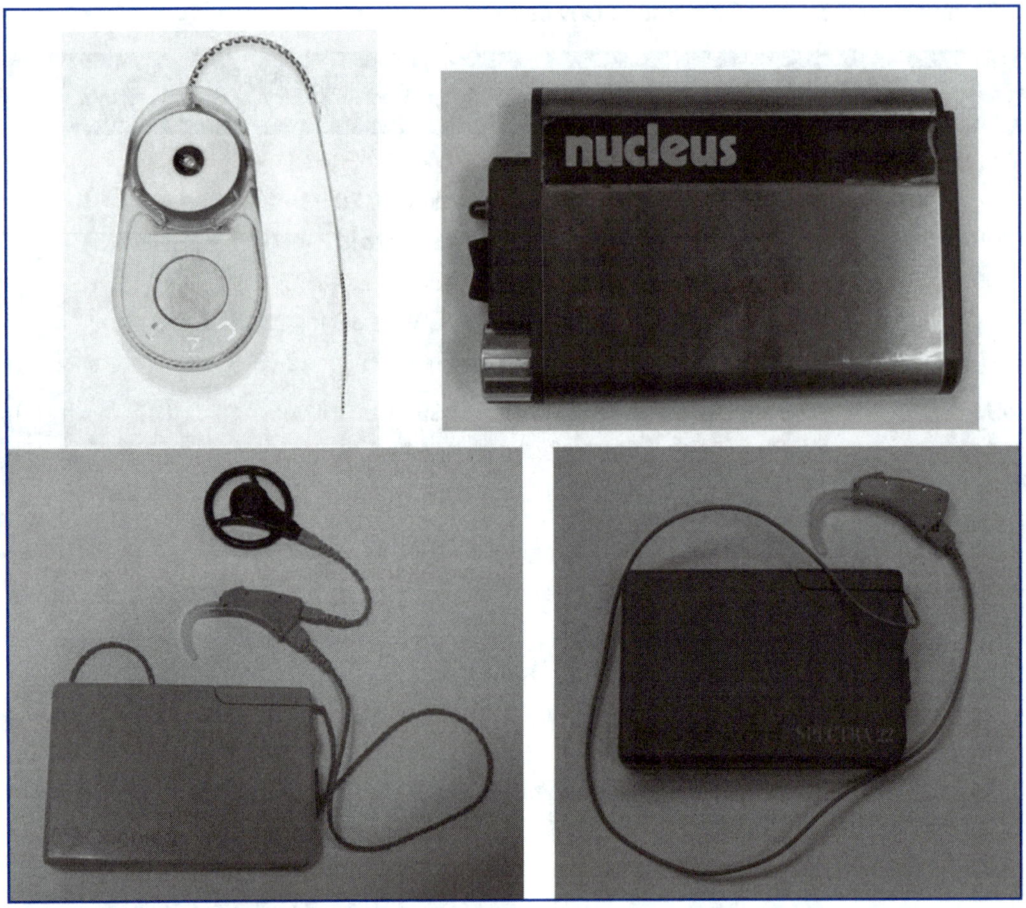


**FIGURE 1–15.** Nucleus 22 internal device (*top left*), Nucleus Wearable Speech Processor (*top right*), Nucleus Mini Speech Processor (*bottom left*), and Nucleus Spectra processor (*bottom right*). Nucleus 22 photo provided courtesy of Cochlear™ Americas, ©2011 Cochlear Americas.

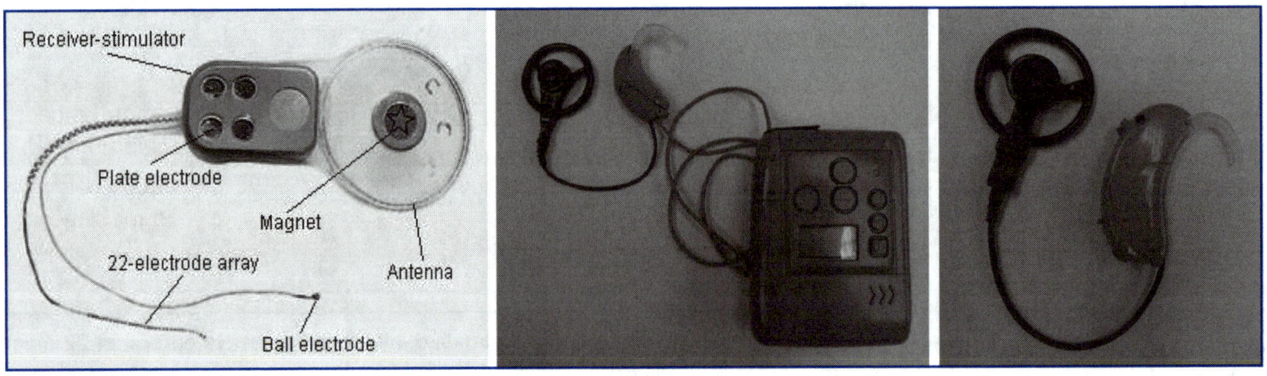


**FIGURE 1–16.** Nucleus CI24M internal device (*left*), SPrint body-worn processor (*middle*), ESPrit ear-level processor (*right*). CI24M photo provided courtesy of Cochlear™ Americas, ©2011 Cochlear Americas.

The CI24M was introduced with the SPrint body-worn sound processor (see Figure 1–16, middle photo). The next processor that was introduced for the CI24M was Cochlear's first ear-level processor, the ESPrit (see Figure 1–16, right photo). (The ESPrit was introduced for the CI24M before the Nucleus 22 version was released.) Two other ear-level processors (ESPrit 3G and Freedom) were later released for the CI24M (see Table 1–2). The Freedom (originally introduced with the fourth-generation internal) and the newer CP810 (introduced with the fifth-generation internal, CI512) are the only processors that are currently supported by the manufacturer; the other three (SPrint, ESPrit, ESPrit 3G) are now obsolete.

### Nucleus CI24R

The Nucleus CI24R was the third-generation internal device released by Cochlear (Figure 1–17). It was approved by the FDA in 2000 for adults and children 12 months and older. This device differs from the CI24M in two primary ways. First, the internal receiver-stimulator is reduced in size for use in younger children. The CI24R has three electrode array designs. The first is a precurved array with half-band electrodes, called the CI24R(CS). The "C" stands for "Contour" and the "S" for "stylet." The stylet holds the array straight for insertion into the cochlea. Once the array is inserted, the stylet is removed to release the curl of the array. The combination of half-band electrodes and curvature of the array was designed to improve modiolar proximity and spatial selectivity within the cochlea. The second array is the same full-band straight array as used in the CI24M; this device is called the CI24R(ST). The third array is the Contour Advance (CI24R(CA)), which is an improvement over the original Contour in that it has a softer, cone-shaped tip for reduction of insertion trauma.

The CI24R was not introduced with a specific processor. The SPrint and ESprit were used with the CI24R until the ESPrit 3G (see Figure 1–17, right photo) was released in 2002. The Freedom and CP810 processors (for next-generation internals) are backward compatible for the CI24R (see Table 1–2).

### Nucleus CI24RE

The Nucleus CI24RE "Freedom" was the fourth-generation internal device from Cochlear (Figure 1–18). It was approved by the FDA in 2005 for adults and children 12 months and older. This device differs from the CI24M and CI24R in two primary ways. First, the internal receiver-stimulator has an upgraded electronics chip for faster stimulation, lower power consumption, and a better amplifier for ECAP recordings. Second, this

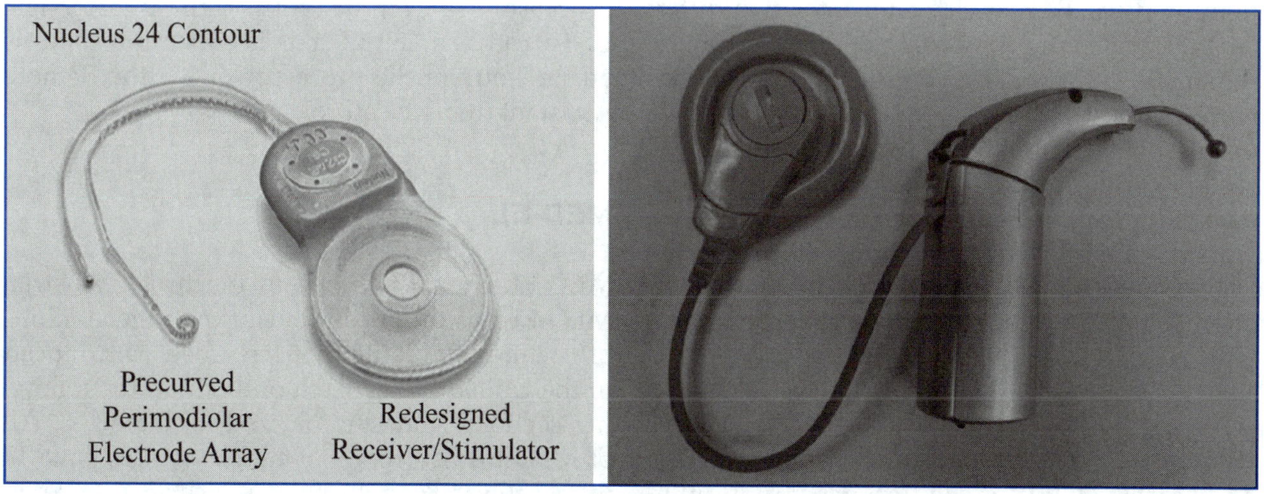


**FIGURE 1–17.** Nucleus CI24R(CS) internal device (*left*) and Nucleus ESPrit 3G ear-level sound processor (*right*). CI24R(CS) photo provided courtesy of Cochlear™ Americas, ©2011 Cochlear Americas.

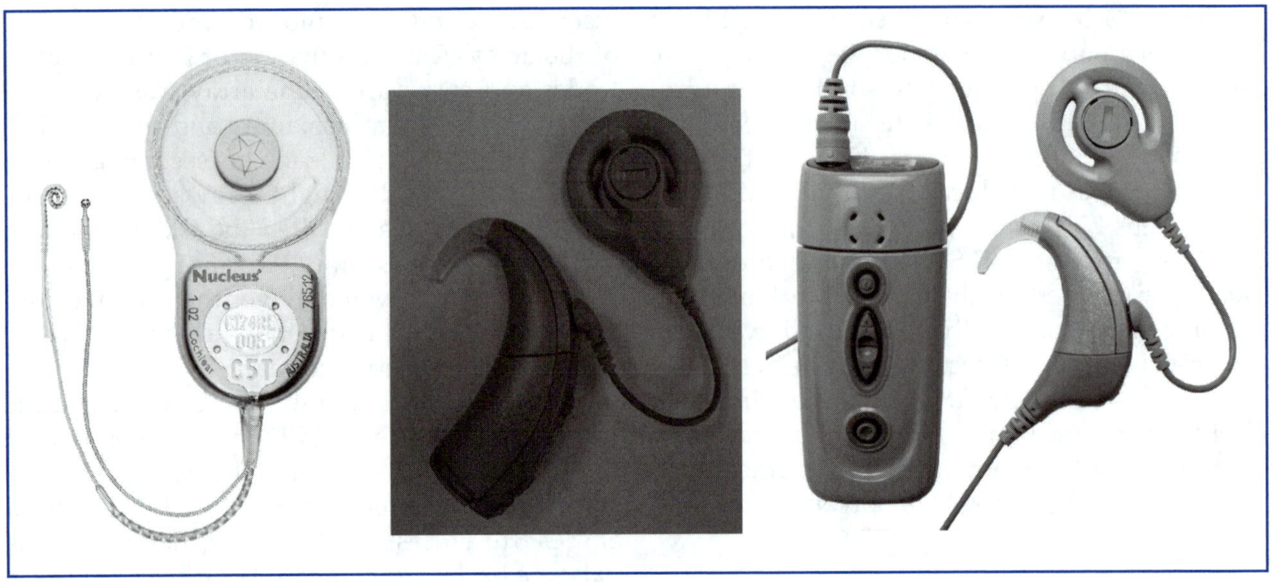


**FIGURE 1–18.** Nucleus 24RE(CA) "Freedom" internal device (*left*), Freedom ear-level processor (*middle*), and Freedom body-worn option (*right*). Nucleus 24RE(CA) photo provided courtesy of Cochlear™ Americas, ©2011 Cochlear Americas.

device was the first to allow for "dual-electrode" mode, where two adjacent electrodes are shorted together to achieve a virtual channel (see Chapter 2; this feature is currently not FDA approved or clinically available). The CI24RE has two electrode array designs: (1) the Contour Advance (CI24RE(CA)), and (2) the same straight array with full-band electrodes as used in the earlier Nucleus 24 devices (called the CI24RE(ST)).

The CI24RE was introduced with the Freedom modular BTE, which allows for two different wearing configurations. In one configuration, the smaller battery pack/controller portion is connected to the processor, resembling a standard BTE processor (see Figure 1–18, middle photo). The second configuration allows for a larger battery pack with the controller worn at the body level, with just the processor and connector behind the ear (see Figure 1–18, right photo). The next-generation sound processor, CP810, is also compatible with the CI24RE internal (see Table 1–2).

### *Nucleus CI512*

The Nucleus CI512 is the fifth-generation internal device from Cochlear (Figure 1–19). It was approved by the FDA in 2009 for adults and children 12 months and older. This device differs from the earlier N24 devices in that the shape of the MP1 electrode is different, and the internal receiver-stimulator and magnet are thinner. Like the CI24RE, the CI512 also allows for "dual-electrode" stimulation (see Chapter 2). The CI512 is only available with the Contour Advance electrode array.

The CI512 was introduced with the CP810 processor (see Figure 1–19, right photo). The CP810 can be manipulated via either user controls on the body of the processor or via the Remote Assistant (remote control).

## MED-EL

MED-EL GmbH is based in Innsbruck, Austria. MED-EL has produced four primary generations of cochlear implants that have been introduced in the United States, each outlined in the following sections, and summarized in Table 1–3. All of MED-EL's currently available devices have 12 intracochlear electrode pairs, which are numbered from 1 to 12, where electrode 1 is most apical. All

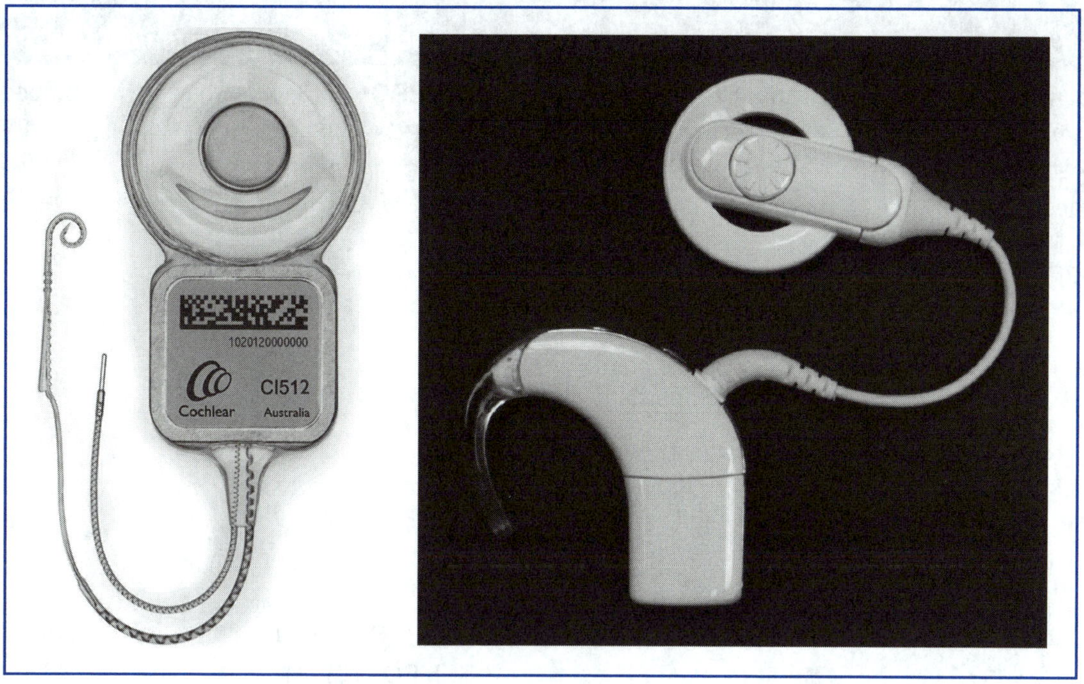


**FIGURE 1–19.** Nucleus CI512 internal device (*left*) and CP810 ear-level processor (*right*). CI512 photo provided courtesy of Cochlear™ Americas, ©2011 Cochlear Americas.

internal devices produce monopolar, pulsatile, sequential stimulation (see Chapter 2). The newer $I^{100}$ series of implants have the capability for simultaneous stimulation, although at this time, simultaneous stimulation is used clinically internationally but is not FDA approved in the United States. All of MED-EL's sound processors are technically forward and backward compatible with all generations of the internal device, although it is unlikely that recipients of newer internal devices would be fit with an older processor.

### *COMBI 40+*

The COMBI 40+ (Figure 1–20, top photo) received FDA approval in the United States in 2001 for adults and children ages 18 months and older. In 2003, the FDA approved expansion to include children down to 12 months of age. The housing of the COMBI 40+ is ceramic, and therefore has a nonremovable magnet. The device is MRI safe for up to 0.2 tesla in the United States, and is additionally MRI safe for 1.0 and 1.5 tesla internationally.

The electrode array consists of 24 electrode pairs that yield 12 channels. The COMBI 40+ contains a separate lead for the extracochlear monopolar electrode. Four electrode array options were available for the COMBI 40+ internal, each of which contained 24 electrodes for 12 channels: (1) standard array, which spaces channels over 26.4 mm, or 2.4 mm apart; (2) medium array, which spaces channels over 20.9 mm, or 1.9 mm apart; (3) compressed array, which spaces channels over 12.1 mm, or 1.1 mm apart; and (4) split array for extensively ossified cochleae, which contains 5 channels on a 4.4-mm lead (1.1 mm apart) and 7 channels on a 6.6-mm lead (1.1 mm apart).

The COMBI 40+ was introduced with the CIS PRO+ body-worn processor (Figure 1–20, bottom left photo) and, later, the TEMPO+ BTE processor (see Figure 1–20, bottom right photo), which has five different on- and off-ear wearing options. Compatible processors (and processing strategies, in parentheses) are listed in Table 1–3. The speech processor listed in boldface is the processor that was introduced with or shortly after the corresponding internal device (but before the next-generation internal was released).

**Table 1–3.** Summary of MED-EL Devices

| *Internal Device* | *Electrode Array* | *Sound Processors (Strategies)* | *Impedance/ ECAP* |
|---|---|---|---|
| **COMBI 40+** (2001)<br>• Ceramic case<br>• Nonremovable magnet<br>• Extracochlear monopolar electrode for all array types | **Standard**<br>• 12 electrode pairs (2.4 mm apart)<br>**Medium**<br>• 12 electrode pairs (1.9 mm apart)<br>**Compressed**<br>• 12 electrode pairs (1.1 mm apart)<br>**Split**<br>• 5 electrode pairs on apical lead<br>• 7 electrode pairs on basal lead (1.1 mm apart) | **CIS PRO+** (CIS, N of M)<br>**TEMPO+** (CIS+)<br>OPUS 1 (HDCIS, FSP)<br>OPUS 2 (HDCIS, FSP) | Impedance telemetry;<br>no ECAP capability |
| **PULSARCI$^{100}$** (2005)<br>• Ceramic case<br>• Nonremovable magnet<br>• Extracochlear monopolar electrode<br>• Capable of simultaneous stimulation | **Standard**<br>**Medium**<br>**Compressed**<br>**Split** | CIS PRO+ (CIS, N of M)<br>TEMPO+ (CIS+)<br>OPUS 1 (HDCIS, FSP)<br>OPUS 2 (HDCIS, FSP) | Impedance telemetry;<br>ECAP capability;<br>Electrical field telemetry |
| **SONATATI$^{100}$** (2007)<br>• Titanium case<br>• Same chip as PULSAR<br>• Nonremovable magnet<br>• Extracochlear monopolar electrode<br>• Capable of simultaneous stimulation | **Standard**<br>**Medium**<br>**Compressed** | CIS PRO+ (CIS, N of M)<br>TEMPO+ (CIS+)<br>**OPUS 1** (HDCIS, FSP)<br>**OPUS 2** (HDCIS, FSP) | Impedance telemetry;<br>ECAP capability;<br>Electrical field telemetry |
| **CONCERT** (2011)<br>• Titanium case<br>• 25% thinner electronics package<br>• Nonremovable magnet<br>• Extracochlear monopolar electrode<br>• Capable of simultaneous stimulation | **Standard**<br>**Medium**<br>**Compressed** | CIS PRO+ (CIS, N of M)<br>TEMPO+ (CIS+)<br>OPUS 1 (HDCIS, FSP)<br>OPUS 2 (HDCIS, FSP) | Impedance telemetry;<br>ECAP capability;<br>Electrical field telemetry |

*Note:* All devices listed are capable of monopolar, sequential, pulsatile stimulation. All intracochlear arrays are numbered from 1-12 in an apical to basal direction. All sound processors are backward and forward compatible with all internal devices (although older processors would not likely be fit for new recipients). Boldface indicates processors that were developed with or shortly after the associated internal device (but before the next-generation internal was released). ECAP = electrically evoked compound action potential. CIS = continuous interleaved sampling. HDCIS = High-definition CIS. FSP = Fine Structure Processing.

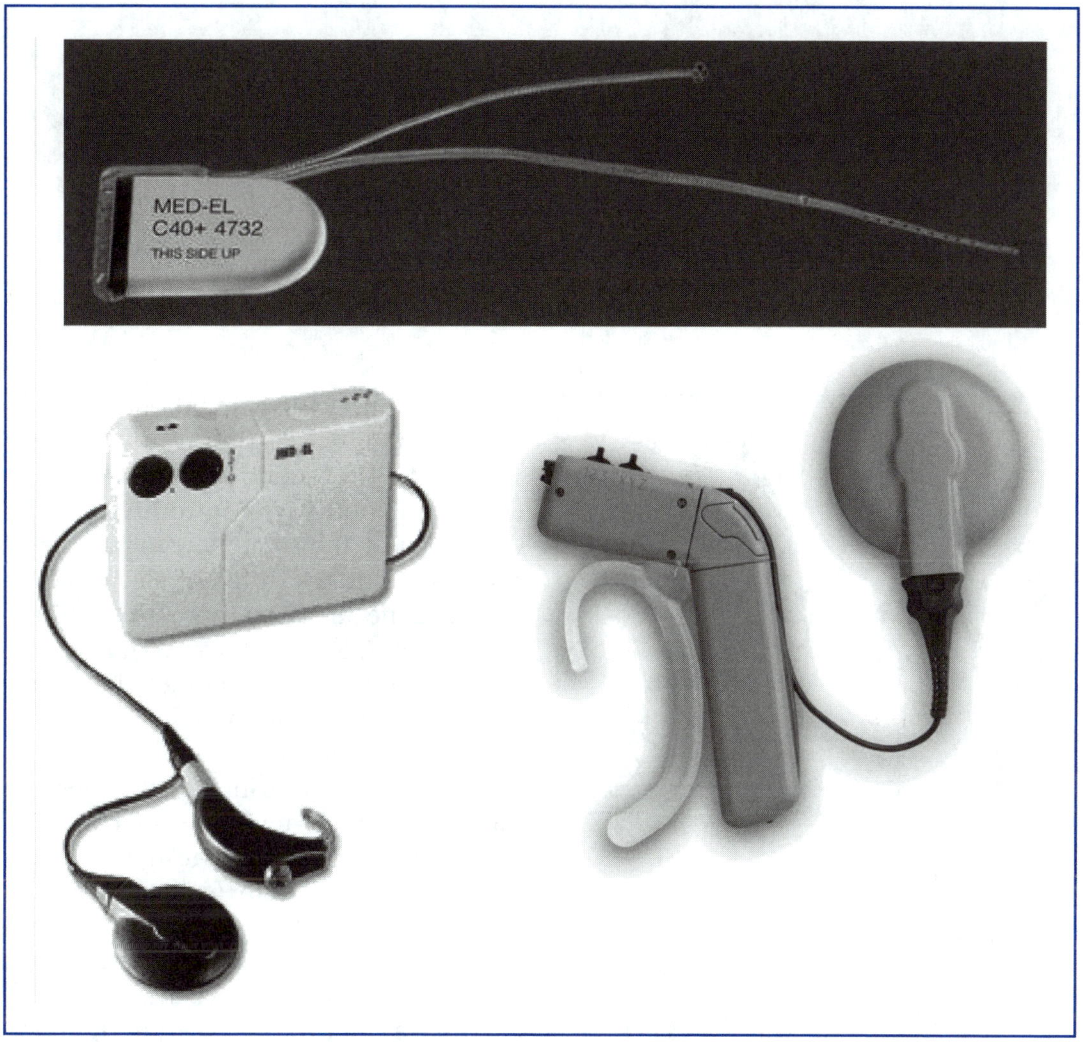


**FIGURE 1–20.** MED-EL COMBI 40+ internal device (*top*), CIS PRO+ body-worn processor (*bottom left*), and TEMPO+ behind-the-ear processor (*bottom right*). Photos courtesy of MED-EL.

### *PULSAR$_{CI}^{100}$*

The PULSAR (Figure 1–21) was FDA approved in 2005 for adults and children ages 12 months and up. Like the COMBI 40+, the PULSAR has a ceramic casing, a separate electrode lead for the monopolar ground, and is MRI safe for up to 0.2 tesla (but is approved for higher MRI strengths in other countries). The PULSAR has an updated electronics package that allows for ECAP telemetry, electrical field telemetry, and simultaneous stimulation (although at this time, simultaneous stimulation is not used clinically in the United States). It also has the capability to deliver pulse shapes other than the traditional biphasic current pulse, such as triphasic and triphasic precision pulses (Hochmair et al., 2006; see Chapter 2). The PULSAR comes with the same four electrode array options as the COMBI 40+. The PULSAR was originally fit with the existing TEMPO+ processor, until the OPUS 1 and OPUS 2 processors were introduced in 2008 and 2009, respectively (described in the next section).

### *SONATA$_{TI}^{100}$*

The SONATA (Figure 1–22, top left photo) was FDA approved in 2007 for adults and children

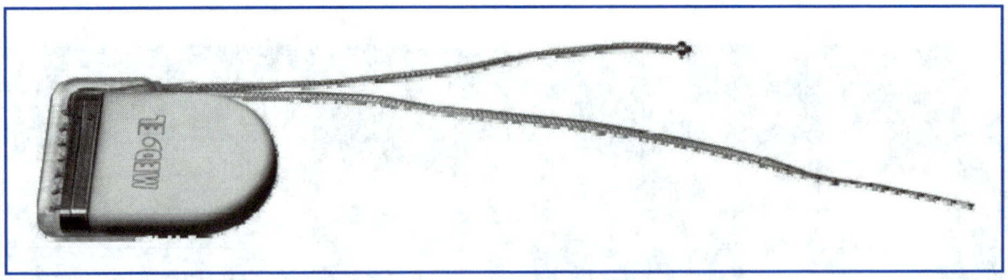

**FIGURE 1–21.** MED-EL PULSAR internal device. Photo courtesy of MED-EL.

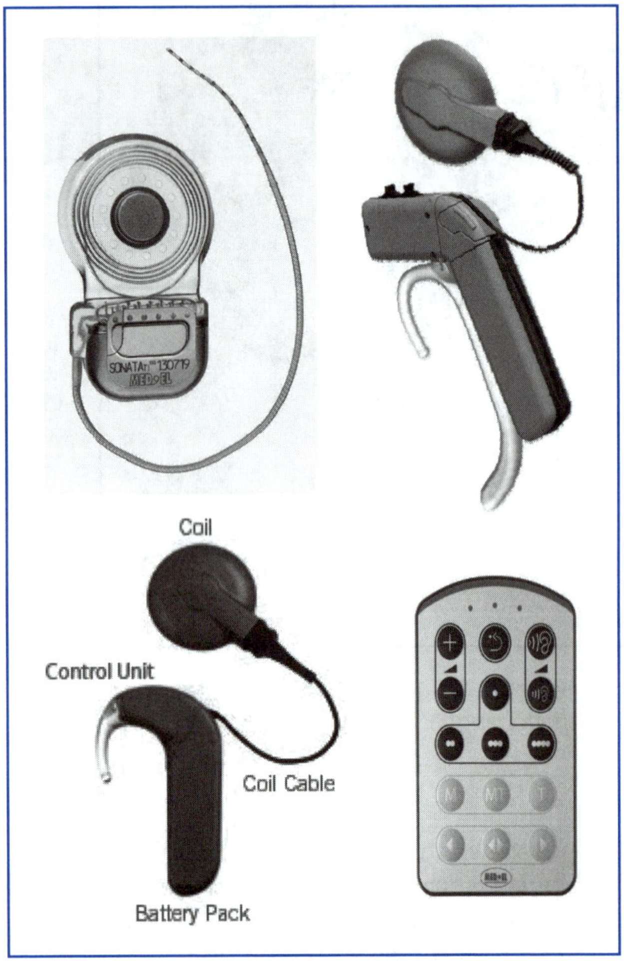


**FIGURE 1–22.** MED-EL SONATA internal device (*top left*), OPUS 1 behind-the-ear processor (*top right*), OPUS 2 behind-the-ear processor (*bottom left*), and remote-control FineTuner (*bottom right*). Photos courtesy of MED-EL.

ages 12 months and up. It has the same I$^{100}$ chip as the PULSAR, but it has a titanium case; the magnet is not removable. The SONATA comes with three of the previously mentioned electrode array options: standard, medium, and compressed.

The OPUS 1 sound processor (see Figure 1–22, top right photo) was introduced in 2008. The OPUS 1 uses the same housing as the TEMPO+ processor, but has different electronics that support the Fine Structure Processing (FSP) and High Definition Continuous Interleaved Sampling (HDCIS) strategies. (Although at this time, FSP is not indicated for prelingually deafened children in the United States.)

The OPUS 2 was introduced later in 2008 (see Figure 1–22, bottom left photo). Unlike the OPUS 1, the OPUS 2 has a redesigned housing, one additional program slot (4 instead of 3), and a few other additional features (telecoil, wireless FM capability). It also has no user controls; the processor is manipulated via the FineTuner remote control (see Figure 1–22, bottom right photo).

### MED-EL CONCERT

The MED-EL CONCERT (Figure 1–23) is the latest-generation internal device from MED-EL. It received FDA approval in July, 2011 for adults and children ages 12 months and up. The CONCERT (called CONCERTO outside the United States) has the same I$^{100}$ chip as the PULSAR and SONATA; however, the internal receiver/stimulator portion is significantly thinner than the previous models (thus called Mi1000). As with the SONATA, the CONCERT has a titanium case and the magnet is not removable. The CONCERT has the same three electrode array options as the SONATA: standard, medium, and compressed. Presently, the CONCERT is fit with the Opus 2 processor.

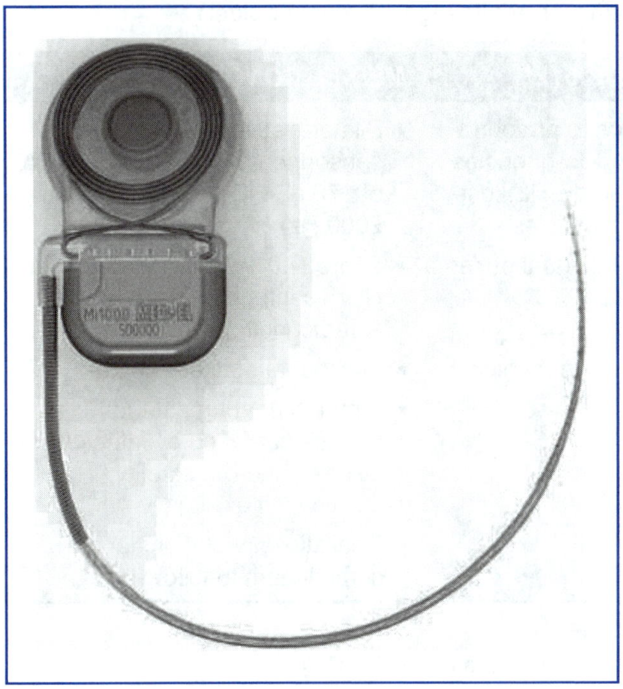

**FIGURE 1–23.** MED-EL CONCERT internal device. Photo courtesy of MED-EL.

## CANDIDACY

When multichannel cochlear implants were first introduced, candidacy criteria were limited to only postlingually deafened adults with profound hearing loss and no measurable benefit from properly fit hearing aids. Outcomes were modest; for some, the implant improved speech reading and closed-set speech understanding. For others, limited open-set word and sentence recognition was achieved (e.g., Dowell, Mecklenburg, & Clark, 1986; Gantz et al., 1988; Parkin, Eddington, Orth, & Brackmann, 1985). However, as technology improved and new speech coding strategies were developed, speech understanding with cochlear implants increased to include open-set speech understanding, and for a subset of recipients, use of the telephone (e.g., Krueger et al., 2008). As performance continues to improve, candidacy criteria have been periodically re-evaluated and refined to include children, individuals with additional disabilities, prelingually deafened individuals, cochlear malformations, and persons with greater amounts of residual hearing (i.e., better audiometric thresholds and/or some speech perception ability).

Specific candidacy criteria vary with each device. All FDA-approved cochlear implants have a specific list of indications for use. Device-specific indications from the respective package inserts are listed in Table 1–4 (adults) and Table 1–5 (children) for currently available FDA-approved devices for each of the three manufacturers in the United States. These devices are the HiRes 90K, manufactured by Advanced Bionics (Sylmar, CA, United States); the Nucleus CI512, manufactured by Cochlear Ltd. (Macquarie, NSW, Australia); and the CONCERT, manufactured by MED-EL GmbH (Innsbruck, Austria).

One important issue to point out regarding Tables 1–4 and 1–5 is that when a percent-correct cutoff is specified regarding speech perception performance, many factors that affect performance are often not specified in the indications. This is problematic because a patient may or may not meet candidacy criteria depending on exactly what parameters or conditions were used for speech perception testing. First, cochlear implant recipients typically perform more poorly when speech is presented at softer levels. As an example, Firszt et al. (2004) and Spahr, Dorman, and Loiselle (2007) showed that recipients performed more poorly on open-set sentences presented in quiet at 50 to 54 dB SPL than at 60 to 64 or 70 to 74 dB SPL. Note that presentation level for speech perception testing is not specified for any of the three devices in Table 1–4 (adults), nor for two of the three devices in Table 1–5 (children). Therefore, a potential candidate may qualify if sentences are presented at 50 dB SPL, but not qualify if speech is presented at 60 dB SPL.

A second factor affecting performance is whether testing is conducted in quiet or noise. Firszt et al. (2004) and Spahr et al. (2007) showed significantly poorer performance on open-set sentences presented at +5, +8, or +10 dB SNR versus in quiet. It may be assumed that the percents listed in Tables 1–4 and 1–5 apply to speech perception testing in quiet, but this important parameter is not explicitly specified.

**Table 1–4.** Manufacturer-Specific FDA-Approved Indications for Adults (age 18 years or older)

| *Advanced Bionics HiRes 90K* | *Cochlear Nucleus CI512** | *MED-EL CONCERT* |
|---|---|---|
| • Bilateral severe to profound sensorineural hearing loss (≥70 dB HL)<br>• Postlingual onset of severe or profound hearing loss<br>• Score ≤50% with recorded HINT sentences using appropriately fit hearing aids. | • Bilateral moderate to profound hearing loss in low frequencies and profound (≥90 dB HL) loss in mid to high frequencies<br>• Pre-, peri-, or postlingual onset hearing loss<br>• Score ≤50% (ear to implant) or ≤60% (best aided) on recorded open-set sentences. | • Bilateral severe to profound sensorineural hearing loss (PTA of ≥70 dB HL at 500, 1000, and 2000 Hz)<br>• Score ≤40% with recorded HINT sentences in the best-aided condition<br>• Functional auditory nerve<br>• 3-month hearing aid trial (unless deafened by infectious disease and/or risk of ossification exists)<br>• Realistic expectations and commitment to follow-up. |

*Note:* HINT: Hearing in Noise Test (Nilsson, Soli, & Sullivan, 1994).

*The CI512 was voluntarily recalled by the manufacturer while this book was in the editing stage.

**Table 1–5.** Manufacturer-Specific FDA-Approved Indications for Children (age 12 months to 17 years)

| *Advanced Bionics HiRes 90K* | *Cochlear Nucleus CI512** | *MED-EL CONCERT* |
|---|---|---|
| • Bilateral profound sensorineural hearing loss (≥90 dB HL)<br>• 6-month hearing aid trial for children ages 2 to 17 years; 3-month trial for children ages 12 to 23 months (waived if evidence of ossification)<br>• For <4 years of age, failure to reach developmentally appropriate auditory milestones (using the MAIS or ITMAIS) or ≤20% on MLNT using live-voice presentation at 70 dB SPL<br>• For ≥4 years, score ≤12% on PBK or ≤30% on HINT-C using recorded materials presented at 70 dB SPL. | • Bilateral profound sensorineural hearing loss (ages 12 to 24 months) or bilateral severe to profound (ages 2 years and up)<br>• For younger children, lack of progress in simple auditory skill development with appropriate binaural hearing aids and 3 to 6 months of aural habilitation<br>• For older children, ≤30% on MLNT or LNT<br>• 3- to 6-month hearing aid trial recommended | • Bilateral profound sensorineural hearing loss (≥90 dB HL at 1000 Hz)<br>• For younger children, lack of progress in simple auditory skill development with appropriately fit amplification and 3 to 6 months of aural habilitation<br>• For older children, <20% on MLNT or LNT<br>• 3- to 6-month hearing aid trial (waived if evidence of ossification)<br>• Functional auditory nerve<br>• Realistic expectations and commitment to follow-up. |

*Note:* HINT-C: Hearing in Noise Test for Children (Nilsson, Soli, & Gelnett, 1996); MAIS: Meaningful Auditory Integration Scale (Robbins, Renshaw, & Berry, 1991); ITMAIS: Infant-Toddler Meaningful Auditory Integration Scale (Zimmerman-Phillips, Osberger, & Robbins, 2000); MLNT: Multisyllabic Lexical Neighborhood Test (Kirk, Pisoni, & Osberger, 1995); LNT: Lexical Neighborhood Test (Kirk et al., 1995).

*The CI512 was voluntarily recalled by the manufacturer while this book was in the editing stage.

A third factor is the specific sentence material used. Some tests consist of shorter, more predictable sentences that are recorded using a slow, deliberate speaking rate (e.g., CUNY or HINT sentences), while others are longer, less predictable sentences that are recorded using a normal speaking rate (e.g., AZBio or IEEE sentences). The result can be poorer scores with more difficult test materials. For example, Spahr et al. (2007) showed significantly poorer performance with AZBio sentences than with CUNY sentences for the same subjects and presentation level. As can be seen in Table 1–4, HINT sentences are suggested for both the Advanced Bionics and MED-EL devices, but no specific test is recommended for the Cochlear device.

Last, hearing configuration (monaural vs. binaural) can also impact speech perception performance. Some candidates perform better when listening with hearing aids in both ears than with either alone (e.g., Boymans, Goverts, Kramer, Festen, & Dreschler, 2008; Day, Browning, & Gatehouse, 1988; Köbler & Rosenhall, 2002). In this case, testing with binaural hearing aids would be considered the best-aided condition. Other candidates perform better with one ear aided than with both aided (e.g., Carter, Noe, & Wilson, 2001; Walden & Walden, 2005); in this case, a monaural hearing aid would represent the best-aided condition. For candidates seeking a second-side cochlear implant, testing in the best-aided condition would typically mean an implant on one side and a hearing aid on the other. For adults (see Table 1–4), both Cochlear and MED-EL specify that speech perception testing is to be done in the best-aided condition. Advanced Bionics specifies using "appropriately fit hearing aids" (for both children and adults), which seems to imply that testing be conducted in the binaural or best-aided condition, although this is not explicitly stated. The package insert for the MED-EL CONCERT simply says "with appropriate amplification" in regard to indications for children.

In summary, the manufacturers' package inserts (listing FDA approval criteria) do not include enough specific information regarding the test conditions that should be used to obtain speech perception results. Scores can vary as a function of presentation level, testing in quiet or in noise, specific sentence materials used, and listening configuration (monaural, binaural, best-aided). It is important for clinicians to realize that the percent-correct cutoffs for speech perception that are reported for candidacy determination therefore have limited utility for their intended purpose.

# 2

# Signal Delivery

This chapter begins with a brief overview of the differences between channels and electrodes, followed by more in-depth descriptions of the various types of signals, stimulus timing, electrode configurations, and electrode designs that are used both clinically and experimentally with cochlear implant recipients. It is essential to have a clear understanding of the types of signals that cochlear implants can employ so that one can better understand how manipulating these signals can affect both perceptual and objective measures with electrical stimulation.

## CHANNELS VERSUS ELECTRODES

The terms "channels" and "electrodes" are often used interchangeably, but they actually refer to two different things. An electrode is the physical structure that injects current into the tissue, whereas a channel is the resulting distinct field of stimulation. Some people further define "channel" as the resulting field of stimulation that produces a distinct percept. An example is shown in Figure 2–1. Figure 2–1A shows an array with six physical electrode contacts (E1–E6). Depending on how the electrodes are coupled, these six electrodes may produce six channels, fewer than six channels, or more than six channels. If monopolar coupling is used (described later in this chapter), then the six electrodes will produce six stimulation channels (C1–C6, Figure 2–1A). If bipolar coupling is used (i.e., adjacent electrodes form the current path), the result would be three channels (C1–C3, Figure 2–1B). Finally, if adjacent electrodes are linked together to form one intermediate virtual channel using either simultaneous or sequential stimulation (explained further in the next section), a total of 11 or more channels would result (6 physical electrodes and at least 5 intermediate channels; Figure 2–1C).

### Virtual Channels

There are three ways that virtual channels are typically produced, based on the specific capabilities of each device. The first is to apply sequential stimulation to adjacent (or nonadjacent) electrodes (Frijns, Kalkman, Vanpouke, Snel Bongers, & Briaire, 2009; Kwon & van den Honert, 2006; McDermott & McKay, 1994; McKay, McDermott, & Clark, 1996; Saoji, Litvak, & Hughes, 2009). With this method, it is critical to use a very short time interval (on the order of less than 0.5 ms) between pulses. This technique is illustrated in Figure 2–2, where the star represents the theoretical tonotopic location of the peak of the field of excitation.

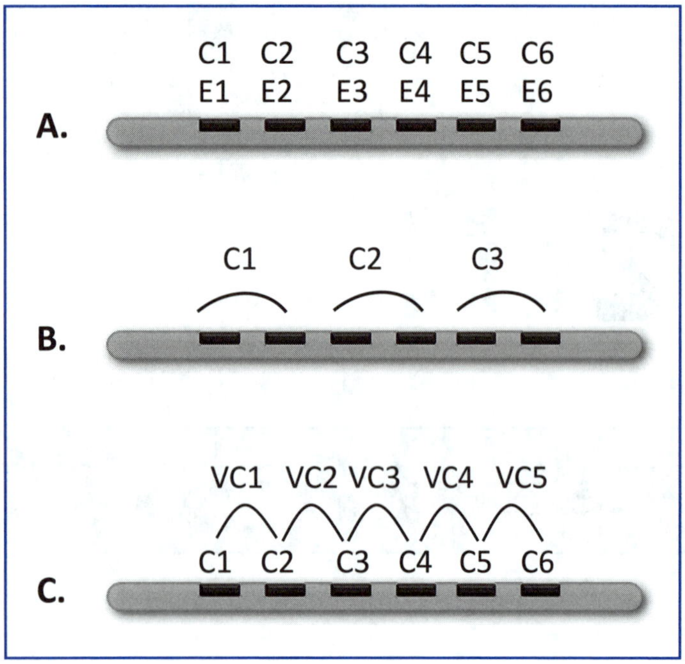


**FIGURE 2–1.** Schematic illustrating the difference between electrodes and channels. **A.** Six physical electrodes (E1–E6) that yield six stimulation channels (C1–C6). **B.** With bipolar stimulation, adjacent electrodes are used for the active and return current path, creating three channels (C1–C3) of stimulation with six electrodes. **C.** With either simultaneous or sequential stimulation of adjacent electrodes, "virtual channels" (VC1–VC5) can be created between adjacent physical electrodes (C1–C6). In this example, one VC is created for each pair of adjacent electrodes, resulting in a total of 11 channels (5 virtual, 6 physical).

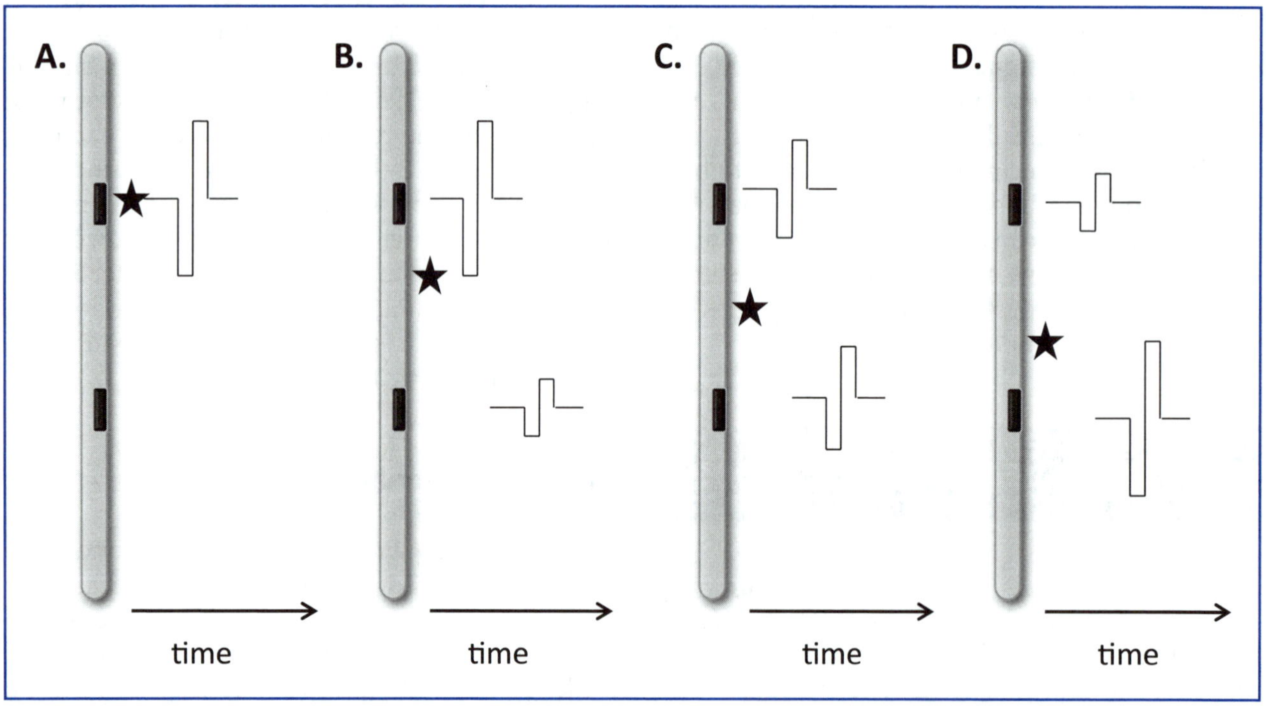


**FIGURE 2–2.** Schematic illustrating the use of sequential stimulation of two adjacent electrodes to achieve intermediate areas of excitation, or channels. The location of the star along the electrode array represents the theoretical tonotopic location of the peak of the field of excitation. As the relative amplitudes change, the locus of excitation changes. **A.** Stimulation on a single electrode alone. **B.** A larger-amplitude pulse is delivered to the first electrode, and a smaller-amplitude pulse is delivered sequentially to the second electrode. The resulting "channel" is between the two physical electrodes, but more heavily weighted toward the electrode with the larger-amplitude pulse. **C.** Equal-amplitude pulses yield a stimulation channel halfway between the adjacent electrodes. **D.** The opposite case as B.

By varying the relative amplitude between the two pulses, intermediate pitch percepts and unique physiological spatial excitation patterns can be achieved. In Figure 2–2B, the resulting "channel" is between the two physical electrodes, but more heavily weighted toward the electrode producing the larger-amplitude pulse. Kwon and van den Honert (2006) used sequential stimulation to measure the number of intermediate pitch percepts between adjacent electrodes, and found that on average, cochlear implant recipients could perceive approximately 3 to 6 intermediate pitches across electrode pairs.

The second method uses a technique called "current steering" (e.g., Bonham & Litvak, 2008; Donaldson, Kreft & Litvak, 2005; Firszt, Koch, Downing, & Litvak, 2007; Frijns et al., 2009, Saoji et al., 2009). With this method, the total amount of current is split between two simultaneously stimulated adjacent (or nonadjacent) electrodes. As the ratio of the current distribution is varied, the locus of the resulting current field will change. This is the method used in Advanced Bionics' HiResolution Fidelity 120 speech processing strategy. Results with this method are consistent with those reported for sequential stimulation; Firszt et al. (2007) reported an average of approximately 4 to 6 intermediate pitch percepts between adjacent electrodes with current steering. This technique is illustrated in Figure 2–3. It is important to note that this method can only be used with devices that have the capability to produce simultaneous stimulation on different electrodes (i.e., having independent current sources for each electrode).

The third method used to produce virtual channels involves electrically coupling two adjacent electrodes (i.e., creating a short circuit between the two electrodes). With this method, the resulting locus of the current field should be different than that produced by either of the single electrodes alone (Busby, Battmer, & Pesch, 2008; Busby & Plant, 2005; Hughes & Goulson, 2011).

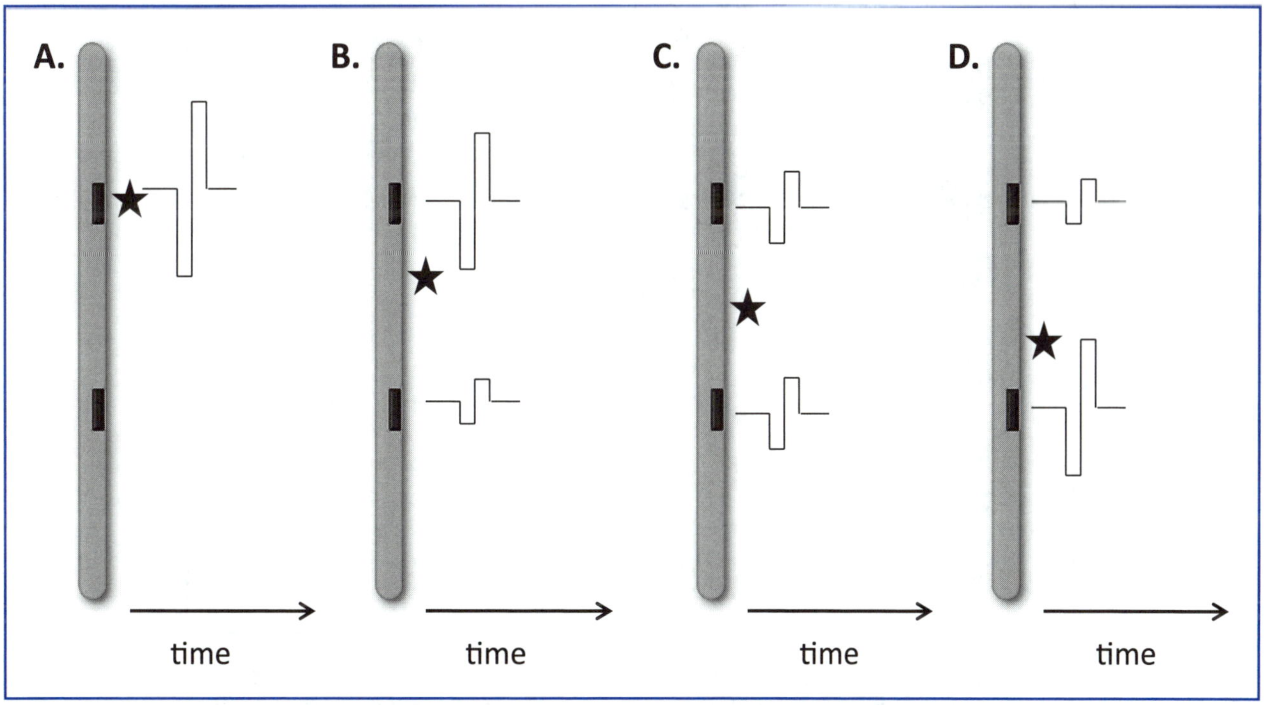


**FIGURE 2–3.** Schematic illustrating the use of simultaneous stimulation (current steering) between two adjacent electrodes to achieve intermediate areas of excitation, or channels. The principles are similar to Figure 2–2 except that current pulses are delivered simultaneously to adjacent electrodes (note that they align along the time axis). The location of the star along the electrode array represents the theoretical tonotopic location of the peak of the field of excitation. As the relative current-pulse amplitudes change, the locus of excitation changes.

This is the method used for the "dual-electrode mode" with newer-generation Nucleus devices (CI24RE and CI512; this feature is presently not commercially available). Unlike the previous two methods, the location of the intermediate channel cannot be manipulated, and no more than one intermediate pitch percept is possible. This method is illustrated in Figure 2–4.

## SIGNAL TYPE

Throughout the history of cochlear implants, two types of signals have been used to represent sound: analog signals and pulsatile signals. Some of the early speech processing strategies (compressed analog, or CA, and simultaneous analog stimulation, or SAS) used analog signals. However the majority of past strategies and all contemporary strategies use pulsatile stimulation.

### Analog Signals

Analog signals are continuous in time (i.e., not discrete). Because of this, the output from each filter band is delivered simultaneously across electrodes. Amplitude variations are created by voltage changes as a function of time. Two early speech processing strategies used analog signals: CA and SAS. The theoretical benefit behind analog signals is that they can provide a truer representation of the speech signal. The two primary drawbacks, however, are that they use up more battery life and produce electrical field interactions because they are continuous signals. Figure 2–5A shows an example of an analog signal.

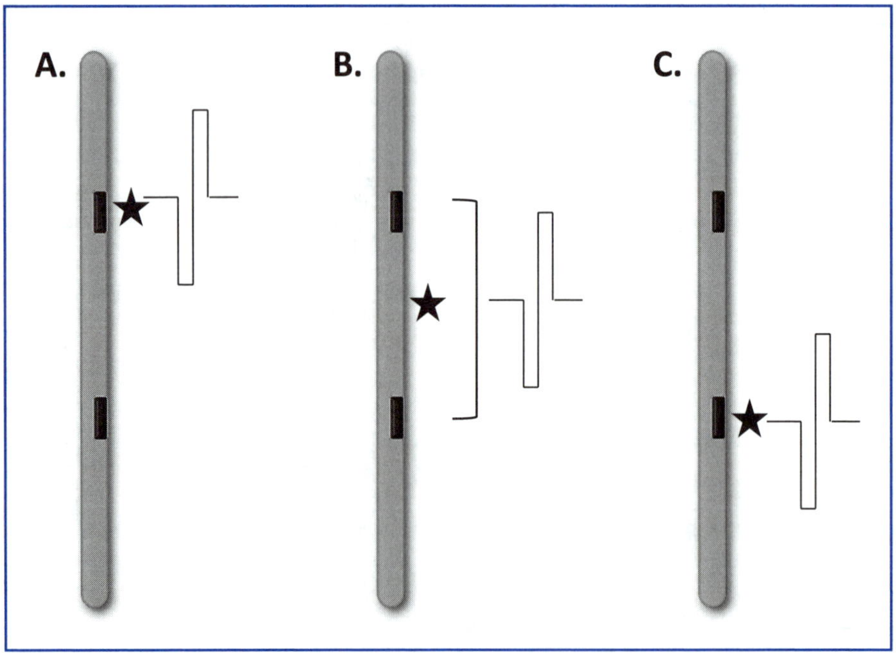


**FIGURE 2–4.** Schematic illustrating the use of electrical coupling (shorting) between two adjacent electrodes to achieve a single intermediate area of excitation, or channel. **A** and **C.** Stimulation of each adjacent electrode separately. **B.** Electrical coupling of the two adjacent electrodes to produce a single intermediate channel. In each segment, the location of the star represents the theoretical tonotopic location of the peak of the field of excitation.

### Pulsatile Signals

In contrast to analog signals, pulsatile signals are discrete. Single pulses are described in terms of the following characteristics:

1. Duration—The duration is how long the pulse is on (Figure 2–5B). Pulse duration is sometimes also referred to as pulse width, and is typically given in microseconds. Shorter pulse durations are more effective for neural excitation (see Abbas & Miller, 2004).
2. Amplitude—Amplitude is the height of the pulse, given in current (see Figure 2–5B).
3. Polarity (anodic or cathodic)—Anodic means that the pulse is positive (see Figure 2–5B), and cathodic means the pulse is negative (Figure 2–5C).
4. Charge balance—"Charge balanced" means that the total charge for the anodic phase equals that of the cathodic phase. If the amplitude of one phase is decreased, then the pulse duration would have to increase to maintain charge balance. It is important that cochlear implants deliver charge-balanced pulses because residual charge that is left in the tissue from asymmetric pulses can be damaging (e.g., Brummer & Turner, 1975; Clark, 2003). Figures 2–5D through 2–5G are examples of charge-balanced pulses.
5. Pulse shape (monophasic, pseudomonophasic, biphasic, or triphasic)—Monophasic pulses consist of a single phase (see Figure 2–5B and 2–5C), and are thus not charge balanced. Pseudomonophasic pulses employ a second, low-amplitude, long-duration phase to provide charge balancing (see Figure 2–5D). Biphasic pulses consist of two opposite phases (see Figure 2–5E). Triphasic pulses (see Figure 2–5F) consist of three phases, where the first and last phases provide the charge balance for the middle phase. Typically, all three phases are the same duration, but the first and third phases are half the amplitude of the second phase.
6. Interphase gap—An interphase gap is a short period of time between cathodic and anodic phases. Thresholds are typically lower for pulses with an interphase gap because the neuron has more time to depolarize in response to the first phase before the charge is removed by the second phase.

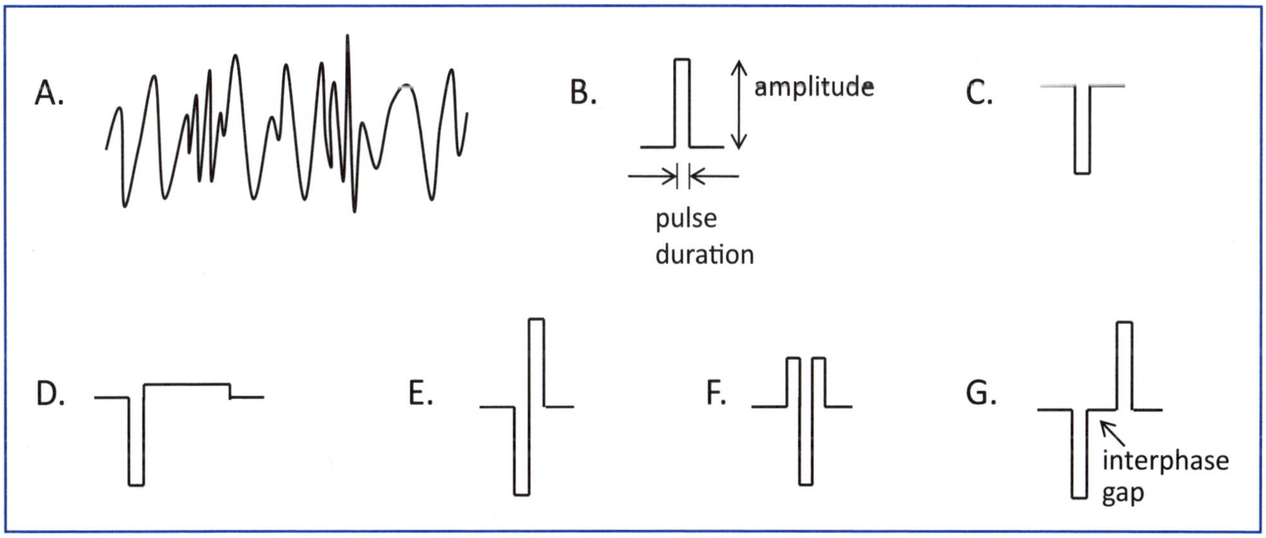


**FIGURE 2–5.** Illustrations of different types of signals. **A.** Continuous analog signal. **B.** Anodic monophasic pulse. **C.** Cathodic monophasic pulse. **D.** Cathodic-leading pseudomonophasic pulse. **E.** Traditional cathodic-leading, charge-balanced biphasic pulse. **F.** Anodic-leading, charge-balanced triphasic pulse. **G.** Cathodic-leading, charge-balanced biphasic pulse with interphase gap.

Single pulses can be used in isolation for evoked potentials, or they can be strung together into pulse trains. Pulse trains are further described by the rate at which individual pulses are delivered (referred to as pulse rate or per-channel stimulation rate), and the overall duration of the pulse train. For example, Figure 2–6A shows a train of six biphasic current pulses. The period is the time from the onset of one pulse to the onset of the next pulse. The pulse rate (like frequency) is the inverse of the period. In this example, if the period is 1 msec, then the pulse rate would be 1000 pps (1/0.001 sec), and the overall duration would be 6 msec.

Simple pulse trains (like the one shown in Figure 2–6A) can also be modulated using the envelope of a sine wave or speech. An example is shown in Figure 2–6B. For sine-modulated signals, the modulation depth is specified.

## STIMULUS TIMING

Stimulus timing refers to the temporal overlap or nonoverlap of stimuli across electrodes in the array. Options include sequential, simultaneous, and partially simultaneous stimulation. All three options have been used with different types of speech processing strategies; the most commonly used is sequential stimulation.

### Sequential Stimulation

Sequential stimulation is when stimuli do not temporally overlap across electrodes (also called nonsimultaneous stimulation). Sequential stimulation can only be achieved with pulsatile stimuli.

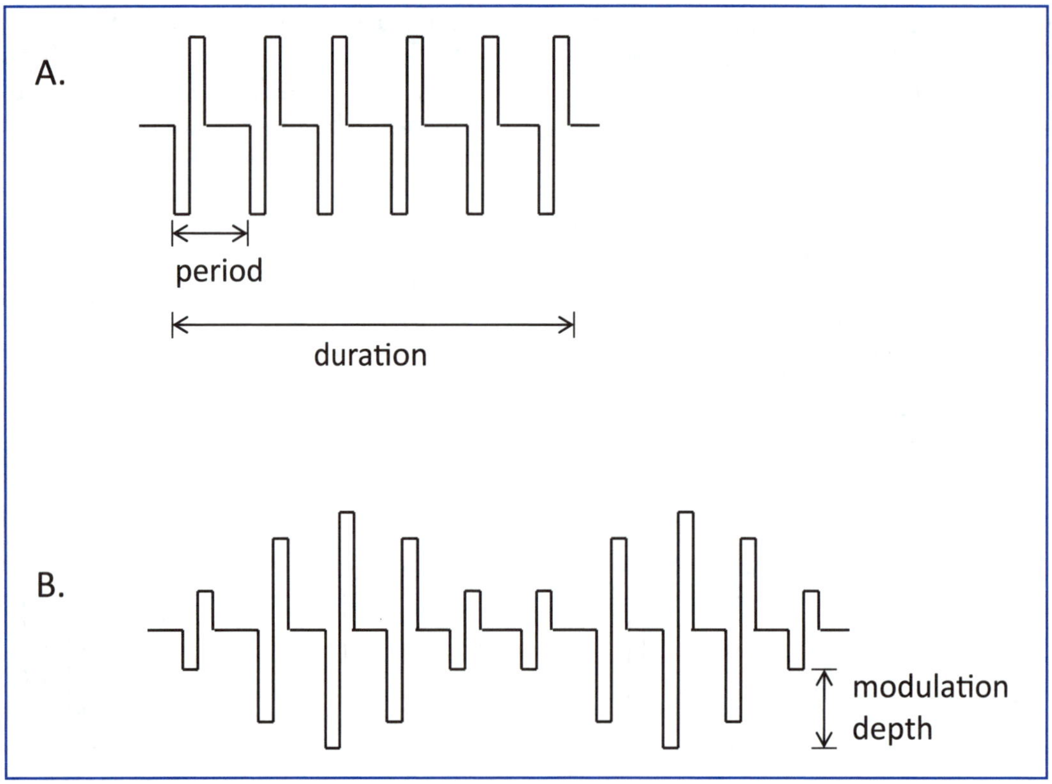


**FIGURE 2–6. A.** Standard equal-amplitude pulse train. Period is the time from onset of one pulse to onset of the next pulse. **B.** Modulated pulse train. Modulation depth is the amplitude difference between the peak and valley of the modulation.

Depending on the time between pulses, sequential stimuli can either have summative effects (for short interpulse intervals) or forward-masking effects (for longer interpulse intervals; see Cartee, van den Honert, Finley, & Miller, 2000). Figure 2–7 shows an example of sequential stimulation across a series of six electrodes. This is the method that most contemporary processing strategies use.

### Simultaneous Stimulation

Simultaneous stimulation is when stimuli are delivered at the same time across all electrodes. Simultaneous stimulation can be achieved with either analog (Figure 2–8A) or pulsatile (Figure 2–8B) stimuli. Devices with independent current sources for each electrode can produce simultaneous stimulation. The primary disadvantage of simultaneous stimulation is that the current fields produced by electrodes that are in close proximity to one another can sum (if in phase) or subtract (if out of phase) prior to neural stimulation (e.g., Abbas & Brown, 1988; Bierer & Middlebrooks, 2004; Boëx, de Balthasar, Kós, & Pelizzone, 2003; de Balthasar et al., 2003; Hughes & Stille, 2009; Stickney et al., 2006). This summation/subtraction can result in either excessive or inadequate stimulation, respectively. This drawback is the primary reason that simultaneous stimulation is not widely used.

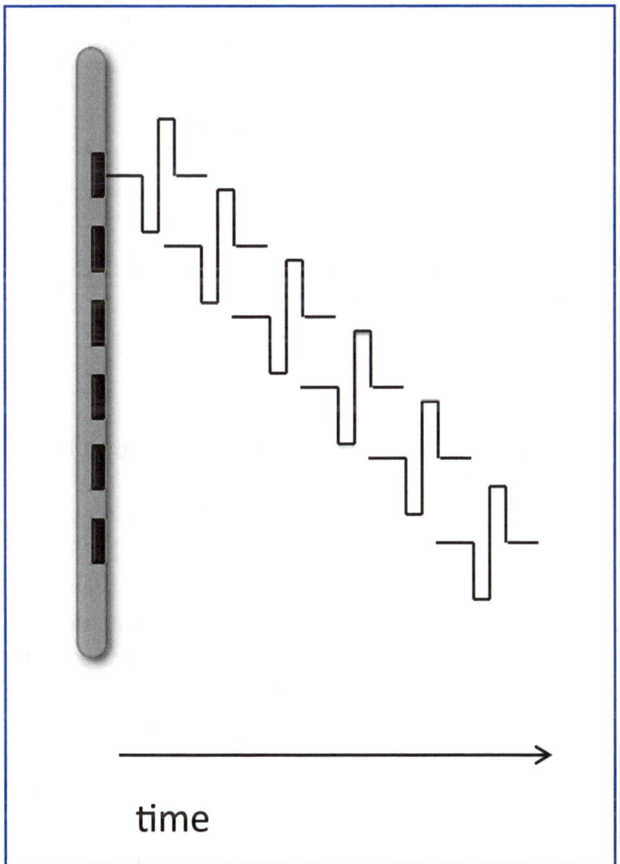


**FIGURE 2–7.** Schematic example of sequential stimulation. Sequential stimulation can only be achieved with pulsatile stimulation (not analog). Note there is no temporal overlap across current pulses delivered to each electrode.

### Partially Simultaneous Stimulation

As its name implies, partially simultaneous stimulation is a cross between sequential and simultaneous stimulus delivery (Figure 2–9). Partially simultaneous stimulation can only be achieved with pulsatile stimuli (to allow for interleaving), and only with devices having independent current sources for each electrode (to allow for simultaneous stimulation). With this method, two (or more) electrodes are stimulated at the same time. The simultaneously stimulated pairs should be widely spaced (e.g., half the array apart) to avoid current field overlap. The timing is sequential across simultaneously stimulated pairs.

## ELECTRODE CONFIGURATION

There are several different ways in which electrodes can be coupled for stimulation. These differences result in different shapes of the current fields and resulting patterns of neural excitation (e.g. Bierer & Middlebrooks, 2002; Landsberger & Srinivasan, 2009; Middlebrooks & Bierer, 2002; van den Honert & Stypulkowski, 1987). In general, broader stimulation modes yield lower thresholds and less selective stimulation patterns because a

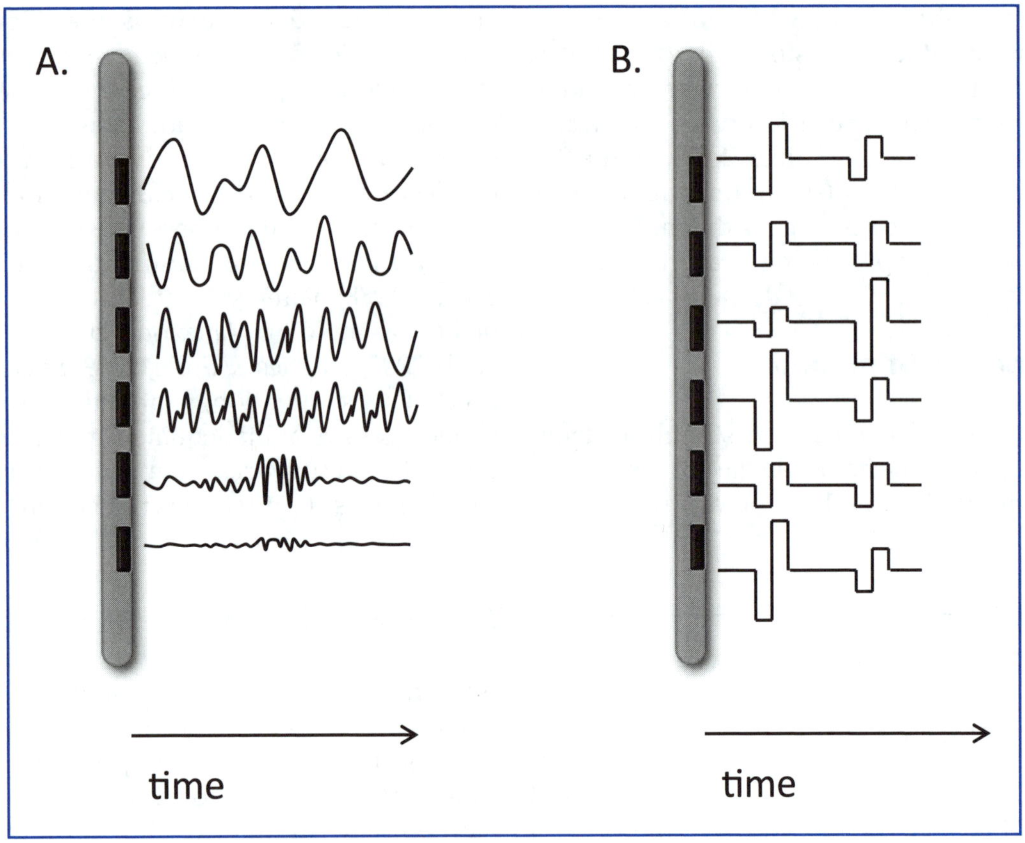


**FIGURE 2–8.** Schematic example of simultaneous stimulation. **A.** Simultaneous stimulation across electrodes with analog stimuli. **B.** Simultaneous stimulation across electrodes with pulsatile stimuli.

larger population of neurons is recruited. Common coupling modes are:

1. Monopolar—Monopolar stimulation involves using a single intracochlear contact as the active electrode and an extracochlear electrode as the return, or ground (Figure 2–10A). This mode typically results in the broadest pattern of excitation (among the modes listed here), given a fixed stimulus level. As a result, lower current levels are needed to achieve threshold. Additionally, thresholds (either physiological or behavioral) and behavioral upper comfort levels tend to be more uniform across the array. Several investigators have described methods to reduce spatial spread for monopolar stimulation, such as using simultaneous stimulation of phase-inverted signals on neighboring electrodes to cancel nondesired portions of the excitatory current field (i.e., Rodenhiser & Spelman, 1995; Van Compernolle, 1985; van den Honert & Kelsall, 2007).
2. Pseudomonopolar—Pseudomonopolar coupling can be used with devices that do not have an extracochlear ground electrode. With this mode, a single intracochlear electrode (typically the most basal) is used as the return (Figure 2–10B).
3. Common ground—With common ground stimulation, a single intracochlear electrode is designated as the active electrode, and all remaining intracochlear electrodes are shorted together to create a single (or common) ground (Figure 2–10C). Because current follows the path of least resistance, the direction of current flow will depend on the

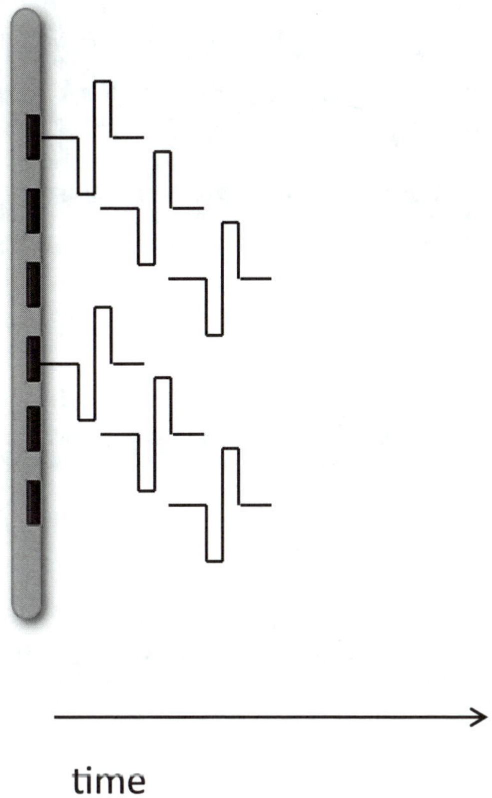


**FIGURE 2–9.** Schematic example of partially simultaneous stimulation. Paired electrodes are stimulated simultaneously, whereas stimulation across pairs is delivered sequentially. Partially simultaneous stimulation can only be achieved with pulsatile stimulation.

weighting of the collective impedances of the shorted electrodes. For example, if the active electrode is near the base, current will flow toward the apex for the return. Conversely, if the active electrode is near the apex, current will flow toward the base for the return. If the active electrode is in the middle of the array, the return path may be split in both basal and apical directions (see Figure 2–10C).

4. Bipolar—Bipolar (BP) stimulation uses one intracochlear electrode as the active electrode, and an adjacent electrode (typically the next apical) as the return (Figure 2–10D). Variations on this coupling mode include bipolar-plus-one (BP+1; Figure 2–10E), BP+2, and so forth, where the "+N" indicates the number of electrodes between the active and return. Of these variations, BP yields the narrowest (or more selective) stimulation pattern, with broader stimulation patterns for wider spacing between the active and return electrodes. Higher current levels are therefore needed for narrower modes to achieve threshold. Additionally, thresholds (either physiological or behavioral) and behavioral upper comfort levels tend to be less uniform across the array for narrower modes, and more likely to reflect local regions of dense versus sparse neural survival.
5. Variable bipolar—This represents a combination of more than one mode of bipolar spacing (e.g., BP and BP+1). Variable bipolar modes are often used clinically in cases where one or more electrodes must be excluded from the processing program (e.g., due to short or open circuits). For example, if electrode 3 has an open circuit, it cannot be used for either the active or return, and would need to be disabled. If the recipient uses a BP program, electrode 2 (which uses electrode 3 as the return in BP mode) would also have to be disabled. However, electrode 2 could be retained in the program if BP+1 mode is designated for that electrode because electrode 4 would be used (instead of electrode 3) as the return.
6. Tripolar—Tripolar stimulation uses one intracochlear electrode as the active electrode, and the two flanking adjacent electrodes as the return (Figure 2–10F). Each of the flanking electrodes return half the total current. Tripolar stimulation has been shown to yield narrower excitation patterns than bipolar or monopolar stimulation (e.g., Bierer & Middlebrooks, 2002; Bonham & Litvak, 2008; Briaire & Frijns, 2000). The drawback, however, is that it can be difficult to achieve adequate stimulation levels without exceeding voltage compliance limits with the device (see Chapter 3).
7. Partial tripolar—Partial tripolar stimulation is a cross between tripolar and monopolar stimulation. With this mode, a fraction of the total current is returned to the extracochlear monopolar electrode, and the remaining fraction

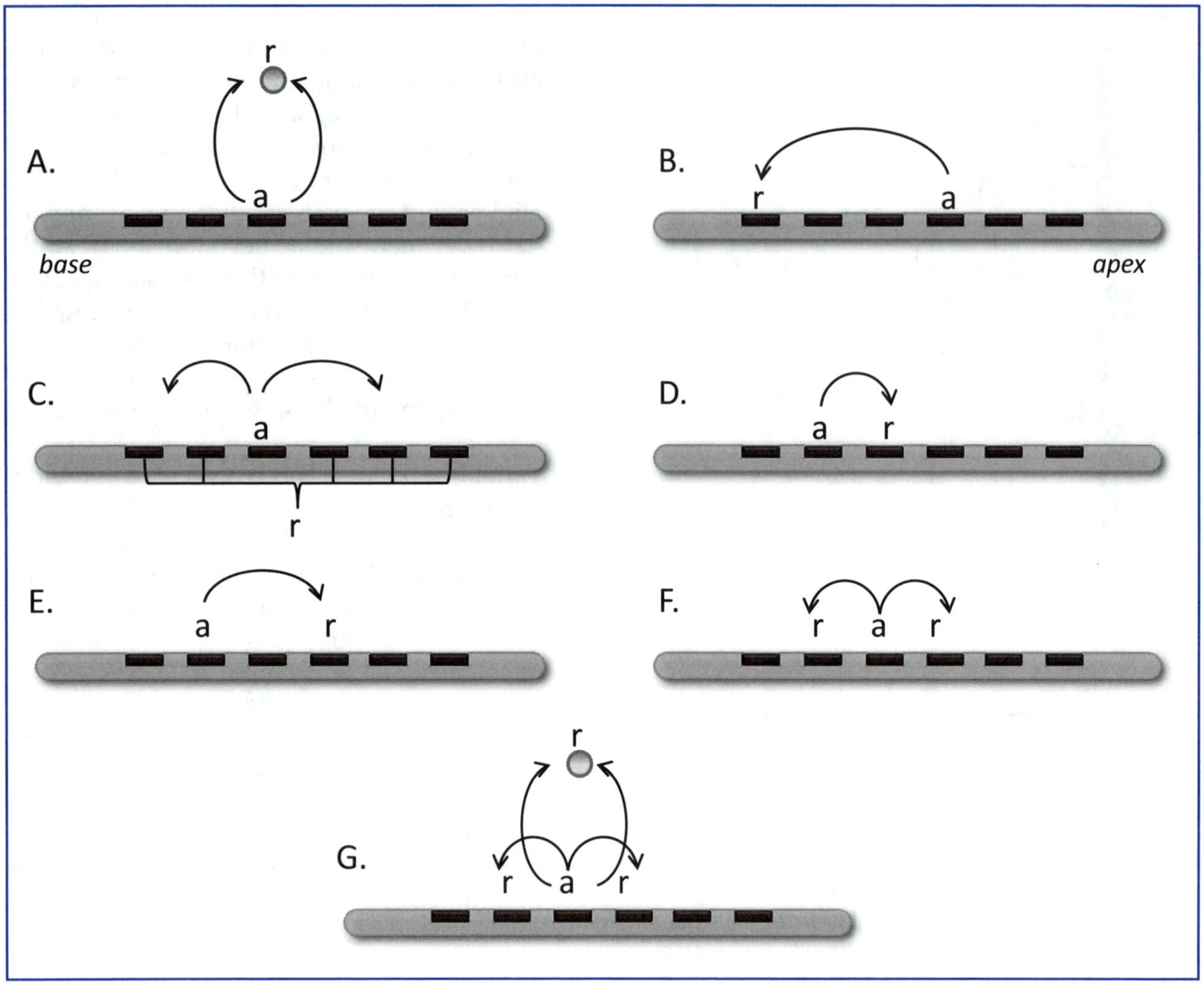


**FIGURE 2–10.** Schematic illustrations of different types of electrode coupling. In all examples, "a" is the active electrode and "r" is the return. **A.** Monopolar, where the return is extracochlear. **B.** Pseudomonopolar. **C.** Common ground. **D.** Bipolar. **E.** Bipolar plus one. **F.** Tripolar. **G.** Partial tripolar.

is split in half and returned in equal portions to the flanking intracochlear electrodes (Bierer & Faulkner, 2010). For example, if half the total current is returned to the monopolar electrode, then one fourth is returned to each of the two flanking electrodes. The ratio can vary from 0 (true monopolar) to 1 (true tripolar). The goal with partial tripolar stimulation is to achieve better spatial selectivity (as with tripolar), but to broaden the stimulation pattern enough to obtain adequate loudness growth and avoid voltage compliance problems.

## ELECTRODE DESIGN

In addition to how electrodes are coupled, the shape and design of each electrode contact can affect the shape of the resulting current fields (e.g., Finley, Wilson, & White, 1990). In general, smaller electrode contacts that face the modiolus will yield more focused stimulation. Figure 2–11 illustrates three different electrode shapes/designs that are currently being used. Figure 2–11A shows

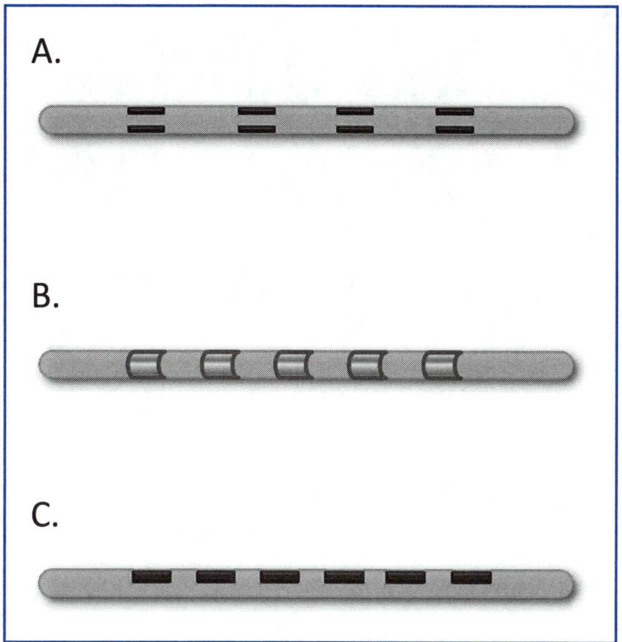


**FIGURE 2–11.** Schematic of different electrode designs. **A.** Radial pairs. **B.** Full-band electrodes. **C.** Half-band or focused electrodes.

an example of pairs of small electrode contacts, similar to those used in MED-EL implants. Figure 2–11B shows an example of full-band electrode contacts, which are composed of rings that encircle the electrode carrier. This design is employed in the Nucleus 22 and 24 generation straight arrays. Finally, Figure 2–11C shows an example of half band contacts, such as those used in the Nucleus Contour arrays. The Advanced Bionics HiFocus arrays are somewhat similar, with pad-shaped contacts that are slightly recessed in the silicone carrier to create a more focused area of stimulation. An example of the older ball-type electrode is shown in Chapter 1, Figure 1–11.

## SUMMARY

This chapter has described the various types of signals, stimulus timing, electrode configurations, and electrode designs that are used both clinically and experimentally with cochlear implant recipients. Key concepts are summarized below:

1. An electrode is the physical structure that injects current into the tissue, whereas a channel is the resulting field of stimulation and/or distinct response resulting from the field of stimulation.
2. Virtual channels can be produced via: (a) varying the relative amplitude of pulses delivered sequentially to adjacent (or nonadjacent) electrodes, (b) varying the relative amplitude of pulses delivered simultaneously to adjacent (or nonadjacent) electrodes ("current steering"), or (c) electrical coupling/shorting of two adjacent electrodes.
3. Analog signals are continuous in time and are therefore presented simultaneously across electrodes for typical cochlear implant use. Analog signals are not used with newer cochlear implant technology.
4. Pulsatile signals can be presented either simultaneously, partially simultaneously, or sequentially across electrodes.
5. Pulsatile signals are described in terms of duration, amplitude, polarity, charge balance, pulse shape, and interphase gap.
6. Different types of electrode coupling can be used to achieve broader (e.g., monopolar) or narrower (e.g., tripolar) stimulation patterns.

# Part II

## Nonphysiological Objective Measures

# 3

# Electrode Impedance

## INTRODUCTION

The next three chapters describe different types of tests that are primarily used to assess the function of the internal device, including that of the individual electrodes: Chapter 3 describes electrode impedance, Chapter 4 describes electric field imaging, and Chapter 5 describes averaged electrode voltages. These assessment tools are designed to measure electrode-specific voltage, impedance, and electrical field (voltage) patterns across the array. As such, these tests can also be used to gain insight into properties of the surrounding tissue, the electrode-tissue interface, and the path of current flow. In contrast to the measures described in Chapters 6 to 10, the tests described in Chapters 3 to 5 are not used to assess the physiological functioning of the auditory pathway. Depending on the specific tools available to the clinician, one or more of these tests may be used to assess device function for the primary purposes of making decisions about: (1) whether or not to exclude specific electrodes from the speech processor program, or (2) whether or not to recommend an explant/reimplant.

This chapter begins with a basic introduction to electrode impedance, which covers Ohm's law, the two primary components of impedance, and different types of abnormal impedance. Next, a brief orientation to the current manufacturers' software for clinically measuring impedance is given. Finally, clinical uses for impedance measures are provided with specific examples.

## THE BASICS OF ELECTRODE IMPEDANCE

Clinically, impedance measures are important for determining whether intracochlear and extracochlear electrodes are functioning appropriately. Impedance measures can also provide information about the properties of the tissue in contact with the electrode's surface (electrode-tissue interface). Impedance can be determined using Ohm's law:

$$V = IR \text{ or } I = V/R,$$

where V is voltage, I is current, and R is resistance (or, more generally, impedance). To better understand the relationship between voltage, current, and resistance, let us begin with a basic definition of each of these three components. Voltage is the difference in potential between two points in an electrical circuit, and is measured in volts. Voltage can be thought of as the amount of work it takes to move electrical charge between two points. Current is similar to velocity; it is the rate at which electric charge (ions or electrons) moves through a medium, and is measured in amperes. Electrical impedance is the opposition to current flow when a certain voltage is applied, and is measured in ohms.

## The Components of Impedance

Impedance and resistance are not exactly the same thing. Impedance is the opposition to current flow for an AC circuit, and includes both magnitude and phase components. Resistance is the opposition to current flow for a DC circuit, and consists of only the magnitude component. In cases where the phase is zero, then impedance and resistance are essentially the same thing. In cochlear implants, impedance is the vector sum of reactance (phase) and resistance (magnitude) components. These two components are described further in the following sections (see also Chapter 4 in Clark, 2003 for a more comprehensive description). Significant changes in impedance over time can indicate substantial changes in either the electrode-tissue interface or electrode function. Separating out these two potential factors requires a better understanding of the two primary components of impedance.

### *Resistance*

The resistance component of impedance is often referred to as "access resistance" (Clark, 2003; Tykocinski, Duan, Tabor, & Cowan, 2001). In an electrical circuit, resistance is the opposition to current flow. In cochlear implants, access resistance results from the size and composition (i.e., type of metal) of the electrode contact and lead wire, as well as the resistivity of the surrounding medium (e.g., perilymph, fibrous tissue, bone; Clark, 2003). An example is illustrated in Figure 3–1A, where $R_a$ represents the access resistance for the electrode lead wire, electrode contact, and fluid/tissue. Each of these components provides some opposition to current flow, and if viewed in terms of an electrical circuit (Figure 3–1B), each can be considered a resistor in series.

### *Reactance*

The source of the reactance component (sometimes called the polarization component) is the interface between the electrode surface and surrounding fluid or tissue (see Figure 3–1). The reactance component of impedance reflects two mechanisms of charge transfer (Clark, 2003). The first is capacitive (represented as "C" in Figure 3–1), in that it stores energy to oppose current flow. A capacitor in an electrical circuit consists of two metal plates, which are separated by an insulating layer. Each plate holds either a positive or negative charge. In simple terms, think of the electrode surface as one of the charged plates of a capacitor, and the adjacent fluid/tissue as the other plate, with opposite charge. It is also important to understand that current flow along a metal surface (i.e., the electrode lead wire and contact) is accomplished via the movement of electrons, whereas current flow within an electrolyte solution (i.e., the perilymph) is accomplished via movement of ions. Thus, the electrode-tissue interface represents the transition of current flow from electrons to ions.

The second mechanism operating at the electrode-tissue interface is faradic ("$R_f$" in Figure 3–1), which transfers charge via chemical reactions (Clark, 2003). In electrical terms, faradic charge transfer is a resistive component. This is the mechanism that is responsible for the formation of a hydride layer (hydrogen atoms) on the surface of the electrode (Brummer & Turner, 1977). It is also the mechanism that can produce toxic substances (such as dissolved metal) in the fluid/tissue if the charge density is too high (Clark, 2003). Thus, the capacitive component is the most ideal for charge transfer from the electrode to the tissue because it is safer (Clark, 2003); this is why all commercial cochlear implants use a net AC current for stimulation. Table 3–1 summarizes the differences between the resistance and reactance components of impedance.

Figure 3–2 illustrates the relative contribution of the resistance and reactance components of impedance. Figure 3–2A shows a biphasic current pulse (i.e., the stimulus) with magnitude "I." Figures 3–2B and 3–2C show the resulting voltage measurements. The access resistance component is reflected in the initial, instantaneous rise in

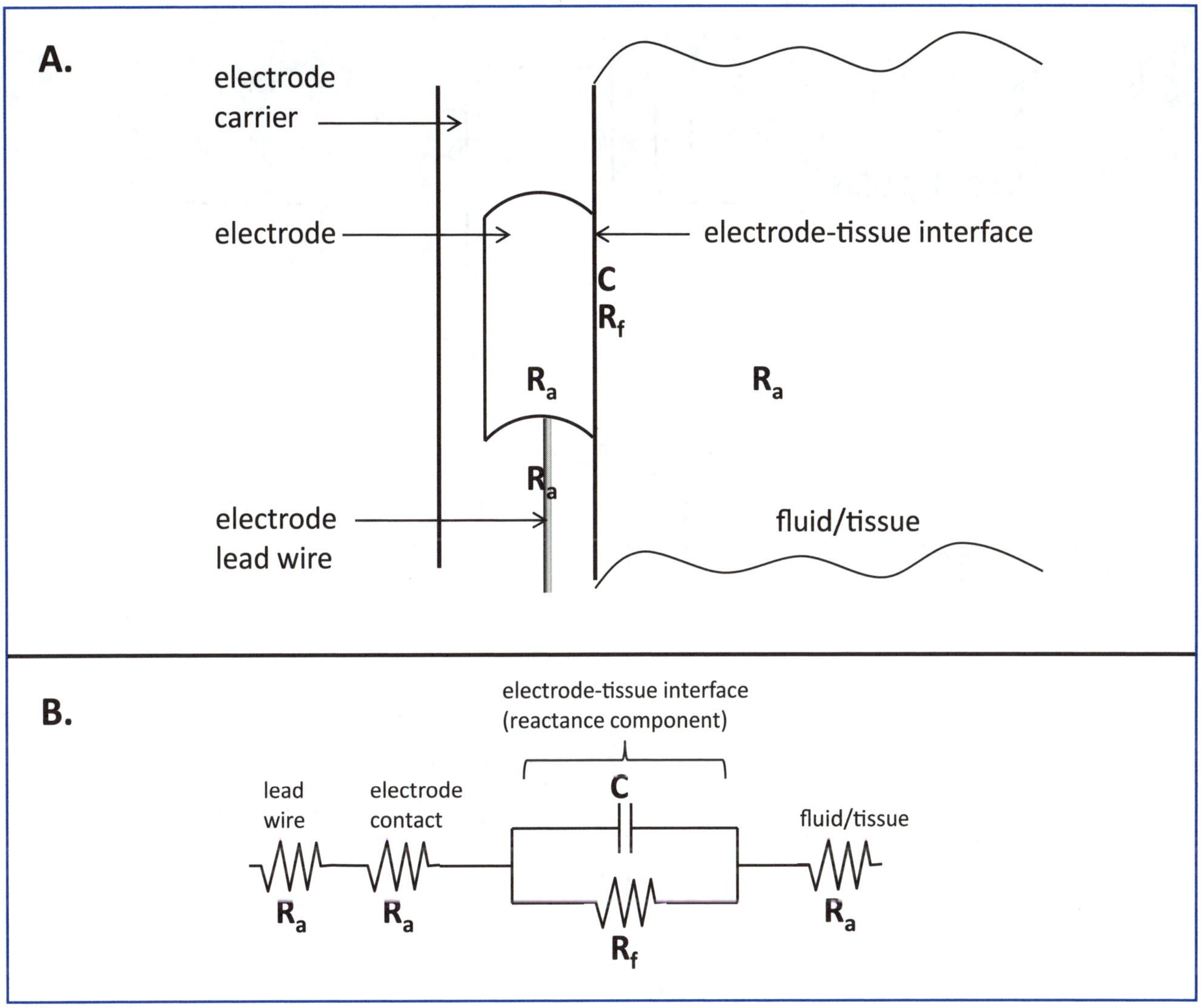


**FIGURE 3–1.** Sources of resistance and reactance components of impedance. **A.** Schematic of electrode contact on a silicone carrier. $R_a$ represents the access resistance (electrode lead wire, electrode contact, fluid/tissue medium); C represents the capacitance (reactance component) at the electrode-tissue interface; $R_f$ represents potential faradic resistance. **B.** Corresponding electrical circuit diagram for panel A.

**Table 3–1.** Comparison of Resistance and Reactance Components of Impedance

| *Resistance* | *Reactance* |
|---|---|
| Opposes current flow | Stores energy to oppose current flow |
| Resistive properties | Capacitive properties |
| Source: electrode contact, lead wire, surrounding fluid/tissue medium | Source: electrode-tissue interface |
| AKA "access resistance" | AKA "polarization component" |

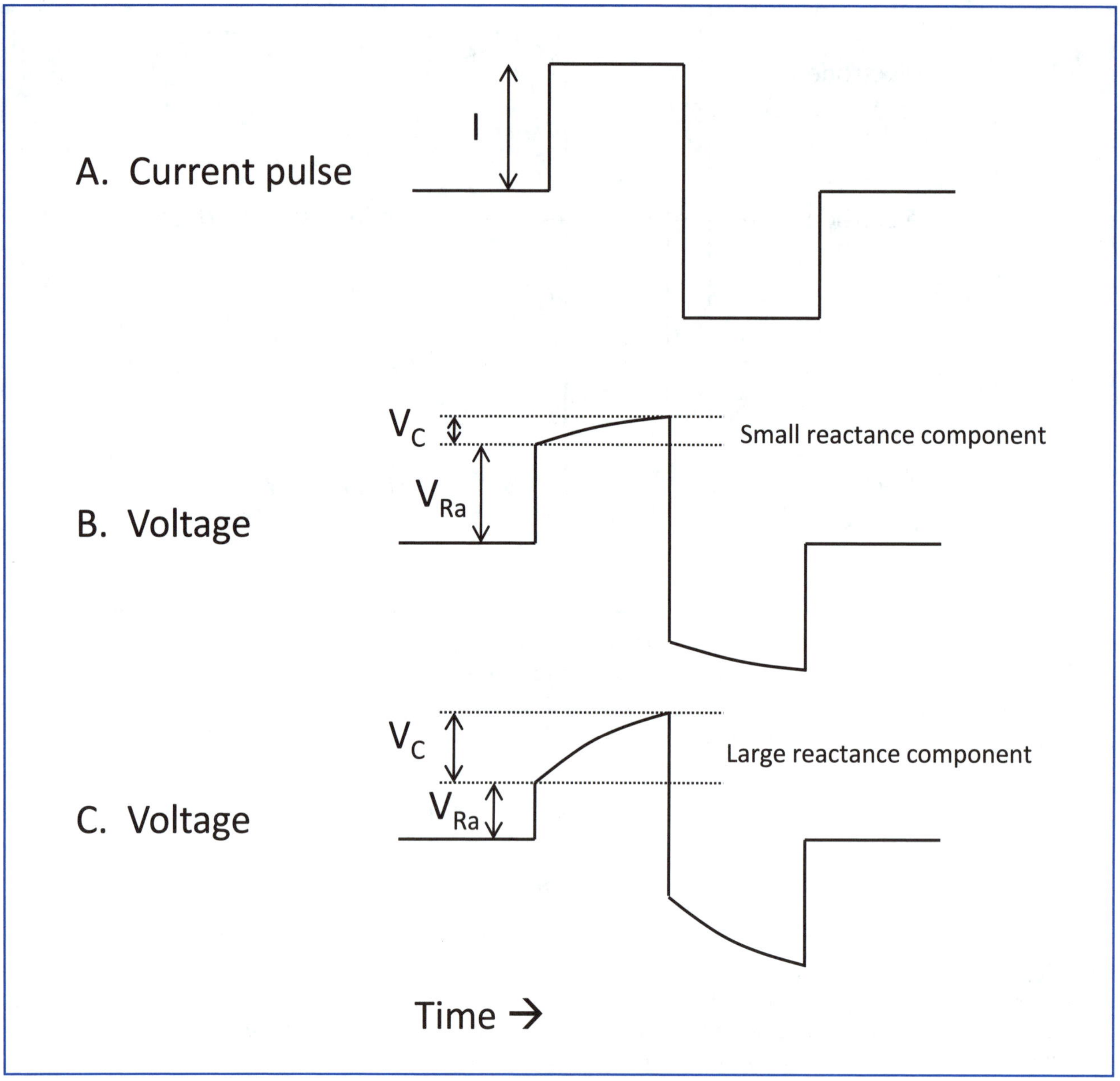


**FIGURE 3–2. A.** Charge-balanced biphasic current pulse (i.e., the stimulus), where I is the amplitude of the pulse. **B.** Resulting voltage waveform showing an example of a relatively small reactance component ($V_C$) and larger resistance component ($V_{Ra}$). **C.** Resulting voltage waveform showing an example of a relatively large reactance component ($V_C$) and smaller resistance component ($V_{Ra}$). Time is represented along the x-axis. Adapted from Newbold et al., 2004, Figure 2; Tykocinski et al., 2001, Figure 1; and Clark, 2003, Figure 4.1.

voltage ($V_{Ra}$). The reactance component ($V_C$) is reflected by the nonlinear slow growth in voltage over the duration of the pulse, and is the result of charging up the capacitive electrode-tissue interface (Tykocinski et al., 2001). Figure 3–2B shows an example of a small reactance component, and Figure 3–2C shows an example of a larger reactance component.

### Geometric Versus Real Surface Area

Because electrode surface area affects impedance, it is important to understand the different ways that electrode area is quantified. Electrodes with larger surface areas typically have lower impedance (e.g., Saunders et al., 2002). The geometric area of an electrode refers to the calculated area based the electrode's dimensions. For example, the area of a rectangular electrode would be the length multiplied by width; or for a spherical electrode, the area would be $4\pi r^2$. The "real" surface area includes the "roughness" of the surface of the electrode (Brummer & Turner, 1977; Tykocinski et al., 2001). Electrode surface area can be "roughened" using a variety of techniques, including etching with lasers or applying electrochemical coatings (De Ceulaer et al., 2003; Paasche, Bockel, Tasche, Lesinski-Schiedat, & Lenarz, 2006; Tykocinski et al., 2001). Additionally, when hydrogen atoms are deposited at the surface of the electrode (hydride layer), the geometric surface area is effectively increased by the "real" surface area. Brummer and Turner (1977) reported that a shiny platinum electrode with a geometric area of 1 $cm^2$ is typically about 1.4 real $cm^2$.

### Impedance Changes Over Time

Clinically, it is not uncommon to see changes in electrode impedance over time. It is therefore important to understand the typical course of impedance changes so that atypical changes can be investigated further and managed appropriately. Impedance is usually lowest at the time of surgery (Busby, Plant, & Whitford, 2002; Hughes et al., 2001) because the medium surrounding the array most likely consists of perilymph. In the 2 to 3 weeks following surgery (Paasche et al., 2006; Tykocinski et al., 2001), impedance increases (e.g., Busby et al., 2002; Hughes et al., 2001; Newbold et al., 2004) due to fibrous tissue encapsulation of the electrode array, which is a by-product of the body's immune response to a foreign body (e.g., Clark, Shute, Shepherd, & Carter, 1995; Newbold et al., 2004; Tykocinski et al., 2001). Several investigators (Newbold et al., 2004; Tykocinski et al., 2001; Xu, Shepherd, Millard, & Clark, 1997) have reported higher impedances for more extensive encapsulation (i.e., more cells surrounding the electrode results in increased electrical resistance). Additionally, Clark et al. (1995) noted increased impedance when inflammatory cells were present within the fibrous tissue sheath. The use of steroids during surgical insertion of the electrode array has been shown to reduce the amount of fibrous tissue encapsulation (by suppressing the response of the immune system) and thus lowering impedance (e.g., De Ceulaer et al., 2003; Paasche et al., 2006).

Once the implant is stimulated, impedance typically decreases and is stabilized within the first few months of device use (Busby et al., 2002; De Ceulaer et al., 2003; Dorman, Smith, Dankowski, McCandless, & Parkin, 1992; Henkin, Kaplan-Neeman, Muchnik, Kronenberg, & Hildesheimer, 2003; Henkin et al., 2006; Hughes et al., 2001; Newbold et al., 2004; Saunders et al., 2002). Newbold et al. (2004) showed a decrease in the number of cells covering the electrode following electrical stimulation for their in vitro experiments. However, they noted that this process of cell reduction does not occur in vivo (e.g., in humans). They suggested that, for humans, the decrease in impedance following electrical stimulation may be due to a reorganization of the fibrous tissue matrix that surrounds the electrode array (e.g., it may become less dense).

Although impedances should typically stabilize within the first few months of device use, it is important to recognize factors that can affect impedance later on (other than defects related to the device, such as short or open circuits, which are described further in the following sections). First, impedance can increase for electrodes that are not stimulated for a period of time (e.g., Hughes et al., 2001; Newbold et al., 2004; Schulman, 1995). For example, if an electrode is excluded from a patient's program (e.g., due to unpleasant pitch percept or change in strategy) then the impedance of that electrode will increase during the period of nonuse. Second, reimplantation has been shown to result in higher impedances for the subsequent array (De Ceulaer et al., 2003). De Ceulaer et al. (2003) proposed that this trend may be due to the additional trauma imposed by removal and reinsertion of a new electrode array. Third, increases in electrode impedance with concurrent increases in programming levels have been observed clinically with concomitant middle ear infection, fluid, otalgia, vertigo, common cold, or other similar processes (Neuburger, Lenarz, Lesinski-Shiedat, & Büchner, 2009). However, there are few published reports that document the time course, process, or underlying mechanism for this observation (e.g., Neuburger et al., 2009). It may be that middle ear fluid, which is an electrically conductive medium, changes the path of current flow, particularly for monopolar stimulation. Once the fluid resolves, the current path may revert back to normal. Alternatively, the presence of inflammatory cells within the cochlea (as may be the case with labyrinthitis) has been shown to result in increased impedance (Clark et al., 1995). These impedance changes would also explain concurrent changes in map programming levels during the time frame that the disease process is active. Finally, the use of fast-rate strategies may lead to greater probability of operating outside of the device's voltage compliance limits (described further below), resulting in impedance increases (Neuburger et al., 2009). Fast-rate strategies naturally require narrower pulse widths, which in turn require increased voltage to generate the charge necessary to achieve adequate loudness levels. Exceeding voltage compliance limits may lead to slight pulse asymmetry, resulting in platinum dissolution (e.g., Brummer & Turner, 1975; Clark, 2003). This may result in further increases in impedance, which subsequently increases the probability of exceeding compliance limits (Neuburger et al., 2009). Neuburger et al. (2009) proposed a simple solution of widening the pulse duration (which reduces the stimulation rate) so that lower-amplitude current pulses can be used.

## Abnormal Impedance

The following subsections describe the various types of abnormal impedance that are seen clinically. The two most straightforward and commonly known impedance abnormalities are open or short circuits. A partial short circuit is less well-known because it is not as straightforward to identify. Finally, although not technically considered abnormal impedance, voltage compliance issues result from electrodes with normal but relatively high impedance. Voltage compliance is included in this section because it is an impedance-related issue that must be managed clinically.

### Open Circuits

An electrical circuit must have an intact loop (source and return path) to allow current to flow. An open circuit is defined as an incomplete path for current to flow, or a discontinuous circuit. Causes might include a broken electrode contact, broken lead wire, or a nonconductive medium surrounding the electrode contact (such as air). In any of these cases, an infinite resistance prohibits the flow of current. True open circuits are characterized by near-infinite impedance values (megohms). Clinical software also flags electrodes with very high impedance (typically on the order of 20 to 30 kilohms or greater for today's cochlear implants) in the same way as true open circuits. Open circuits can be identified using any of the usual electrode coupling modes that are clinically available (see Chapter 2).

Figure 3–3 illustrates how three different coupling modes are effective at identifying open circuits. The left column illustrates the "normal" path of current flow for monopolar (A), common ground (C), and bipolar (E). The right column illustrates how current flow is not possible (dashed line) with any of the three modes shown (B, D, and F). In all three cases, there is a discontinuity between the stimulating electrode and return path, which prohibits the flow of current. The net result is a very high impedance measure.

### Short Circuits

A short circuit is defined as low resistance between two points in a circuit that differ in potential. The result is an increase in current flow (for a fixed voltage). Short circuits are typically caused by conductive electrical components coming into contact with one another. Examples would include two electrode contacts that are touching because the array is kinked or curled back on itself within

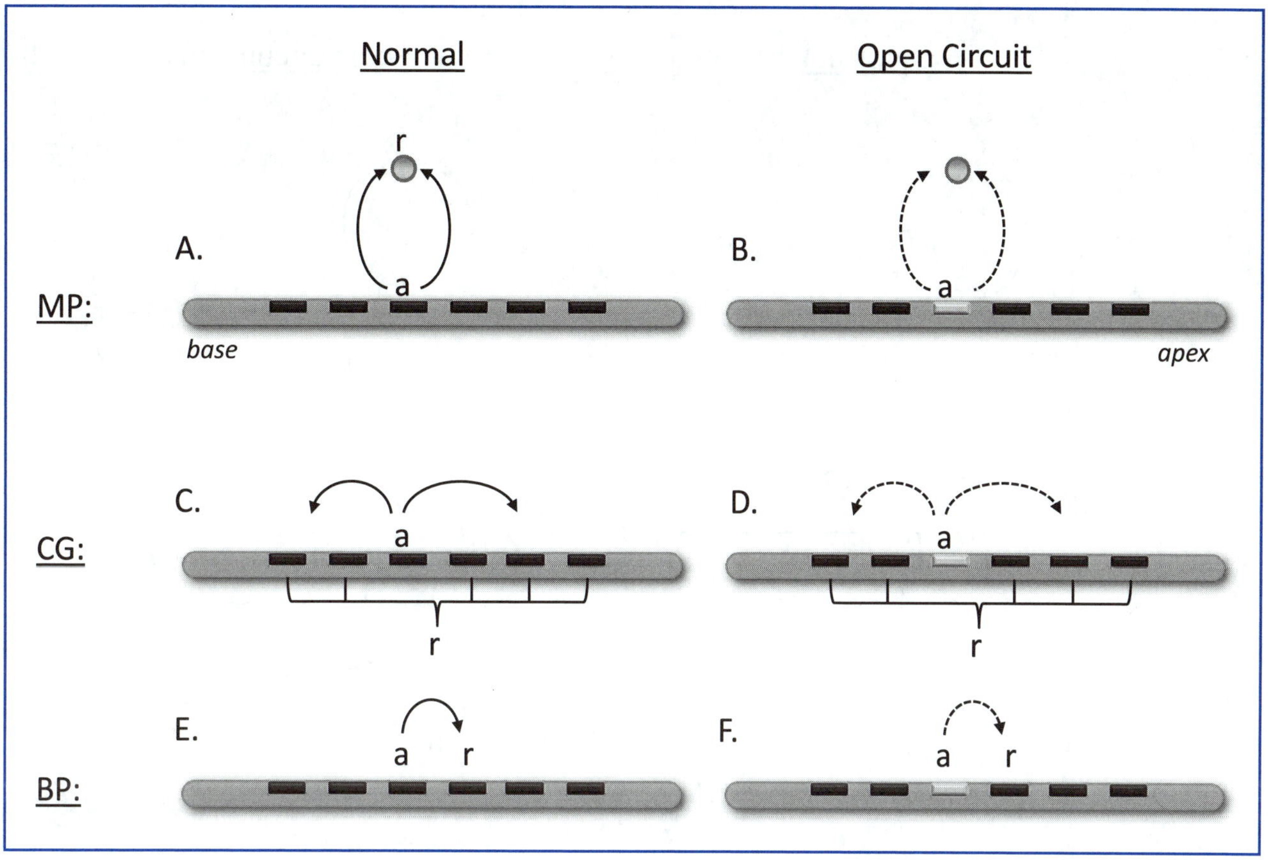


**FIGURE 3–3.** Illustration of how different coupling modes are effective at identifying open circuits. Left column: "normal" path of current flow for monopolar (*A*), common ground (*C*), and bipolar (*E*) stimulation. Right column: current flow is not possible with any of the three modes shown (*B*, *D*, and *F*). Dashed arrows indicate no current flow; "a" is the active electrode, which in this case has an open circuit (shown as a grayed-out electrode contact); "r" is the return electrode. In the case of common ground coupling (*C* and *D*), all return electrodes are shorted together (indicated by brackets) to form a single ground.

the cochlea, or two electrode lead wires that are touching within the electrode carrier because of compromised insulating layers. Short circuits can be identified by very low impedance values. The short circuit limits are slightly different across manufacturers due to differences in electrode sizes across devices. Typically, these values are on the order of about 1 kilohm or less.

Short circuits between two intracochlear electrodes can be identified with common ground or various bipolar coupling modes, but not reliably with monopolar coupling. The exception is if an intracochlear electrode is shorted to an extracochlear monopolar electrode. In that rare case, monopolar impedance testing would be the only way the short circuit would be detected. Figure 3–4 illustrates how different coupling modes can identify or miss a short circuit. In this example, the two most basal electrodes are shorted together for the arrays shown in the right column. For normal monopolar stimulation (Figure 3–4A), a single intracochlear electrode serves as the active and the extracochlear (monopolar) electrode serves as the return. When a single intracochlear electrode is shorted to another intracochlear electrode (Figure 3–4B), current flows between the two intracochlear electrodes. However, current still has a path to flow to the extracochlear return. In this case, monopolar coupling will typically not identify the short circuit between the two intracochlear electrodes because the overall path remains intact.

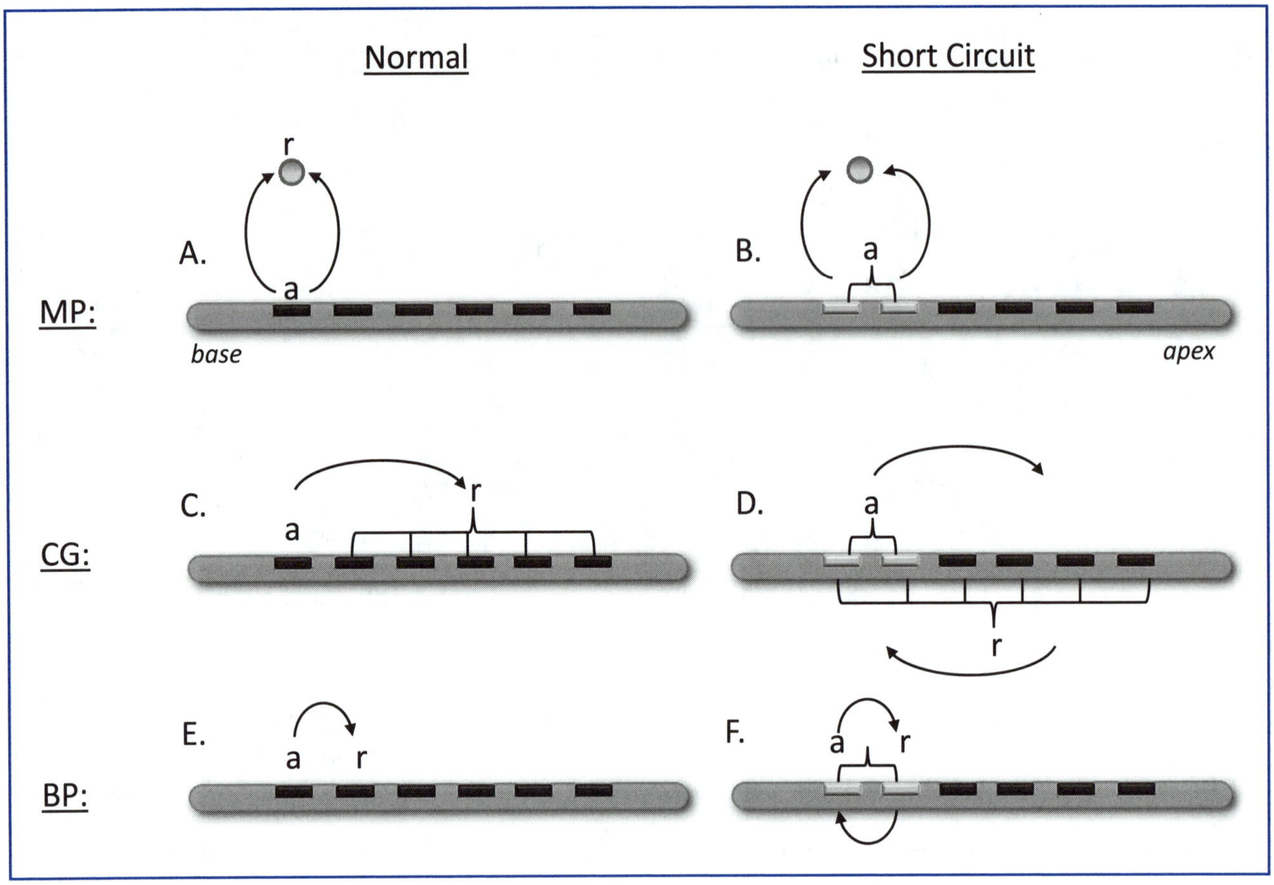


**FIGURE 3–4.** Illustration of how different coupling modes are effective (or ineffective) at identifying short circuits. Schematic is laid out similar to Figure 3–3, where "a" is the active electrode and "r" is the return. Electrodes with unintentional short circuits are indicated in the right column (*B*, *D*, and *F*) by the two most basal grayed-out electrode contacts. Brackets indicate electrodes that are shorted together (intentionally for common ground mode, and unintentionally for the two basal electrodes in the right column). The double arrows going in opposite directions in examples *D* and *F* indicate increased current flow. In this case, common ground (CG) and any bipolar (BP) coupling will be effective in identifying a short circuit (*D* and *F*), but monopolar (MP) will not (*B*).

In contrast, common ground and bipolar modes are more effective in identifying short circuits. For normal common ground stimulation (Figure 3–4C), a single intracochlear electrode serves as the active electrode and the remaining intracochlear electrodes are shorted together to yield a single return "electrode" (or a common ground). When two intracochlear electrodes are shorted together (Figure 3–4D), current flows between the two electrodes. This means that when the "remaining" electrodes are shorted together for the return, the entire electrode array is shorted together, thus yielding an overall low impedance result. Similarly, for bipolar stimulation (Figures 3–4E and 3–4F), if the active and return electrodes are shorted together, the result is increased current flow between the active and return, and therefore low impedance.

### Partial Short Circuits

A partial short circuit is characterized by relatively low resistance resulting in increased current flow, but less so than for a true short circuit. Partial short circuits present as impedances that are lower than that of nonaffected electrodes, but not low enough to be flagged by the clinical software as a true short circuit. Partial short circuits can result from small tears or fractures in the silicone surrounding the electrode fantail or lead. Partial short circuits have also been referred to as "atypical impedances" or "insulation damage" (Carlson et al., 2010).

Figure 3–5 illustrates how a partial short circuit works. The top panel shows the normal condition, where current (I) is delivered to the middle lead wire, which is connected to the middle electrode. The resulting current field is shown below

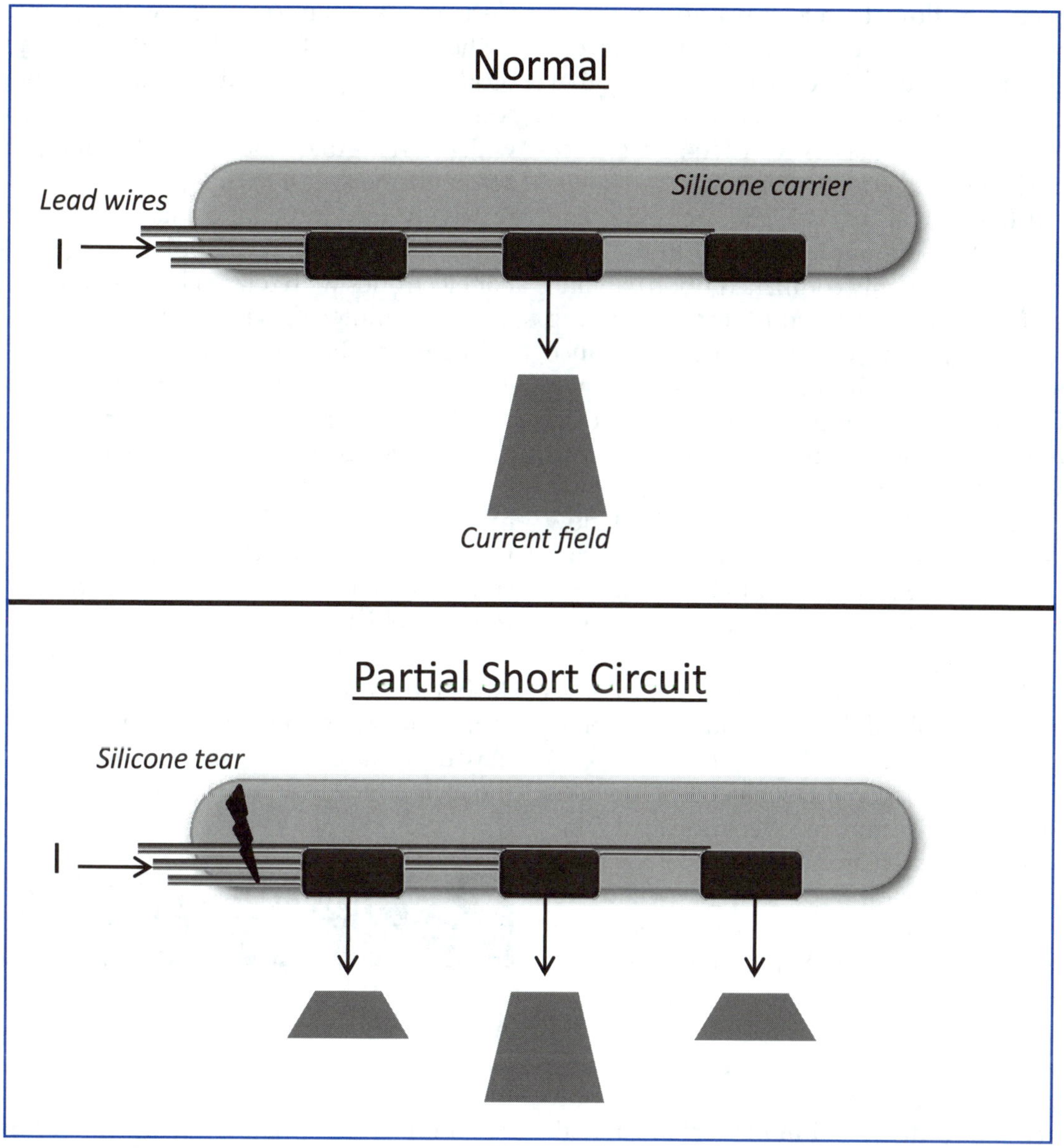


**FIGURE 3–5. Top:** In a normally functioning cochlear implant, current flows down the lead wire to a specific electrode contact. The surrounding silicone provides insulation. The shaded area below the electrode contact indicates the theoretical resultant current field. **Bottom:** Schematic of a partial short circuit caused by a small fracture or tear in the silicone, causing a portion of the current to shunt away from the intended electrode toward adjacent electrodes. This results in less current flow to the intended electrode, which can manifest clinically into elevated thresholds and upper comfort levels due to insufficient current. Current that is shunted to adjacent electrodes can functionally result in pitch confusions, distortion, or reduced speech perception.

the activated electrode. In the case of the partial short circuit (bottom panel), a small tear allows for fluid ingress into the silicone carrier, altering the impedance path of the current intended for the middle electrode. In this example, the silicone tear extends across all three lead wires. Because fluid is more conductive than silicone, there is less resistance to current flow, thereby resulting in lower impedance for the middle electrode and current leakage to the electrodes connected to the other involved lead wires. In this scenario, the result would be lower impedances for each of the three electrodes, when tested individually.

Identification of partial short circuits can be difficult while the implant is still in use. The problem is typically only confirmed upon explant. There are two key components for identifying suspected partial short circuits using impedance measures. The first is that impedances (common ground is the preferred mode) will decrease over time. When silicone fractures are small, it can take time for fluid ingress to occur. As more fluid fills the fracture, the resistance to current flow decreases, and impedance measures will drop. Second, impedance changes should be examined relative to the impedances of other electrodes in the array. If the impedances for only certain electrodes systematically decrease over time, whereas others remain stable, this may be an indication of a partial short circuit.

For certain models of Cochlear Ltd. devices, the even- and odd-numbered electrode lead wires are bundled separately from each side of the internal receiver-stimulator. Depending on where silicone fractures occur, the result can present as an alternating or zigzag pattern in the impedance measures. An example is shown in Figure 3–6 for common ground, MP1, MP2, and MP1+2 test modes. In this example, impedances for the even-numbered electrodes are lower than for odd-numbered electrodes, resulting in a characteristic alternating pattern across all test modes with the lowest impedance measures obtained for common ground (circles).

### Voltage Compliance

Most cochlear implants are constant current devices, where a fixed amount of current is specified in the software, and the amount of supply voltage (from the battery) is varied depending on the impedance of the electrode and surrounding tissue. Because impedance can change over short or long time intervals (as well as with the type of stimulus), dynamically varying the voltage results in a consistent amount of current that is injected from the electrode. So, let us consider "voltage compliance" in the context of Ohm's law, where voltage is the product of impedance times current. The current sources in the implant are fed by a supply voltage, which can regulate the electrode voltage between zero and the supply voltage. For electrodes with relatively low impedance, larger current values can be used before the supply voltage is reached. For electrodes with relatively high impedance, the device is limited to smaller current values before voltage compliance is reached (i.e., more voltage is needed to achieve the desired current level).

It is important to consider that the surface area of the electrode contact will affect voltage compliance limits. Smaller contacts typically have higher impedances because of their smaller surface areas (e.g., Saunders et al., 2002). As a result, smaller contacts (with higher impedance) will be more likely to exceed voltage compliance limits than larger contacts (with lower impedance). Also, electrodes with higher impedances require more voltage for a specified current level, which may translate clinically into shorter battery life for the recipient.

## HOW IMPEDANCE IS MEASURED CLINICALLY

All three manufacturers have incorporated impedance measures into their clinical software. For older devices that do not have back-telemetry capabilities (see Chapter 1), impedance measures cannot be made using the clinical software. In these cases, other measures such as averaged electrode voltages (AEVs; see Chapter 5) can be used. The following sections provide a brief overview of each manufacturer's clinical impedance measures. In all cases, a fixed current is applied to a given electrode, and the voltage is measured between the active and return electrodes at the output of the

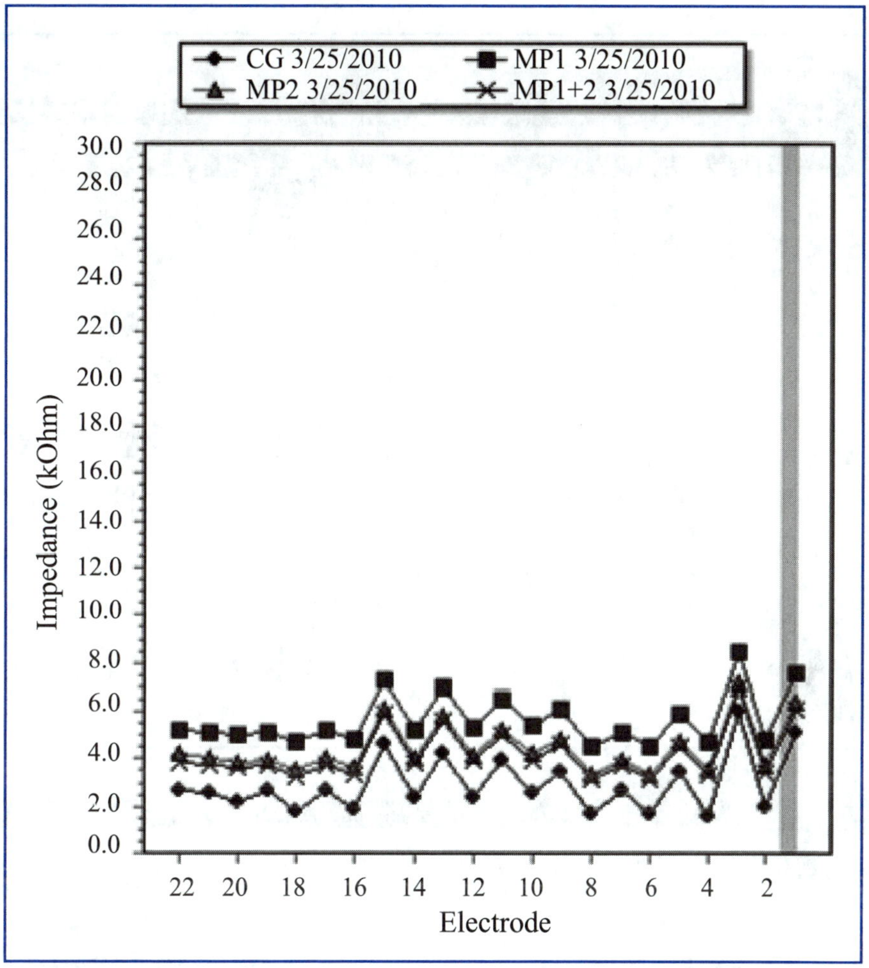


**FIGURE 3–6.** Example of zigzag impedance pattern in a Nucleus 24R(CS) recipient. Impedances for even-numbered electrodes are lower than for odd-numbered electrodes. Note the pattern is evident with all modes of stimulation (CG = common ground, MP1 = ball monopolar electrode, MP2 = case monopolar electrode, MP1+2 = MP1 shorted to MP2).

current source. The known values for current and voltage then allow for impedance to be calculated. The stimulus used for the impedance measures is typically a low-level biphasic current pulse; however, it may be audible for some recipients.

## Advanced Bionics

For Advanced Bionics devices, impedance is tested only in monopolar mode. Figure 3–7 shows screen shots of impedance results for two recipients, measured with the SoundWave clinical programming software. Impedance values are shown in the numerical grid in the upper section of each panel. Each row represents a different test occurrence. The results shown in the top panel of Figure 3–7 indicate short circuits on electrodes 9 and 14, with impedance values of 2.7 kilohms (see the top highlighted row). The example in the bottom panel shows open circuits on electrodes 3, 4, 7, 8, 12, and 13, measured intraoperatively. These open circuits were likely the result of air bubbles introduced during the surgery because all open circuits were resolved postoperatively.

SoundWave automatically runs impedance measurements every time the processor headpiece is connected to the implant (via the software).

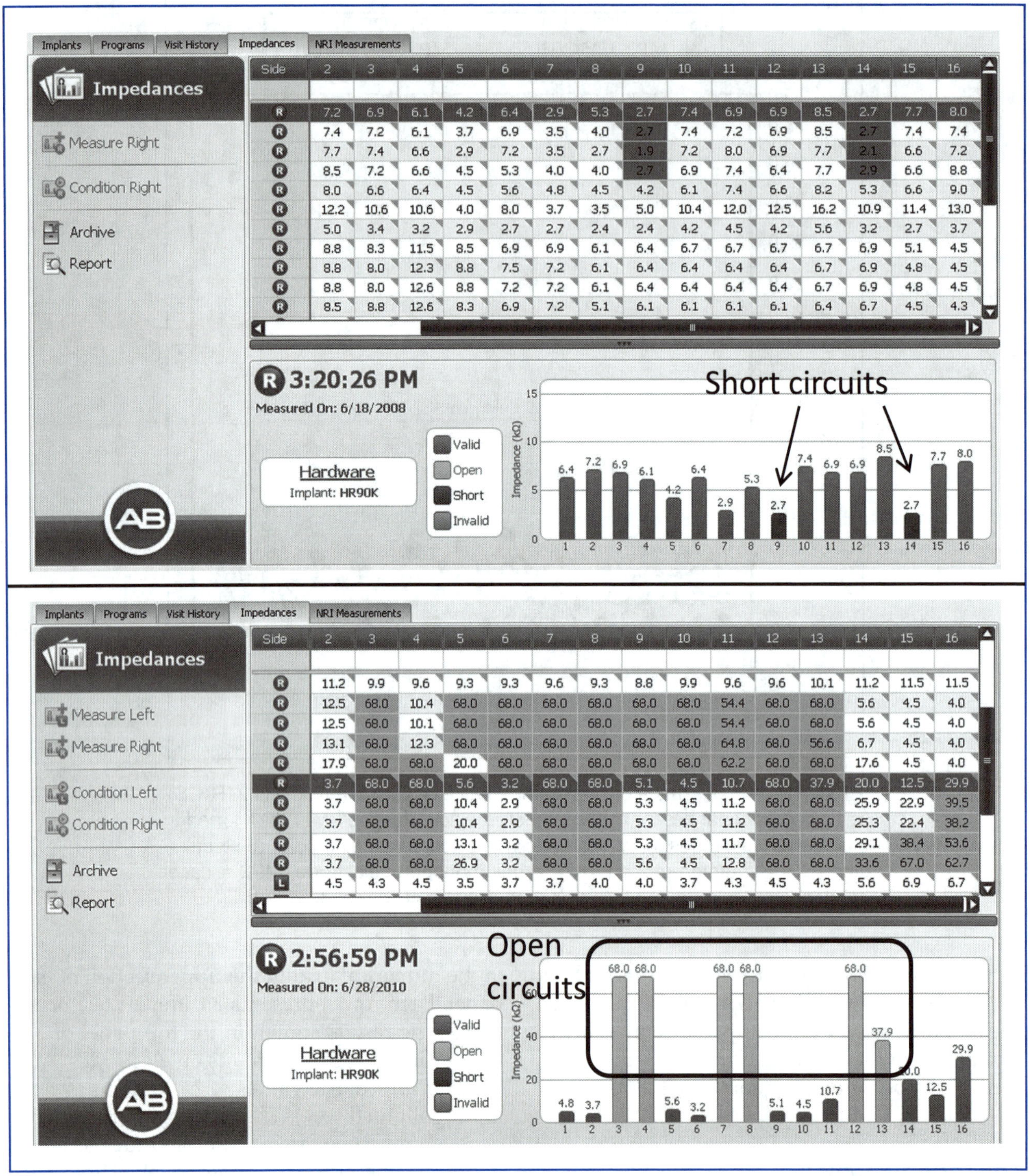


**FIGURE 3–7.** Screen shots of impedance results obtained with Advanced Bionics' SoundWave software. **Top:** Example of results for a recipient with short circuits on electrodes 9 and 14. **Bottom:** Results for a recipient with open circuits or high impedance on electrodes 3, 4, 7, 8, 12, and 13.

Impedance values are color coded (although not discernible in Figure 3–7) according to whether they are valid, open circuit, short circuit, or invalid. Valid measurements represent normally functioning electrodes, and will typically have impedances between 0.5 kilohms and 30 kilohms. However, it is important to make the distinction that valid measures occur between 0.5 and 30 kilohms, but not all values between 0.5 and 30 kilohms are necessarily valid/normal, as is seen for the 2.7-kilohm short circuit in Figure 3–7 (explained further in Chapter 4). Open circuits are indicated for impedance values greater than 30 kilohms. Invalid measures represent an error condition where impedance values are 0.5 kilohms or less (P. Chellakumar, Advanced Bionics, personal communication, 2011). This may occur for a loss of lock between the headpiece and internal device, or other telemetry failure.

Because Advanced Bionics devices are equipped with independent current sources for each electrode, electrodes cannot be shorted together to assess impedance in common ground mode. Recall that monopolar coupling does not accurately identify short circuits (see Figure 3–4B). Therefore, SoundWave runs a version of electrical field imaging and modeling (EFIM; see Chapter 4) behind the scenes to identify short circuits. Briefly, with EFIM, a single intracochlear electrode is stimulated in monopolar mode, which generates a voltage gradient along the length of the cochlea. This voltage gradient is recorded simultaneously by all electrodes in the array, including the stimulating electrode (Vanpoucke, Zarowski, Casselman, Frijns, & Peeters, 2004; Vanpoucke, Zarowski, & Peeters, 2004). The resulting voltage gradients can be used to calculate impedance and determine short circuits by matching impedance values between the stimulated electrode and other nonstimulated electrodes (explained further in Chapter 4).

## Cochlear Ltd.

For Cochlear Ltd. devices, impedance is tested at the end of the first phase of the biphasic current pulse using a voltage-measuring circuit (B. van Dijk, Cochlear Ltd., personal communication, 2011). The software default tests in four coupling modes: common ground, monopolar relative to MP1, monopolar relative to MP2, and monopolar relative to MP1 and MP2 shorted together (MP1+2; see Chapter 2). This latter condition is the default ground for clinical programs. MP1+2 creates a redundancy for the ground in the event that one of the ground electrodes were to fail. For example, if an open circuit were to occur for MP1, current naturally takes the path of least resistance, and would return to MP2.

In Custom Sound and Custom Sound EP, short and open circuits are automatically flagged. Valid impedances for the Contour array range from 0.565 kilohms to 30 kilohms. Impedances less than 0.565 kilohms are flagged as a short circuit and impedances greater than 30 kilohms are flagged as an open circuit. For the straight array, valid impedances range from 0.7 kilohms to 20 kilohms. Figure 3–8 shows two examples of impedance results measured with the Custom Sound (top) and Custom Sound EP (bottom) clinical software. The software provides impedance information in both graphical (shown) and numeric (not shown) form. The four plots in each graph represent the four test (coupling) modes. The top panel shows an example of short circuits on electrodes 5 and 11. It is important to note that the impedance is only abnormal in common ground (diamond symbols); the remaining three monopolar modes show lower impedance for these two electrodes but they are still within the normal range. The bottom panel shows open circuits for five electrodes (10, 13, 15, 17, and 20), which is evident in all four test modes.

## MED-EL

For MED-EL devices, impedance is tested at the end of the second phase of the biphasic current pulse using only monopolar coupling (see "Telemetry" section of the Maestro software Help Menu). The Maestro software uses a tool similar to Advanced Bionics' EFIM (see Chapter 4), where each electrode is stimulated and the voltage is recorded by all electrodes to generate a voltage

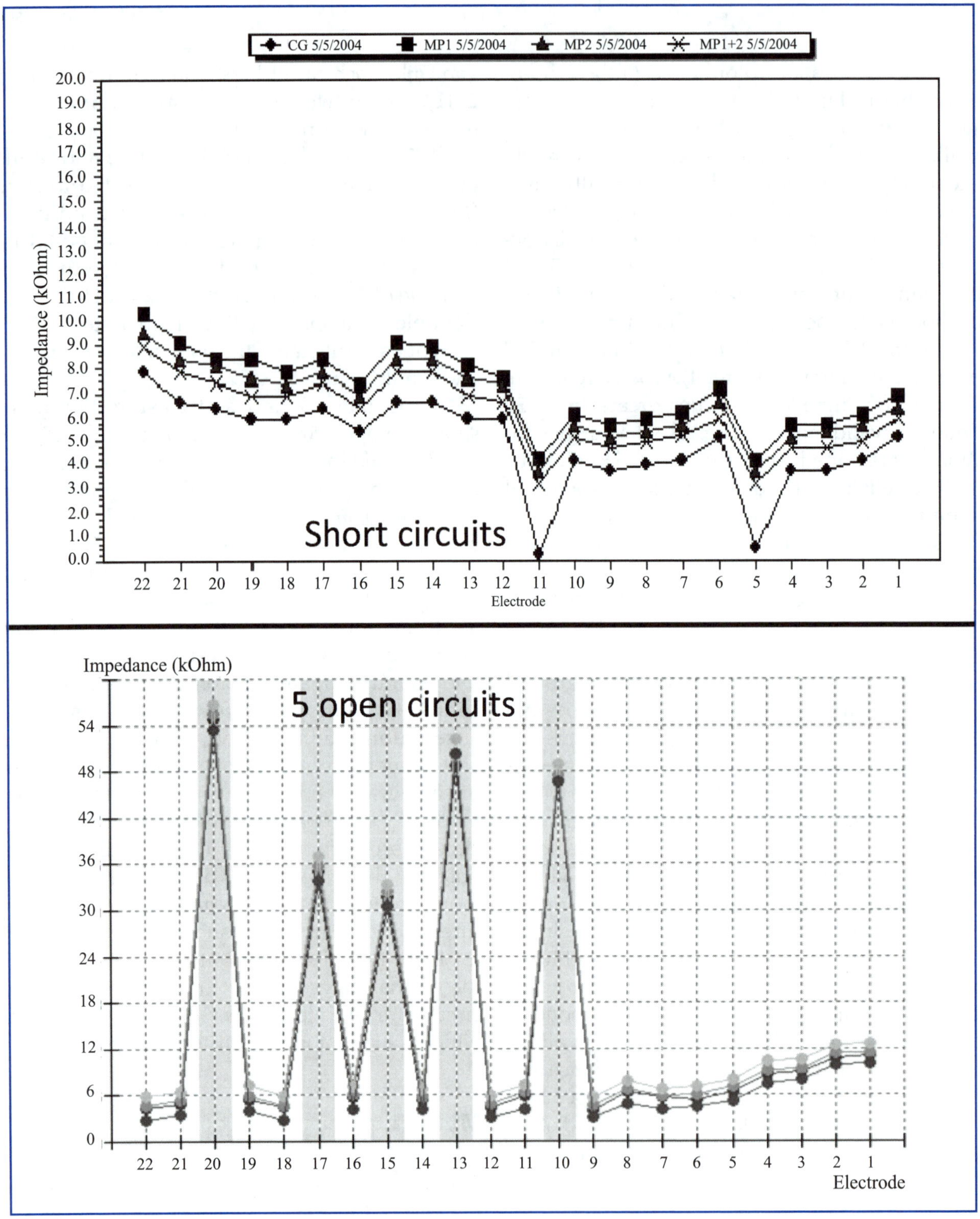


**FIGURE 3–8.** Screen shots of impedance results obtained with Cochlear's Custom Sound software. **Top:** Example of results in common ground, MP1, MP2, and MP1+2 for a recipient with short circuits on electrodes 5 and 11. Note that the short circuits only deviate from the manufacturer's limits with common ground stimulation; impedances for all monopolar modes are reduced relative to neighboring contacts, but are still within normal limits. **Bottom:** Results with Custom Sound EP for a recipient with open circuits on electrodes 10, 13, 15, 17, and 20. All four sets of impedance measures represent the same four test modes listed above. Note that the open circuits are identified in all four modes.

table (Figure 3–9). Values along the diagonal represent voltage measures across the stimulated channels, and thus should be the largest values in each row. For the graphical pane (see Figure 3–9, lower panel), the bar height represents normalized voltages where the voltages in each row are divided by the value obtained from the stimulated electrode (i.e., bar height = 100% along the diagonal). Values in the voltage table are compared across electrodes to identify short circuits, similar to the

| Stimulated Channel \ Measured Channel | 1 | 2 | 3 | 4 | 5 | 6 | 7 | 8 | 9 | 10 | 11 | 12 |
|---|---|---|---|---|---|---|---|---|---|---|---|---|
| 1 | 2.30 | | | | | | | | | | | |
| 2 | 0.30 | 2.04 | | | | | | | | | | |
| 3 | 0.32 | 0.23 | 2.25 | | | | | | | | | |
| 4 | 0.30 | 0.25 | 0.30 | 2.35 | | | | | | | | |
| 5 | 0.30 | 0.30 | 0.30 | 0.32 | 2.32 | | | | | | | |
| 6 | 0.30 | 0.30 | 0.20 | 0.23 | 0.23 | 2.04 | | | | | | |
| 7 | 0.30 | 0.32 | 0.32 | 0.30 | 0.25 | 0.30 | 2.18 | | | | | |
| 8 | 0.30 | 0.32 | 0.30 | 0.32 | 0.32 | 0.30 | 0.32 | 2.25 | | | | |
| 9 | 0.23 | 0.25 | 0.23 | 0.30 | 0.25 | 0.23 | 0.32 | 0.32 | 2.18 | | | |
| 10 | 0.25 | 0.23 | 0.23 | 0.25 | 0.30 | 0.23 | 0.23 | 0.23 | 0.30 | 2.06 | | |
| 11 | 0.30 | 0.30 | 0.30 | 0.30 | 0.23 | 0.23 | 0.25 | 0.30 | 0.30 | 0.30 | 2.16 | |
| 12 | 0.30 | 0.25 | 0.30 | 0.32 | 0.30 | 0.32 | 0.30 | 0.32 | 0.25 | 0.30 | 0.25 | 2.30 |

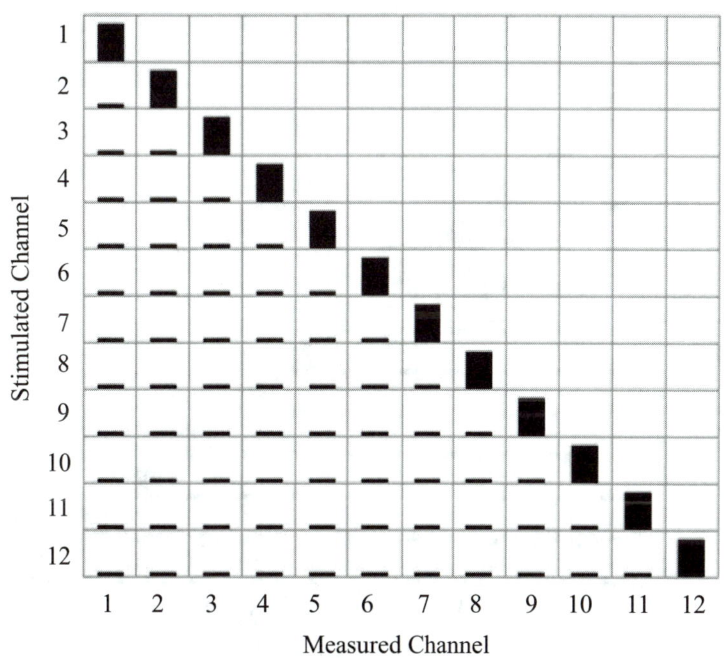


**FIGURE 3–9.** Screen shot of MED-EL's voltage table in numerical format (*top*) and graphical format (*bottom*). Example is for a normally functioning device. Rows indicate the stimulated channel and columns indicate the channel at which the voltage measurement was made. For a normally functioning implant, numerical values (*top*) and bar height (*bottom*) along the diagonal should be the maximum value for each row/column.

method that SoundWave uses (see Chapter 4). Impedances that are similar to the maximal values along the diagonal are flagged as a short circuit. An example is shown in Figure 3–10, showing a short circuit between electrodes 4 and 5.

Figure 3–11 shows screen shots of impedance results for two recipients, measured with the Maestro clinical programming software. The voltage measured at the same electrode that was stimulated yields the impedance value shown in the clinical software. Impedance values for the 12 intracochlear electrode pairs are shown in the numerical grid at the top of each panel. The bottom box in each panel summarizes the number of normal, open-circuit, and short-circuit electrodes in the array. The results shown in the top panel of Figure 3–11 indicate short circuits on electrodes 4 and 5, with impedance values of 5.27 kilohms and

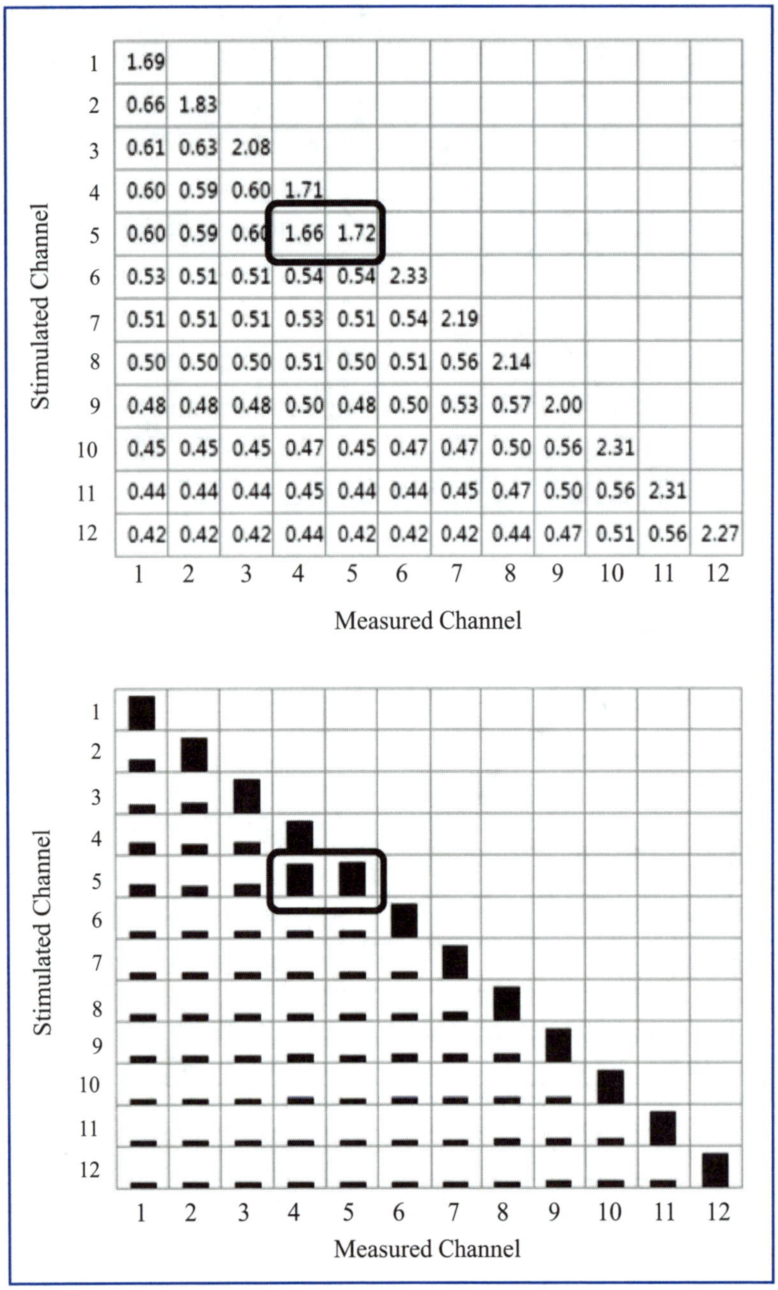

| Stimulated Channel \ Measured Channel | 1 | 2 | 3 | 4 | 5 | 6 | 7 | 8 | 9 | 10 | 11 | 12 |
|---|---|---|---|---|---|---|---|---|---|---|---|---|
| 1 | 1.69 | | | | | | | | | | | |
| 2 | 0.66 | 1.83 | | | | | | | | | | |
| 3 | 0.61 | 0.63 | 2.08 | | | | | | | | | |
| 4 | 0.60 | 0.59 | 0.60 | 1.71 | | | | | | | | |
| 5 | 0.60 | 0.59 | 0.60 | 1.66 | 1.72 | | | | | | | |
| 6 | 0.53 | 0.51 | 0.51 | 0.54 | 0.54 | 2.33 | | | | | | |
| 7 | 0.51 | 0.51 | 0.51 | 0.53 | 0.51 | 0.54 | 2.19 | | | | | |
| 8 | 0.50 | 0.50 | 0.50 | 0.51 | 0.50 | 0.51 | 0.56 | 2.14 | | | | |
| 9 | 0.48 | 0.48 | 0.48 | 0.50 | 0.48 | 0.50 | 0.53 | 0.57 | 2.00 | | | |
| 10 | 0.45 | 0.45 | 0.45 | 0.47 | 0.45 | 0.47 | 0.47 | 0.50 | 0.56 | 2.31 | | |
| 11 | 0.44 | 0.44 | 0.44 | 0.45 | 0.44 | 0.44 | 0.45 | 0.47 | 0.50 | 0.56 | 2.31 | |
| 12 | 0.42 | 0.42 | 0.42 | 0.44 | 0.42 | 0.42 | 0.42 | 0.44 | 0.47 | 0.51 | 0.56 | 2.27 |



**FIGURE 3–10.** Screen shot of MED-EL's voltage table in numerical format (*top*) and graphical format (*bottom*). Example is for a device with short circuits on electrodes 4 and 5. Note that when electrode 5 is stimulated, the voltage measured at electrode 4 is similar to that measured at electrode 5.

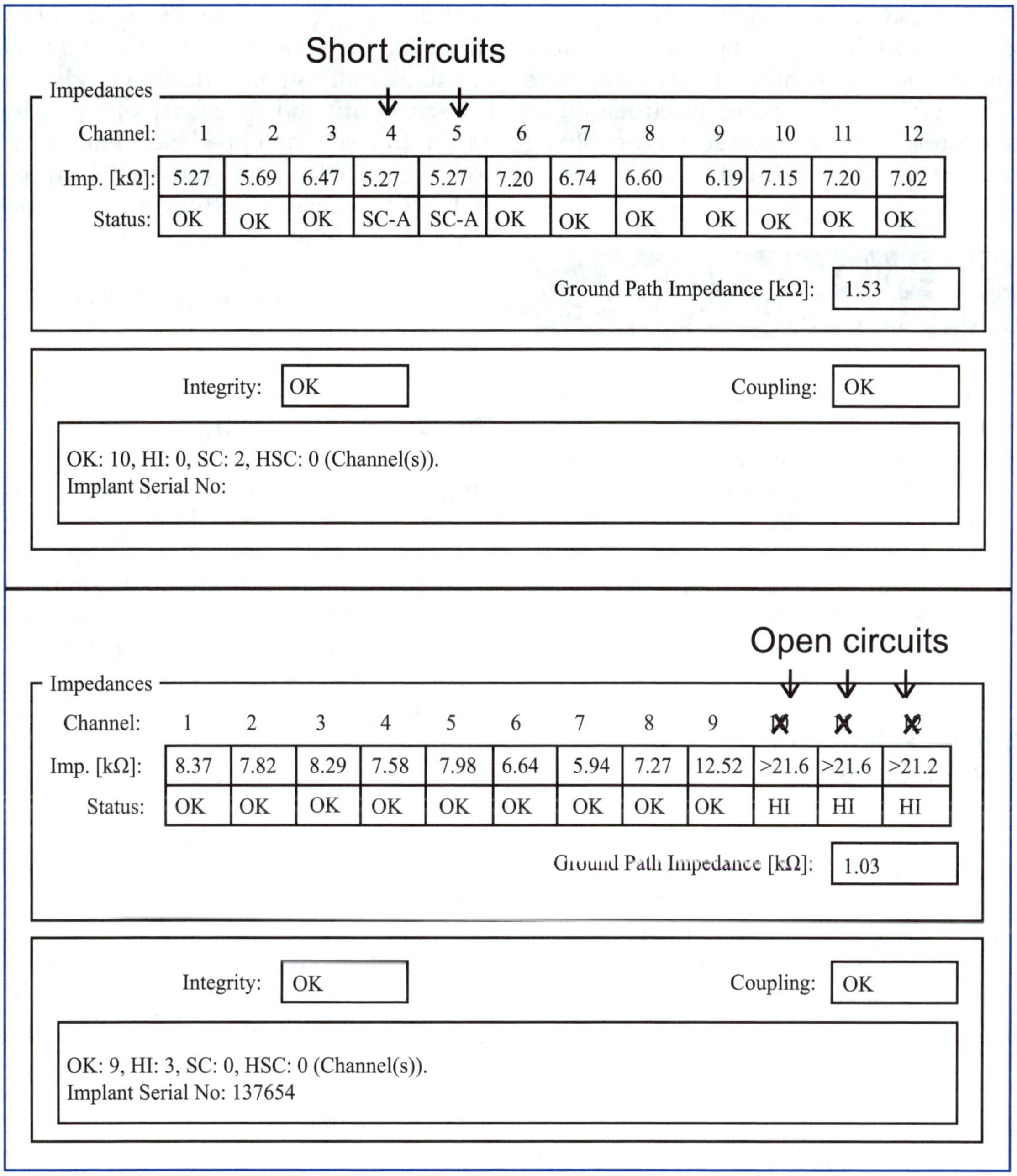


**FIGURE 3–11.** Screen shots of impedance results with MED-EL's Maestro software. **Top:** Example of results for a recipient with short circuits on electrodes 4 and 5. **Bottom:** Results for a recipient with open circuits or high impedance on electrodes 10 to 12.

the short-circuit indicator "SC-A." The software will designate short circuits as A, B, C, D, E, or F to indicate separate short circuits. For example, if electrodes 4 and 5 are shorted together and electrodes 10 and 11 are shorted together in a separate short circuit, the software will indicate 4 and 5 as SC-A and 10 and 11 as SC-B. The example in the bottom panel shows abnormally high impedances (may be considered open circuits) on electrodes 10, 11, and 12, with impedance values >21.6 and >21.2 and the open-circuit indicator "HI." In these cases, the ">" symbol reflects saturation of the current source, so the impedance value displayed represents the minimal possible value. Because the software looks at relative differences across the voltage tables for assessing electrode integrity, there is not a specific cutoff set for identifying short or open circuits for MED-EL devices.

## CLINICAL USES FOR IMPEDANCE MEASURES

Impedance measures can serve a number of clinical uses, including identification of the prevalence of individual electrode failures, identification of electrode failures for purposes of programming the sound processor, verification of voltage compliance, and monitoring of impedances over time so that appropriate decisions can be made for clinical management. Each of these issues is discussed further in the following sections.

### Identify Prevalence of Electrode Failures

The prevalence of short or open circuits among CI users is not well documented. Device manufacturers closely monitor all failure modes for explanted devices; however, individual electrode failures (i.e., short or open circuits) are usually not cause for explantation (unless of course there are a large number of electrode failures in a single device). Individual electrode failures are typically managed clinically by disabling electrodes from patient maps. As a result, the device manufacturers cannot easily track and report this information.

Several investigators have reported on individual electrode failures by retrospectively assessing clinical records. In a review of 636 Nucleus (24 and 24RE) and Advanced Bionics (CII and 90K) devices for which impedance records were available, Carlson et al. (2010) found 57 devices (9%) with at least one electrode failure. Of those 57 devices, 36 (63%) had at least one open circuit, 17 (30%) had at least one short circuit, and 4 (7%) exhibited a pattern of low impedances on alternating electrodes, which is a common pattern seen with partial short circuits. The prevalence of electrode failures was slightly higher for children (12%) than for adults (8%), but this difference was not statistically significant. In a study assessing the sensitivity and specificity of AEVs by comparing to electrode impedance, Hughes, Brown, and Abbas (2004) reported 26 of 197 Nucleus 24M and 24R(CS) devices (13%) with at least one electrode failure. In contrast to the findings of Carlson et al. (2010), the prevalence of electrode failures was slightly higher for adults (16%) than for children (10%).

### Device Programming

The most obvious clinical use for impedance measures is to ensure that malfunctioning electrodes are not included in a recipient's map. All manufacturers' clinical software applications make it easy to quickly measure impedances and disable electrodes that are found to be operating outside of specification. Because impedances can change over time, and short or open circuits can occur at any time, it is essential to measure impedances at every visit. In the case of a short or open circuit that resolves, the clinician may consider reactivating that electrode if the impedance remains normal over several visits. However, if a short or open circuit is intermittent (i.e., resolves, returns to short or open, resolves again, etc.) the clinician should consider keeping these electrodes programmed out of the map because the short or open circuit may return while the device is in use and immediate access to the clinic is not possible. Additionally, repeated intermittencies may be indicative of impending device failure.

### Ensure Voltage Compliance

Fortunately, newer versions of the clinical software calculate voltage compliance based on the impedance measures, and some can limit current levels by automatically increasing the pulse width. The programming software for MED-EL and Advanced Bionics devices does this automatically. For Cochlear devices, the voltage compliance limits are indicated for each electrode within the software; however, pulse width is not automatically adjusted. In the current version of Custom Sound, the clinician has the ability to manually set map levels above the compliance limits indicated by the software.

## Monitor Electrode Function Over Time

As stated previously, it is important to measure impedances at every visit to monitor potential changes over time. Any changes beyond the typical pattern discussed earlier may be an indication of potential problems with the device or anatomical changes that could affect performance. Impedance changes, especially when examined in conjunction with other measures such as map levels, neural measures, and/or performance outcomes, can provide valuable information regarding clinical management.

### *Intraoperative to Postoperative Changes*

Intraoperative impedance measures are useful for providing a baseline indication of normal or abnormal electrode function, and can provide the clinician with preliminary information regarding what to expect at the initial stimulation. Several scenarios are possible. First, if all impedances are normal intraoperatively, then it is expected that all impedances should be normal at the initial programming visit. One exception would be for an incomplete insertion of the array. Intraoperatively, basal electrode contacts that are sitting outside the cochleostomy (in the middle ear) may be bathed in fluid from the surgical procedure, and thus present with normal impedances. Once the fluid resolves, the uninserted basal electrodes will likely present with open circuits postoperatively. Postoperative imaging can be used to confirm whether this is the case. Another exception would be for electrodes that otherwise incur a delayed malfunction after surgery. In a recent records review at Boys Town National Research Hospital, only 6 of 3,430 electrodes (0.17%) presented with abnormal impedance (all open circuits) at the initial postoperative visit following normal impedances measured intraoperatively (Hughes, Goehring, Baudhuin, & Lusk, 2012).

Alternatively, it is not uncommon for abnormal intraoperative impedances (particularly open circuits) to resolve by the initial programming visit. Hughes et al. (2012) found that 64 of 78 electrodes (82%) with abnormal intraoperative impedance resolved by the initial postoperative visit; 62 of those had open circuits intraoperatively. If several contiguous electrodes present with open circuits intraoperatively, the cause is likely to be air bubbles introduced during the insertion process. Open circuits in these cases have a high likelihood of resolving by the time of the initial stimulation as the air is absorbed by the tissue (Hughes et al., 2012; Schulman, 1995). However, if only a single electrode is affected intraoperatively, there is a higher likelihood that it is a true open circuit that will not resolve postoperatively.

### *Changes Across Postoperative Intervals*

As stated previously, impedances typically stabilize within the first month or two of device use (e.g., Busby et al., 2002; Hughes et al., 2001). Substantial increases or decreases in electrode impedance beyond this initial period may be associated with a number of different factors that need to be managed clinically. First, nonuse of the implant can result in impedance increases (e.g., Newbold et al., 2004; Schulman, 1995), which may necessitate map changes when implant use is resumed. Second, middle ear infection/fluid, otalgia, com mon cold, labyrinthitis, or other inflammation/infection processes have been associated with impedance increases (Clark et al., 1995; Neuburger et al., 2009). In those cases, impedance changes are typically transitory and likely return to normal after the episode is resolved. Map changes are typically necessary while the inflammation/infection is active, and again after it has resolved.

If impedance increases do not appear to be associated with inflammation/infection, then it is important to examine the recipient's map levels to ensure that the device is operating within voltage compliance limits. Operating out of voltage compliance can produce asymmetric current pulses, which can lead to platinum dissolution (e.g., Brummer & Turner, 1975; Clark, 2003), and further increases in impedance. As Neuburger et al. (2009) reported, recipients using fast-rate strategies demonstrated significant impedance increases over time. The investigators postulated that impedance increases were the result of the device possibly operating outside of its voltage compliance limits, due to higher pulse amplitudes that are needed to compensate for narrower pulse widths. In the cases that Neuburger et al. (2009) presented, impedances typically returned to normal after the pulse width was expanded, resulting in a slower rate and lower pulse amplitudes.

Finally, impedance decrements over time may be indicative of partial short circuits. As discussed earlier, fractures in the silicone coating can cause fluid to ingress slowly over time. For some recipients, hearing performance is adversely affected; for others it is not. In rare cases, nonauditory sensations can occur with partial short circuits, such as pain or facial nerve stimulation. As discussed previously, identifying suspected partial short circuits while in situ is difficult. A working diagnosis is typically made using a combination of impedances, map levels, subjective perceptions, and performance over time. Because fluid ingress can happen slowly over time, it is most important to look at longitudinal changes; measurements from a single time interval are not sufficient. The following criteria are used for a working diagnosis of partial short circuits:

1. Decrease in impedances of affected electrodes over time.
2. Decrease in impedances of affected electrodes relative to the impedances of other (unaffected) electrodes in the array.
3. Increase in map levels for affected electrodes. This is because a portion of the current is shunted away from the intended electrode. Current levels must therefore be increased to achieve threshold and upper loudness comfort levels.
4. Reduction in speech perception scores or other overall decrement in performance with the device.
5. Poor sound quality (distorted, hum, static, buzz, etc.).
6. Reduced pitch discrimination or pitch reversals.
7. Reduced loudness growth.
8. Pain, headaches, facial twitch, or other nonauditory sensation.
9. Refusal to wear the sound processor.

Three examples of items (1) and (2) are shown in Figure 3–12 for common ground stimulation. For recipient A, impedances dropped significantly on electrodes 2 to 4, 13 to 16, and 19 to 22 at later visits (5 and 10 months post) when compared with the 2-week and 1.5-month visits. For recipient B, a zigzag pattern emerged after the 6-year visit, involving the even-numbered electrodes between 6 and 12. Finally, recipient C developed a more pronounced zigzag pattern between the 5.5- and 7.5-year visits on almost all of the even-numbered electrodes.

Recipients with partial short circuits may present with none, some, or all of the symptoms listed above. It is also important to recognize that many of the symptoms listed above are consistent with other problems (such as external equipment malfunction or physiological changes), which must also be ruled out. Clinical management in these cases typically begins with programming out the affected electrodes, and then using outcome measures (if possible) to verify whether the programming changes were effective. In cases where numerous electrodes are affected (as in Figure 3–12C), it is best to begin with programming out every other affected electrode (e.g., if all odd-numbered electrodes demonstrate low impedance, then disable electrodes 1, 5, 9, 13, etc.). If programming changes do not improve performance, then reimplantation may be warranted.

## SUMMARY

This chapter has described the basics of electrode impedance, what constitutes abnormal measures, and clinical uses for impedance and voltage compliance measures. Key concepts are summarized below:

1. Impedance is the vector sum of the resistance and reactance. Resistance opposes current flow (resistor), and reactance stores energy (capacitor).

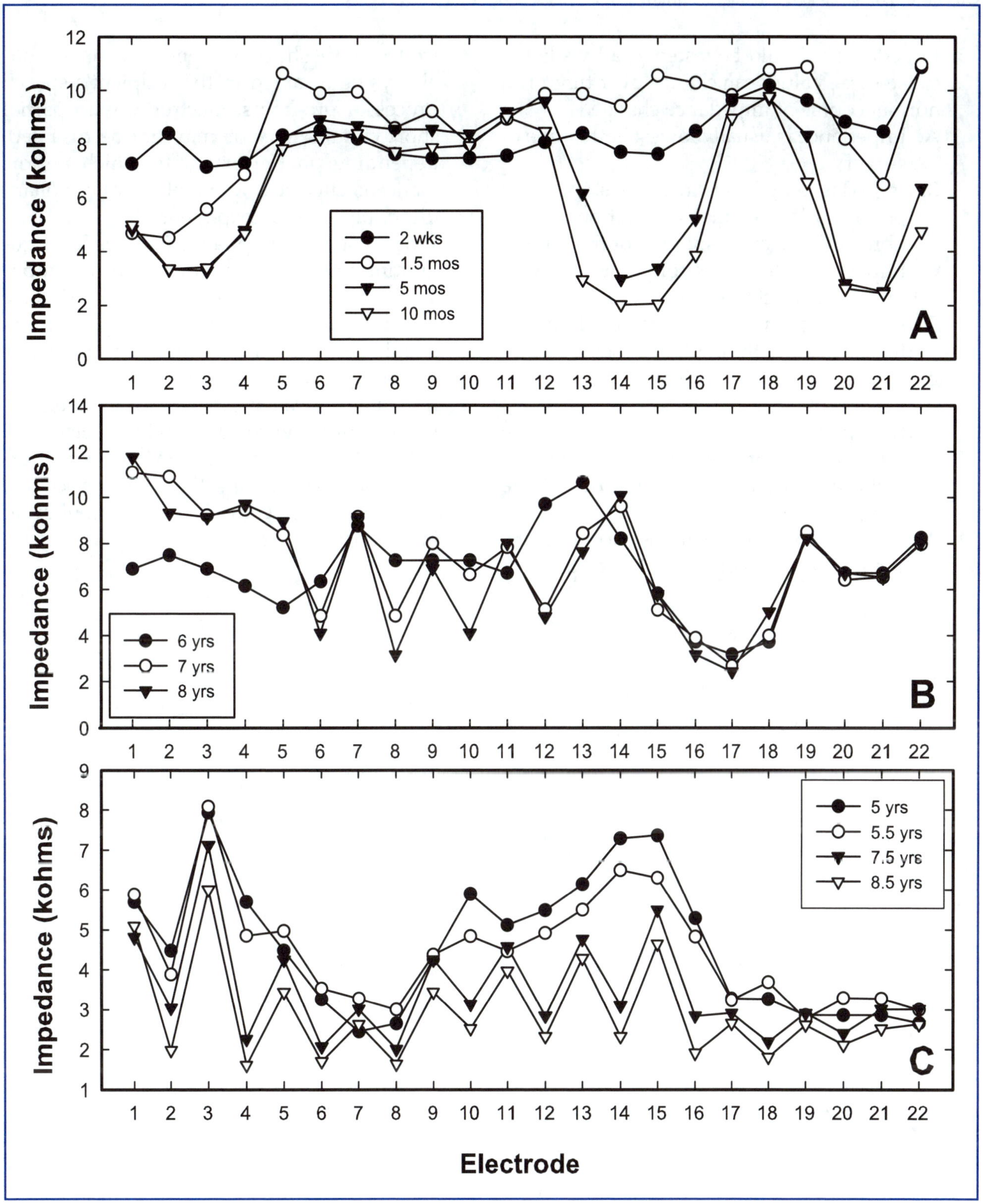


**FIGURE 3–12.** Common ground impedance measures over time for three recipients with suspected partial short circuits. Each panel represents measures from a different recipient. **A.** Significant drop in impedances between 1.5 months and 5 months for electrodes 2 to 4, 13 to 16, and 19 to 22. **B.** Impedance decrement between the 6- and 7-year visits, resulting in a zigzag pattern with low impedances on the even-numbered electrodes from 6 to 12. **C.** Impedance decrement between the 5.5- and 7.5-year visits on even-numbered electrodes from 2 to 20.

2. Impedances should be tested at all visits because these values can change over time. The normal course of impedance change is:
   A. Impedance is usually lowest at the time of surgery,
   B. Impedance increases in the postoperative period (prior to initial stimulation) due to fibrous tissue encapsulation of the array,
   C. Impedance decreases following stimulation of the electrode,
   D. Impedances are usually stable within the first 1 to 2 months of device use.
3. Impedance can increase because of:
   A. Periods of nonuse
   B. Reimplantation
   C. Inflammation or infection
   D. Operating the device outside of voltage compliance limits
4. Abnormal impedance includes short circuits, open circuits, and partial short circuits. Electrodes with short or open circuits should always be disabled in the recipient's speech processor programs. Electrodes with partial short circuits may or may not be disabled, depending on the extent to which performance is affected and whether or not nonauditory percepts are experienced.
5. When voltage compliance is exceeded, programming changes such as reducing upper stimulation levels (map C or M levels), increasing pulse duration, changing electrode coupling to a broader stimulation mode, or disabling the electrode should be used.
6. Impedance measures are useful for identifying the prevalence of individual electrode failures, identifying electrode failures for purposes of programming the sound processor, verifying voltage compliance, and monitoring impedances over time.

# 4

# Electrical Field Potentials

Chapter 3 discussed the clinical importance of electrode impedance measures for assessing the function of intra- and extracochlear electrodes. Although the access resistance and reactance components can provide some insight into the properties of the electrode-nerve interface and surrounding medium, clinical impedance measurements do not provide comprehensive information about these specific components or about spatial spread of current throughout the cochlea. This chapter describes a tool that is presently used with Advanced Bionics (AB) devices (called Electrical Field Imaging and Modeling, or EFIM) and MED-EL devices to assist with calculating impedance for monopolar stimulation, and to generate voltage tables for constructing intracochlear electrical field potentials. In this chapter, electrical field potentials are defined, the method for measurement is described, and the clinical uses are discussed.

## BASIC DESCRIPTION

Electrical field potentials are essentially a collection of impedance (or voltage) measures that, when combined into a matrix, can provide information about the distribution of electrical current within the cochlea. The difference between an individual electrode impedance measure (Figure 4–1, top) and electrical field potentials (Figure 4–1, bottom) is that individual electrode impedances are obtained by measuring the voltage across only the *stimulated* electrode pair. For electrical field potentials, voltage measurements are recorded across the entire array (all electrodes) for a single stimulated electrode pair.

Electrically evoked compound action potentials (described in Chapter 7) have been used to examine neural activation patterns within the cochlea (e.g., Abbas, Hughes, Brown, Miller, & South, 2004; Cohen, Richardson, Saunders, & Cowan, 2003; Cohen, Saunders, & Richardson, 2004; Eisen & Franck, 2005; Frijns, Briaire, de Laat, & Grote, 2002; Grolman et al., 2008; Hughes & Stille, 2010). However, those measures reflect both the spread of the stimulus current within the cochlea (which affects the population of neurons recruited) and the volume conduction of the neural response along the length of the fluid-filled cochlea (which affects the *measurement* of the neural response). Alternatively, three-dimensional modeling can be used to better understand current spread and neural recruitment patterns throughout the cochlea; however, present models do not account for recipient-specific anatomical variations that will likely affect electrical field distributions and subsequent neural recruitment patterns (Vanpoucke,

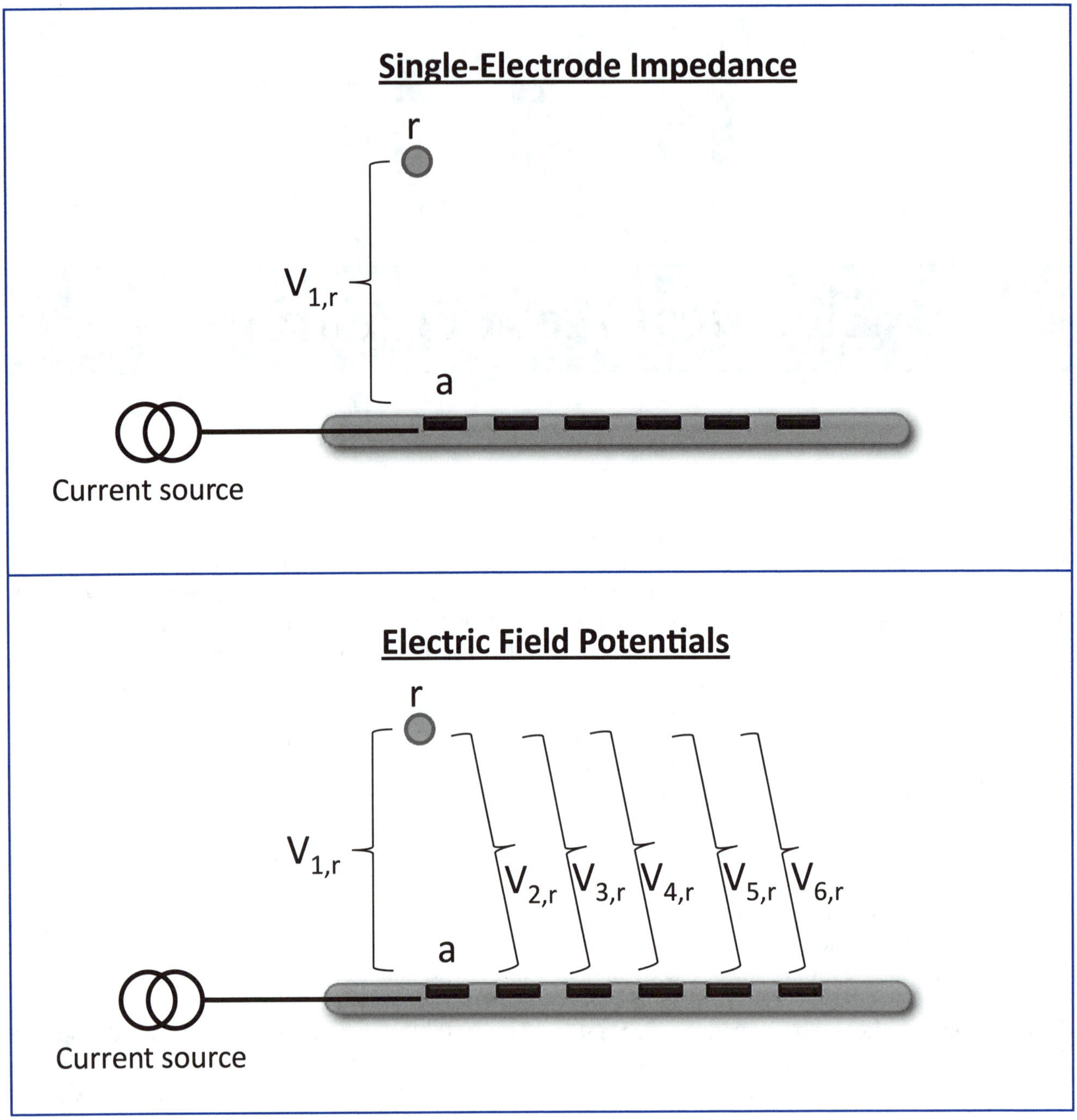


**FIGURE 4–1. Top:** Schematic of how impedance is measured for a single electrode. A fixed current is applied to intracochlear electrode 1 (labeled "a" for active), with the extracochlear monopolar electrode as the return (r). The voltage (V) is measured across the active and return electrodes ($V_{1,r}$). **Bottom:** Schematic of how electric field potentials are derived from a series of impedance measures. A fixed current is applied to intracochlear electrode 1 (a), with the extracochlear monopolar electrode as the return (r). The voltage (V) is measured across each intracochlear electrode and the extracochlear return electrode ($V_{1\text{-}6,r}$).

Zarowski, Casselman, et al., 2004). Electrical field potentials are therefore a potentially useful tool to add to three-dimensional modeling data for parsing out the effect of current spread throughout the cochlea, independent of associated neural responses.

## MEASUREMENT

Electrical field potentials are generated by a low-level stimulus delivered to an electrode pair. The stimulus is typically a single biphasic current pulse (a sine wave or pulse train can also be used) presented in monopolar mode. The resulting voltage can be measured from all contacts in the array, including the stimulating electrode, relative to an extracochlear return. Intracochlear electrical field potentials are quite large (~1 V), so it is not necessary to employ signal averaging as is done with physiological measures.

Similar to the individual electrode impedance measurement, the voltage across the measured electrodes can be divided by the amount of current injected by the stimulated electrode to obtain an impedance value. The result is a collection of impedances measured across the array. Recall from Chapter 3 (see Figure 3–1) that impedance encompasses the following components: (1) the resistive components of the stimulating electrode lead wire and contact (i.e., access resistance), (2) the capacitive component of the interface between the stimulating electrode and surrounding tissue (i.e., reactance or polarization component), and (3) the resistive components of the fluid/tissue medium between the active and return electrodes (also part of the access resistance). When the voltage is measured across *nonstimulating* electrodes, component (3) is the only component of the impedance measure. Components (1) and (2) are not relevant because current is not flowing through the recording contact.

Figure 4–2 shows a typical/normal example of electrical field potentials using the EFIM research tool for Advanced Bionics devices. Electrical field potentials for all 16 stimulating electrodes are shown in the figure. The peak of each function (impedances ~3.5 to 7 kilohms) occurs at the *stimulated* electrode and represents the impedance for that electrode (i.e., derived from the voltage measured across the stimulated electrode pair). The lower portion (or tails) of each function represents the electrical field potential distributions (i.e., derived from the voltage measured across each *nonstimulated* electrode and the return electrode). For better viewing of the field potential distributions (i.e., tail portions), the peak of each function can be replaced by extrapolated values from neighboring electrodes (Figure 4–3). As can be seen in Figure 4–3, the gradient of each function is relatively shallow, which reflects the high conductivity of the fluid-filled cochlea. There is a larger voltage drop (reflected by the larger change in impedance) from apex to base than from base to apex. This pattern reflects current flow along the length of the fluid-filled cochlea toward the base (Vanpoucke, Zarowski, Casselman, et al., 2004).

A number of factors will affect the shape of the field distributions, including the position of the electrode contacts within the cochlea, and the nature of the tissue within the cochlea (fluid, fibrous tissue, bone). The path of current flow from the intracochlear electrode to the extracochlear (monopolar) return can differ across the cochlea and across recipients. Potential current pathways include the internal auditory canal, vestibular structures, facial nerve canal, and potentially the middle ear (Vanpoucke, Zarowski, Casselman, et al., 2004; Vanpoucke, Zarowski, & Peeters, 2004).

## CLINICAL USES FOR ELECTRICAL FIELD POTENTIALS

In its simplest form, electrical field potentials can be used to identify malfunctioning electrodes. As discussed in Chapter 3, monopolar stimulation is not very effective for identifying short circuits. For MED-EL and Advanced Bionics devices, which use only monopolar coupling for impedance measures, voltage/impedance matrices are generated for all combinations of stimulating and recording contacts to assist with the identification of short circuits. Advanced Bionics runs a version of EFIM

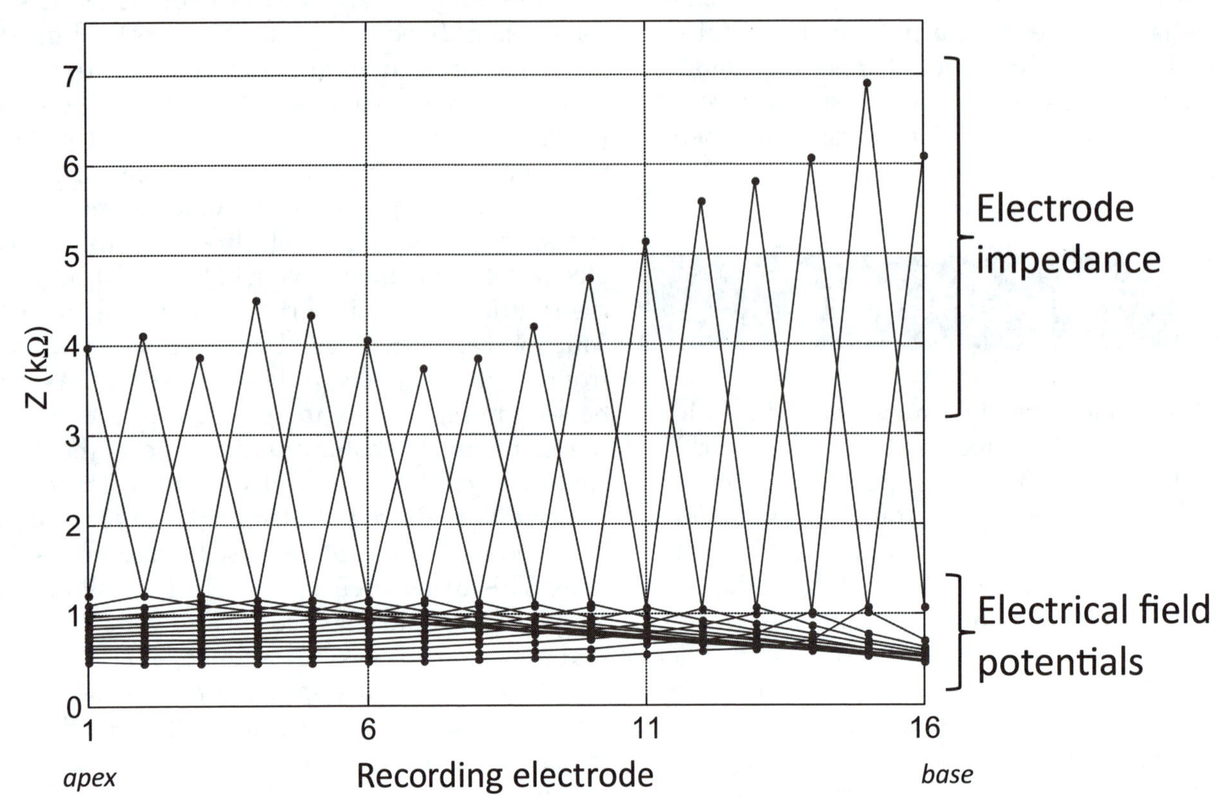


**FIGURE 4–2.** Typical example of electrical field potentials using the Electrical Field Imaging and Modeling (EFIM) research tool (Advanced Bionics). Data are from a recipient implanted with the HiFocus electrode array, with uneventful electrode insertion and no malfunctioning electrodes. Electrodes are numbered 1 to 16, apex to base. The stimuli were 40 μA, 66 msec/phase biphasic current pulses delivered relative to the case ground on the receiver/stimulator package. Peak values represent the impedance for the stimulated electrode, and therefore reflect the access resistance (lead wire, electrode, fluid/tissue between active and return electrodes) and the reactance/capacitive component of impedance (electrode-tissue interface). The lower portions of each function (~1 kilohm or less) represent measurements at the nonstimulated electrodes, and therefore reflect the resistance of the fluid/tissue between the active and return electrodes). Data courtesy of Filiep Vanpoucke, Advanced Bionics European Research Laboratory.

behind the scenes in the clinical software; MED-EL's clinical software displays the resulting voltage matrix. Data from these matrices can be used to determine whether short circuits exist. (They can also identify open circuits, but simple impedance measures in monopolar mode are effective for that purpose.) An example using EFIM is shown in Figure 4–4. In this example, impedances for electrodes 7 and 8 indicate a short circuit. (As an aside, electrodes 11 and 16 demonstrate relatively high impedances because they were deactivated in the recipient's map. Recall from Chapter 3 that impedance is higher for nonused electrodes.)

Criteria for detecting a short circuit are that: (1) two electrodes that are shorted together will have similar impedance values, and (2) the overall impedance for shorted electrodes will be roughly half that of the normally functioning electrodes (i.e., impedance decrease is proportional to essentially doubling the electrode surface area). MED-EL's voltage tables use a similar concept for identifying short circuits; *relative* voltage values

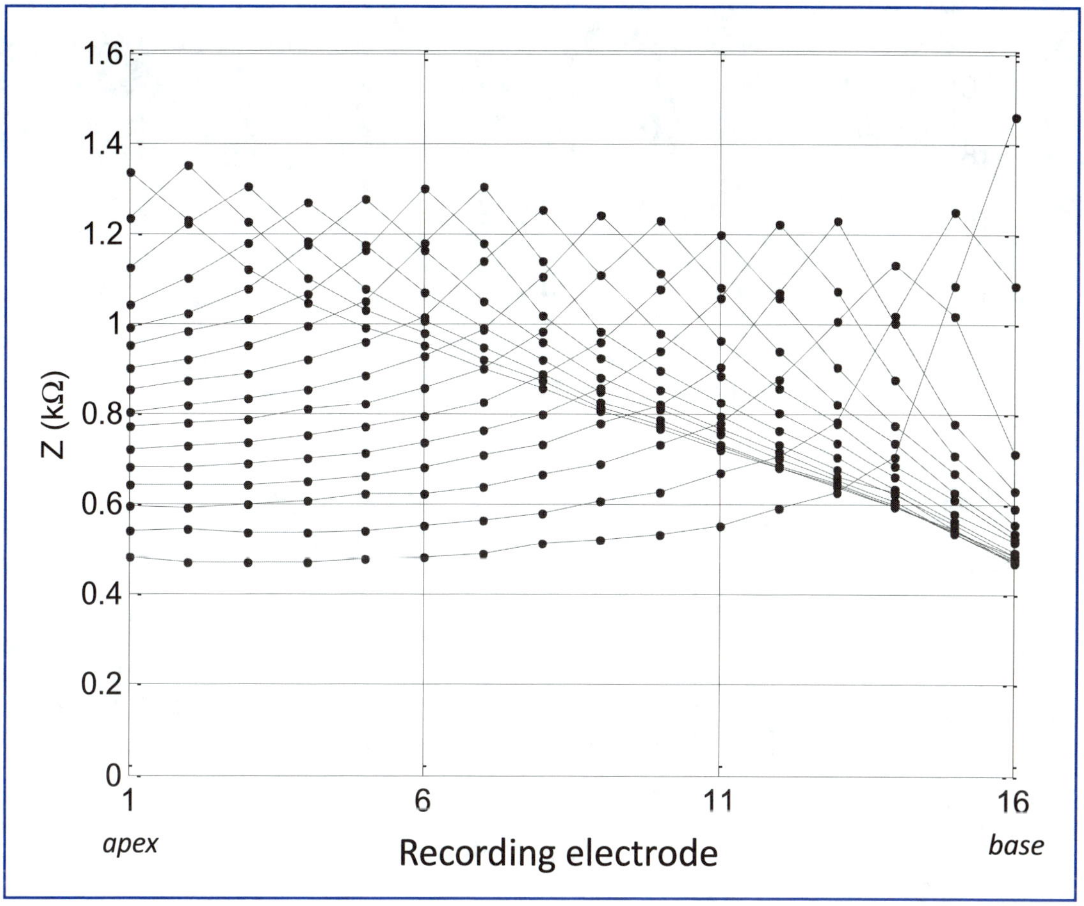


**FIGURE 4–3.** Data from Figure 4–2 with impedance peaks (value for stimulus and recording on the same electrode) extrapolated from the values on neighboring electrodes. This allows for better visualization of the "tail" portions of the functions. These portions represent the impedance of the fluid/tissue medium between the active and return (stimulating) electrodes. Data courtesy of Filiep Vanpoucke, Advanced Bionics European Research Laboratory.

are examined across the matrix (see Figure 3–10). For this reason, specific kilohm values for MED-EL and Advanced Bionics devices are not used as a criterion for identifying a short circuit, but rather, relative differences across the matrix are used.

Electrical field potentials can also be used in conjunction with computer modeling for more complex applications. Vanpoucke, Zarowski, Casselman, et al. (2004) used a resistive ladder network model to evaluate the relative contributions of longitudinal versus transverse resistance to determine whether the bulk of current flow is along the scala tympani (longitudinal) or through a different low-impedance path at some point in the cochlea (transverse). Subjects that exhibited a reduction in the transverse impedance at a given electrode also showed a reduced slope of the tail of the EFIM function at the same electrode. Taken together, these results suggested that current must have exited the cochlea transversally (i.e., through the walls of the cochlea rather than along the length of the scala). High-resolution computed tomography (CT) scans verified that the electrode with reduced transverse impedance was also the closest electrode to the bony wall separating the scala tympani from the facial nerve canal. These results suggested that a relatively large percentage of current was exiting the cochlea toward the

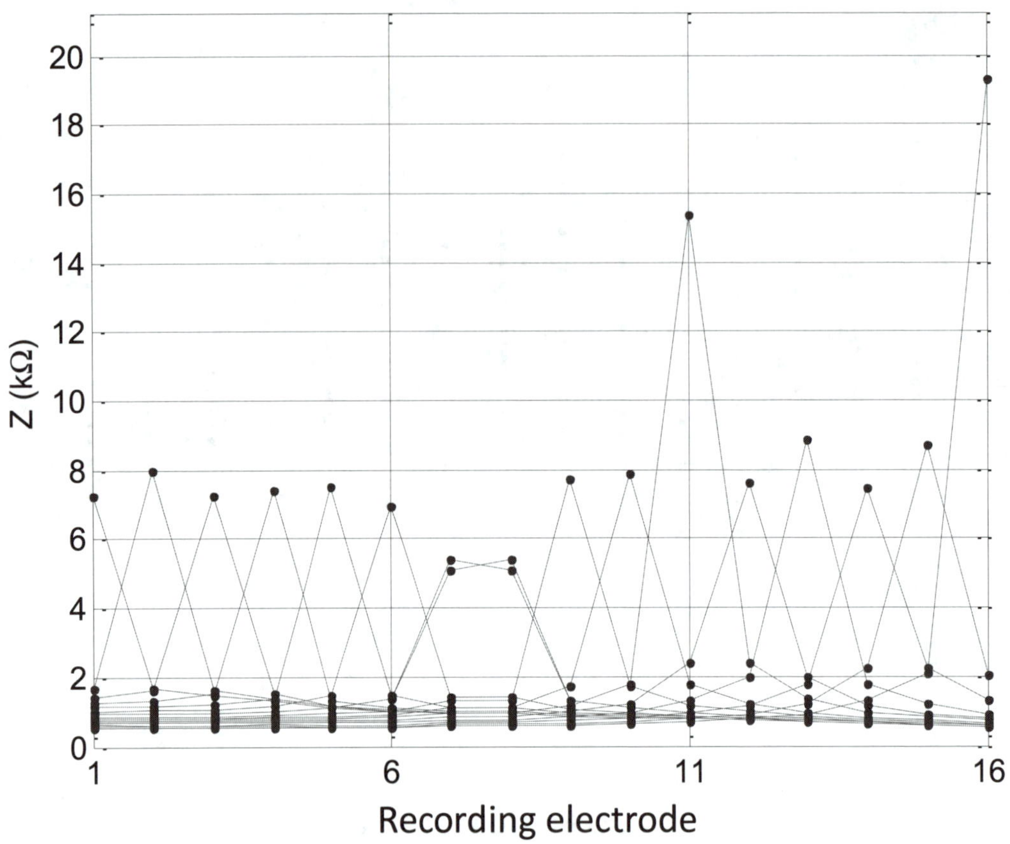


**FIGURE 4–4.** Example of short circuit between electrodes 7 and 8, as exhibited by nearly identical impedances and overall reduced impedance compared with neighboring electrodes. This example also illustrates higher impedances on electrodes 11 and 16, which had been deactivated from the recipient's map. Data courtesy of Filiep Vanpoucke, Advanced Bionics European Research Laboratory.

low-impedance facial nerve canal. For four of the five Advanced Bionics CII/HiFocus subjects in that study, the reduction in transverse impedance occurred at either electrode 7 or 8, which corresponded to approximately 270° from the base; this is also where the facial nerve canal is typically closest to the scala tympani.

Similar modeling techniques that incorporate electrical field potentials can also be used to detect fold-over of the electrode tip or evidence of ossification (Vanpoucke, Boermans, & Frijns, 2009, 2012). Finally, because electrical field potentials are noninvasive and quick and easy to obtain, they can be used to document potential intracochlear changes over time, such as fibrous tissue growth or ossification (Vanpouke, Zarowski, & Peeters, 2004). Ideally, modeling techniques that incorporate electrical field potentials should be integrated into future iterations of clinical software for improved patient management.

## SUMMARY

This chapter has described the basics of electrical field imaging. Key concepts are summarized below:

1. Electrical field potentials represent the spatial distribution of current spread within the cochlea.

2. Electrical field potentials are measured by stimulating an intracochlear electrode relative to an extracochlear ground (monopolar coupling), and measuring the voltage across each electrode relative to the monopolar ground. A matrix is generated from all stimulating/recording combinations to assess electrical field patterns and to identify malfunctioning electrodes.
3. Individual electrode impedances are derived from the voltage measured across only the stimulated electrode pair. When the voltage is measured across the nonstimulating electrodes (as in EFIM), the resistive component of the fluid/tissue medium is the only component of the impedance measure.
4. Electrical field potentials can be coupled with more sophisticated modeling techniques to evaluate more specific paths of current flow within the cochlea.

# 5

# Averaged Electrode Voltages

As with impedance measures (Chapter 3) and electrical field imaging (Chapter 4), averaged electrode voltages (AEVs) can be used to assess the function of the internal device and individual electrodes. Because impedance measures and electrical field imaging use intracochlear electrodes to measure voltages, these measures can only be made with devices that have reverse telemetry capabilities. Reverse telemetry allows for transmission of the measured voltage or impedance information back across the skin to the processor, then to the processor interface, and finally to the computer. AEVs are far-field measurements (recorded with scalp electrodes) of the artifact associated with stimulating an intracochlear electrode; therefore, AEVs can be measured with devices that either do or do not have reverse telemetry capabilities. This chapter begins with a basic description of what AEVs are, how they are measured, and what normal patterns should look like. Examples of atypical waveforms are presented, along with some cases that demonstrate clinical uses for AEVs.

## BASIC DESCRIPTION

Averaged electrode voltages are a measure of the artifact associated with stimulating an intracochlear electrode. If the stimulus is a biphasic pulse, then the AEV generally looks like a biphasic pulse. AEVs are similar to electrical field potentials (see Chapter 4). The primary difference is that AEVs are recorded with surface/scalp electrodes, whereas electrical field potentials are recorded with the intracochlear electrodes. As stated above, electrical field potentials require the device to have reverse telemetry capabilities, whereas AEVs do not. Thus, AEVs may be particularly useful for individuals with older technology that cannot support impedance measurements. As with impedance and electrical field potentials, AEVs are not neural measures and do not require active participation on the part of the recipient.

## MEASUREMENT

### Stimulus

Figure 5–1 illustrates the stimulus and recording setup for AEV measures. The stimulus used for AEVs is typically a single, negative-leading, charge-balanced, biphasic current pulse delivered through the implant. Stimuli are delivered to the recipient in the same way as for programming the device. The recipient is connected to a standard headpiece and sound processor, which is connected to the stimulating computer via a

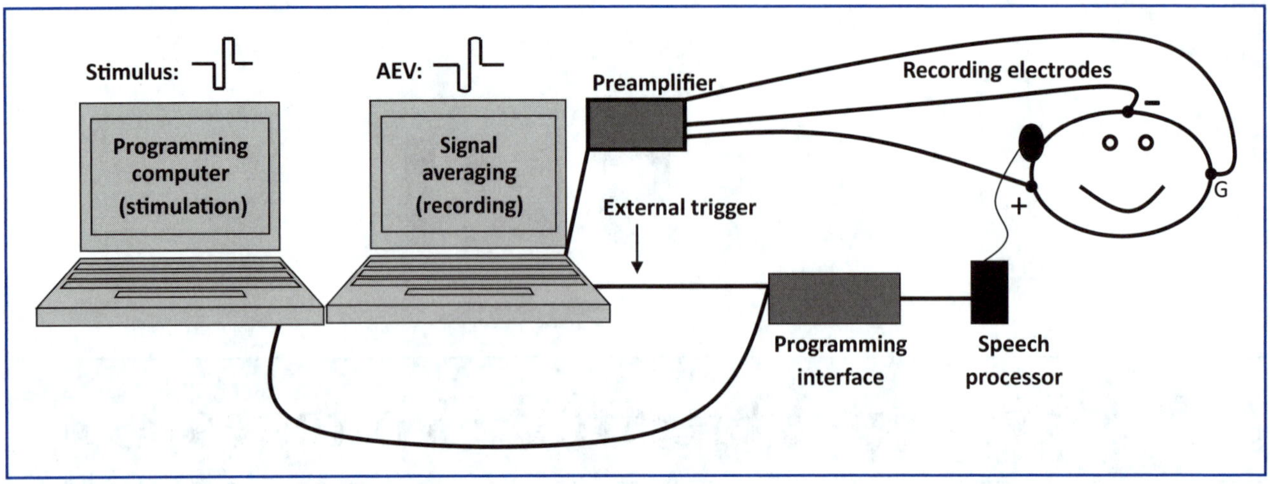


**FIGURE 5–1.** Schematic illustrating the equipment setup and recording for averaged electrode voltages (AEVs). The stimulus (a biphasic current pulse) is delivered via a standard transmitting coil/headpiece connected to a speech processor, which is connected to the stimulating computer via a programming interface. Surface recording electrodes are applied to the mastoid ipsilateral to the implant, contralateral to the implant, and high forehead. In this schematic, + is positive, − is reference, and G is ground. The surface recording electrodes are connected to a preamplifier that is connected to standard signal averaging (evoked potentials) equipment. A trigger pulse is delivered by the programming interface to activate the recording computer to begin averaging responses.

programming interface. Clinical (or specialized manufacturer-specific) hardware and software are used to control the stimulus parameters (i.e., pulse duration, amplitude, electrode coupling, and presentation rate) and deliver the stimulus. A trigger pulse from the programming interface is used to synchronize the signal averaging equipment for recording. Stimuli are typically delivered at a low current level that is near or below behavioral threshold. Higher stimulus levels are not needed because AEVs are relatively large potentials; however the stimulus level depends on the specific electrode coupling mode used (described further below). A slow stimulation rate (~50 to 250 pps) is used to allow for signal averaging.

AEVS should be tested using all available coupling modes that the device is capable of producing. Each mode can provide unique information that, when combined, can provide a comprehensive picture of device function. It should be noted that the examples shown in this chapter are exclusively from Cochlear Corp. devices because those devices are capable of a wider range of electrode coupling modes (common ground, bipolar, variable bipolar mode, monopolar). The principles described herein for monopolar coupling can be applied to MED-EL and Advanced Bionics devices, since monopolar is the standard coupling mode for those manufacturers' devices. Table 5–1 summarizes specific stimulus and recording parameters used in previous studies to measure AEVs.

## Recording

Surface recording electrodes (cup or disc) are applied to the ipsilateral mastoid (positive), high forehead or vertex (reference), and contralateral mastoid (ground). Alternative montages are detailed in Table 5–1. The electrodes are plugged into a preamplifier, which is connected to signal averaging equipment (e.g., a clinical evoked potentials system). A low-pass filter in the amplifier is typically needed to eliminate effects from the radio frequency (RF) pulses that the implant uses to transmit information across the skin to the internal receiver/stimulator. If signal averaging equipment is not available, AEVs can be visualized on an oscilloscope (an isolation amplifier is necessary; Shallop, Kelsall, Caleffe-Schenck, & Ash, 1995).

**Table 5–1.** Summary of Stimulus and Recording Parameters for Studies Measuring Averaged Electrode Voltages

**STIMULUS**

| *Study* | *Device* | *Current Level* | *Coupling* | *Pulse Width (μsec/phase)* | *Stimulation Rate* |
|---|---|---|---|---|---|
| Cullington & Clarke (1997) | Nucleus 22 | 50 CL<br>80 CL | CG<br>BP+1<br>PMP | 200 | 100 pps |
| Hughes et al. (2003) | Nucleus 24 | 100 CL (76 μA)<br>50 CL (28 μA) | CG<br>MP | 100 | 49 pps |
| Mahoney & Proctor (1994) | Nucleus 22 | 126 CL (300 μA) | BP+1 | 200 | 250 pps |
| Mens et al. (1994a, 1994b) | Nucleus 22 | 50 CL (65 μA) | CG<br>VM | 205 | 667 pps |
| Shallop et al. (1995) | Nucleus 22 | 126 CL (300 μA)<br>50 CL (65 μA) | BP+1<br>VM | 200 | 250 pps |

**RECORDING**

| *Study* | *Electrode Montage* | *# Sweeps* | *Gain* | *Filter* |
|---|---|---|---|---|
| Cullington & Clarke (1997) | Ipsi earlobe (+)<br>Contra earlobe (–)<br>Wrist (G) | 100 | 50 mV | 20 Hz–10 kHz |
| Hughes et al. (2003) | Ipsi mastoid (+)<br>Forehead ( )<br>Contra mastoid (G) | 200 | 10,000 | 10 Hz–10 kHz |
| Mahoney & Proctor (1994) | Ipsi earlobe (+)<br>Contra earlobe (–)<br>Forehead (G) | 200 | 5000 | 1 Hz–10 kHz |
| Mens et al. (1994a, 1994b) | Ipsi mastoid (+)<br>Contra mastoid (–)<br>Arm (G) | 256–2048 | 20–50 mV | 100 Hz–6 kHz |
| Shallop et al. (1995) | Ipsi mastoid (+)<br>Contra mastoid (–)<br>Forehead (G) | Not reported | Not reported | Not reported |

*Note:* CL = Nucleus current-level units; CG = common ground; MP = monopolar; BP = bipolar; PMP = pseudomonopolar; VM = variable bipolar mode; pps = pulses per second.

AEVs are typically quite large (relative to evoked auditory neural potentials). As a result, myogenic artifacts are generally not a problem, so recipients do not need to sleep or be sedated for testing. Including application of electrodes, AEVs should only take approximately 20 to 30 minutes to complete.

## FACTORS AFFECTING AEV MEASURES

The exact shape and size of the AEV will depend on several factors. First, AEV amplitudes increase as the amplitude of the stimulus current pulse increases (Cullington & Clarke, 1997; Shallop, 1993; Shallop, Carter, Feinman, & Tabor, 2003). The AEV resembles a biphasic current pulse because the stimulus is a biphasic current pulse, and the AEV represents the artifact associated with electrode stimulation. Thus, the larger the stimulus current pulse, the larger the AEV will be.

Second, AEV amplitudes increase as the distance between the active and return electrodes increases (see Figure 5–4, variable mode, explained further below; Cullington & Clarke, 1997; Hughes, Brown, & Abbas, 2004; Mens, Oostendorp, & van den Broek, 1994a, 1994b; Shallop et al., 1995). Recall that voltage is the product of current and resistance (Ohm's law). Larger distances between active and return electrodes will yield a larger resistance component (i.e., more tissue for current to travel through), and thus a larger voltage potential is generated. Similarly, AEV amplitudes are affected by the impedance of the electrode and surrounding fluid/tissue medium (e.g., cochlear fluid is much more conductive than bone).

Third, AEV amplitudes increase as the distance between the active electrode and the surface recording electrodes decreases (Mahoney & Rotz Proctor, 1994; Mens et al., 1994b). The presumed current pathway in the typical cochlea is through the cochlear fluid along the scala typmani, toward the basal end (Mens et al., 1994b). The basal end represents a lower-impedance path due to the higher fluid volume and more conductive round window/modiolus. Thus, the cochlea can be considered a closed tube (encased in insulating bone) with an open end at the base. If the recording electrodes are closer to the stimulating electrode, the AEVs will be larger. Head size and/or orientation of the array within the cochlea can affect the distance between stimulating and recording electrodes. Mahoney and Rotz Proctor (1994) reported slightly larger AEVs for children than for adults (presumably due to slightly smaller average head sizes for children), and much more variability in the pediatric data than for adult data (likely due to larger variation in pediatric head sizes across the age range of 2.5 to 15 years).

Finally, the polarity of the recorded AEV depends on the direction of current flow relative to the surface recording electrodes (Cullington & Clarke, 1997; Mens et al., 1994b; Shallop et al., 2003). Typically, when the path of current flow between the active and return electrodes is in an apical direction, then the negative-leading biphasic current pulse typically produces a negative-leading biphasic AEV. However, if the dipole is reversed (e.g., current flows in a basal direction), then the polarity of the recorded AEV is reversed. This concept is explained further in the following sections, in the context of specific electrode coupling modes.

## TYPICAL PATTERNS

As with any test, it is important to have a good working knowledge of the typical or normal pattern so that a framework is in place to detect or diagnose atypical measures. Figures 5–2 through 5–5 show normal AEV patterns for four different modes of stimulation. The underlying mechanisms that produce each pattern are described in the following sections.

### Common Ground

Figure 5–2 shows normal AEV patterns for common ground stimulation (left) and schematics

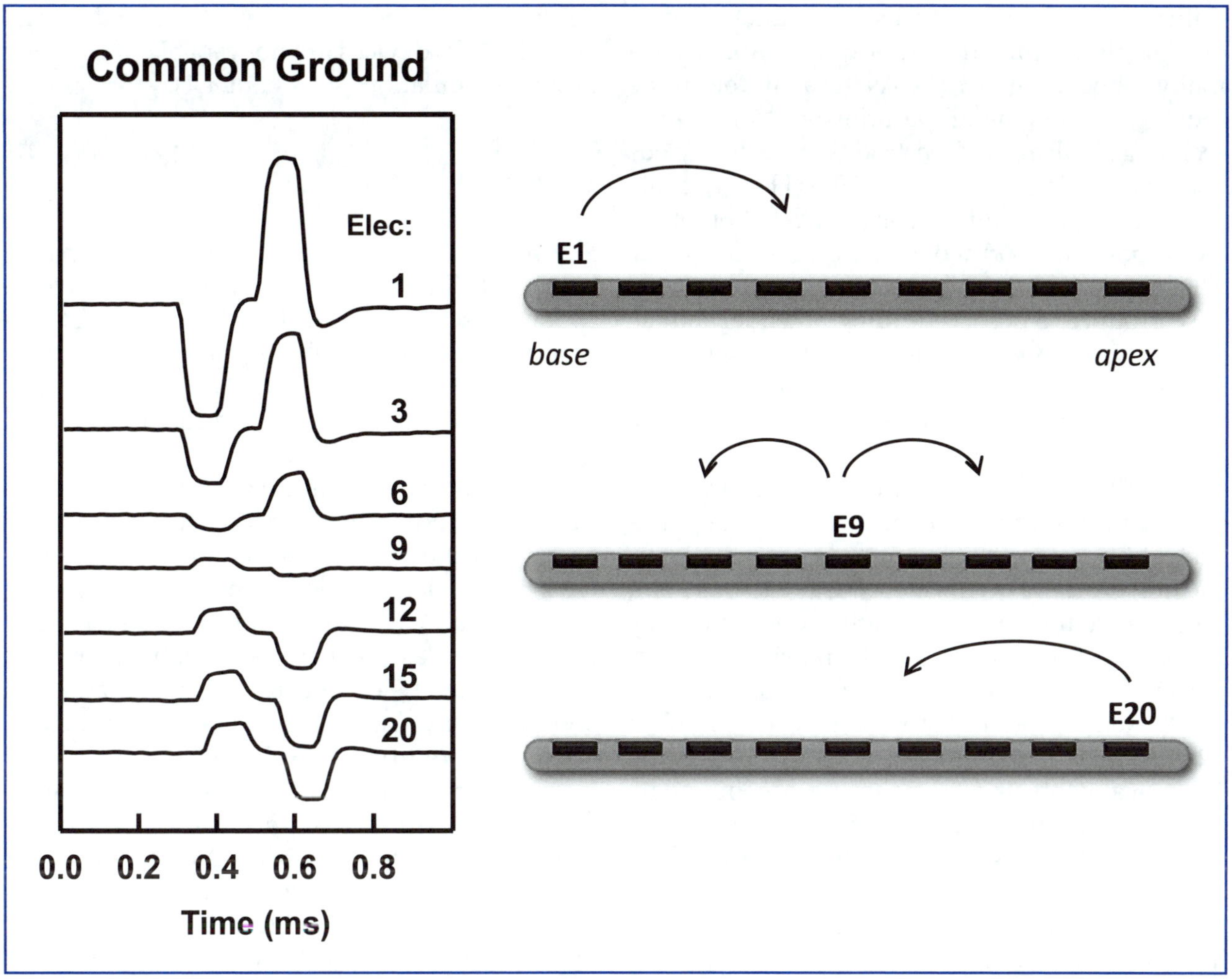


**FIGURE 5–2. Left:** Normal AEV patterns for a Nucleus 22 recipient with common ground stimulation. **Right:** Corresponding schematics illustrating the path of current flow (*arrows*) for active electrodes 1, 9, and 20. The active electrode is labeled on each waveform and schematic. Note that relative (not absolute) electrode locations are labeled in the schematics on the right. Adapted with permission from Figure 1, Hughes et al. (2004), "Sensitivity and specificity of averaged electrode voltage measures in cochlear implant recipients," *Ear and Hearing*, *25*, 431–446, Lippincott, Williams & Wilkins.

indicating the path of current flow (right). Data are from a Nucleus 22 recipient (adapted from Hughes et al., 2004, Figure 1). With common ground coupling, an intracochlear electrode is selected as the active while all remaining intracochlear electrodes are shorted together for the return (see Chapter 2). For brevity, only active electrodes 1, 3, 6, 9, 12, 15, and 20 are shown in the left panel of Figure 5–2, and relative (not absolute) electrode locations are labeled in the schematics on the right.

In the normal condition, the AEV for the most basal electrode (E1) should be negative leading with the largest amplitude. The negative-leading polarity reflects current flow in an apical direction, and the largest amplitude reflects: (1) closest proximity of the active (stimulating) electrode to the far-field recording electrodes and (2) maximal current flow in the same direction because all remaining electrodes for the return are located apical to the active electrode (i.e., the dipole is not split).

Both phases should generally be symmetric; however, slight asymmetry is not uncommon in normally functioning devices. As the active electrode moves apically, the amplitude should decrease, reaching a null around electrodes 6 to 9 in Nucleus devices (Cullington & Clarke, 1997; Hughes et al., 2004). This null point reflects a cancellation of the two dipoles, as recorded by the surface electrodes. That is, the portion of current flowing toward the base produces a positive-leading potential and the portion of current flowing toward the apex produces a negative-leading potential. Depending on the ratio of the size of the two dipoles, averaging these opposite potentials yields a reduced-amplitude AEV or a null (around E9 in Figure 5–2). Although electrode 11 is numerically the "middle" electrode in the 22-electrode Nucleus array, the null typically occurs more basally to this point because the return current path is determined by the collective impedances of the remaining return electrodes. For stimulation of E11, the collective electrode surface area of return electrodes 12 to 22 will be smaller than electrodes 1 to 10 because the apical contacts are smaller (to accommodate the reduced cross-sectional size of the tapered cochlea). After the null point, the polarity of the AEV will invert and the peak-to-peak amplitude may increase slightly (see E12–20 in Figure 5–2). The positive-leading polarity represents current flow predominately in a basal direction. The overall amplitude increases because a greater proportion of the return electrodes are located basal to the active electrode. However, as the active electrode moves apically, the amplitude increase may be somewhat offset by the increased distance of the active electrode from the base of the cochlea. As a result, the amplitude change across active electrodes in the apical portion of the array is not as great as the amplitude change across active electrodes in the basal portion (prior to the null point).

One of the drawbacks of common ground AEV measures is that it may be difficult to accurately assess electrodes in the null region because the amplitudes are no larger than the noise floor. Another disadvantage is that it is not unusual for common ground AEVs to be asymmetric, which is a common diagnostic factor for malfunctioning electrodes (see "Atypical Patterns" section below). Finally, common ground AEVs can only be obtained in Nucleus devices; Advanced Bionics and MED-EL devices are not capable of common ground stimulation (see Chapter 1).

## Bipolar+1

Figure 5–3 shows the normal AEV patterns for bipolar+1 (BP+1) stimulation (left) and corresponding schematics of the relative path of current flow (right). Stimulating electrode pairs 1–3, 3–5, 6–8, 9–11, 12–14, 15–17, and 20–22 are shown. Data are from a Nucleus 22 recipient (adapted from Hughes et al., 2004, Figure 1). With BP+1 coupling, an intracochlear electrode is selected as the active, and an electrode two positions in an apical direction serves as the return (see Chapter 2). If an electrode is functioning abnormally, an abnormal AEV will result when that electrode is designated as the active as well as the return. For example, if electrode 6 is malfunctioning, an abnormal AEV will be recorded for electrode pair 4–6 (6 as the return) and 6–8 (6 as the active). BP+1 is typically used instead of BP because it results in a larger AEV (recall that greater spacing between active and return electrodes results in a larger AEV). Even broader bipolar coupling modes could potentially be used (BP+2, BP+3, etc.), but broader coupling limits the use of the most apical electrodes as the active (i.e., can only be assessed as the return electrode).

In typical cases, the AEV for the most basal electrode pair (E1–3 in Figure 5–3) should have the largest amplitude because it is closest to the basal end of the cochlea and the far-field recording electrodes. As the active electrode moves toward the apex (farther from the recording electrodes), the overall amplitude decreases. The polarity for all waveforms should remain negative leading, which reflects the apical direction of current flow between the active and return (i.e., with BP+1, the return is always apical to the active electrode).

The primary disadvantage of testing AEVs in BP+1 is that the amplitudes for the apical half of the array are typically within the noise floor (~5 to 10 μV; Hughes et al., 2004). It can help to increase the stimulus level for better visualization of AEVs for middle and apical electrodes (Shallop et al., 2003). However, loudness tolerance levels would

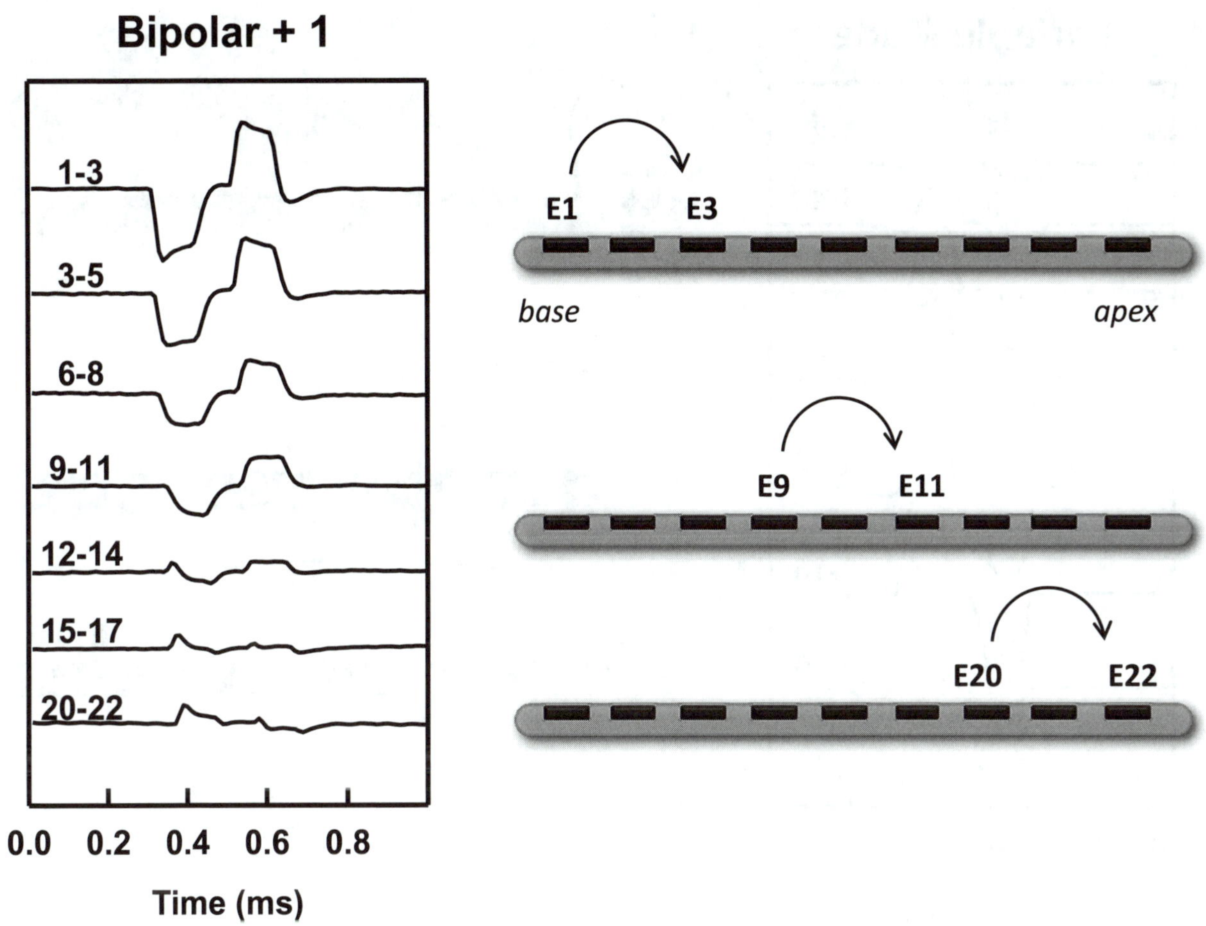


**FIGURE 5–3. Left:** Normal AEV patterns for a Nucleus 22 recipient with bipolar+1 stimulation. **Right:** Corresponding schematics illustrating the path of current flow (*arrows*) for active electrodes 1, 9, and 20. The active-return electrode pair is labeled on each waveform and schematic. Note that relative (not absolute) electrode locations are labeled in the schematics on the right. Adapted with permission from Figure 1, Hughes et al. (2004), "Sensitivity and specificity of averaged electrode voltage measures in cochlear implant recipients," *Ear and Hearing*, *25*, 431–446, Lippincott, Williams & Wilkins.

have to be more closely monitored, and AEVs may still be in the noise floor for the most apical few electrodes.

## Variable Bipolar Mode

Figure 5–4 shows the normal AEV patterns for variable-mode stimulation (left) and current path illustrations (right). Data are from a Nucleus 22 recipient (adapted from Hughes et al., 2004, Figure 1). With variable mode, the most basal electrode (E1 in this case) is used as the active, and progressively larger bipolar spacing (e.g., BP, BP+1, BP+2) is used for the return. The normal AEV pattern for variable mode is that the smallest AEV amplitude will be recorded for the smallest bipolar spacing (E1–2), with progressively larger amplitudes as the bipolar spacing is increased. The polarity for all waveforms should be negative leading, which reflects the apical direction of current flow.

A variation of variable bipolar mode is called pseudomonopolar mode. With pseudomonopolar

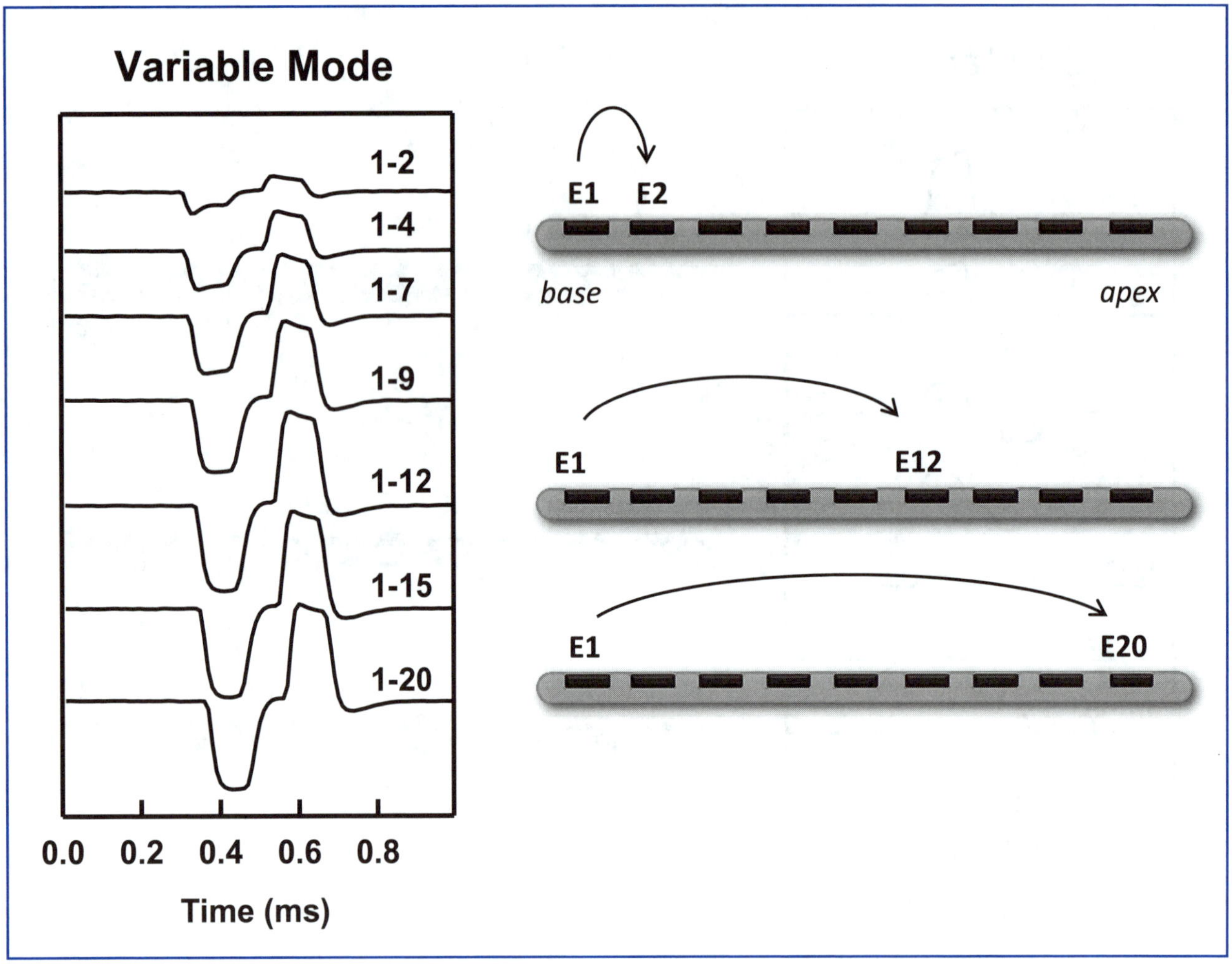


**FIGURE 5–4.** **Left:** Normal AEV patterns for a Nucleus 22 recipient with variable bipolar mode stimulation. Electrode 1 is the active for all traces. **Right:** Corresponding schematics illustrating the path of current flow (*arrows*) for return electrodes 2, 12, and 20. The active return electrode pair is labeled on each waveform and schematic. Note that relative (not absolute) electrode locations are labeled in the schematics on the right. Adapted with permission from Figure 1, Hughes et al. (2004), "Sensitivity and specificity of averaged electrode voltage measures in cochlear implant recipients," *Ear and Hearing*, *25*, 431–446, Lippincott, Williams & Wilkins.

mode, the most basal electrode is fixed as the *return* (instead of fixed as the active). The same pattern is observed as in variable mode, where the smallest amplitude is recorded for the most basal pair (E2–1) because the electrode spacing is smallest, and the amplitude increases as the spacing is progressively widened (E22–1). The only difference between variable mode and pseudomonopolar mode is that the polarity is reversed. For pseudomonopolar AEVs, the waveform is positive leading, which reflects the basal direction of current flow (see Figure 3.14 in Shallop et al., 2003). One disadvantage of pseudomonopolar or variable mode is that loudness percepts increase as the bipolar spacing widens, which increases the possibility of overstimulation. It should be noted that the nomenclature for variable bipolar and pseudomonopolar modes have not always been used consistently in the literature (e.g., Hughes et al., 2004; Shallop et al., 2003).

## Monopolar

Figure 5–5 shows the normal AEV patterns for monopolar stimulation (left) and corresponding

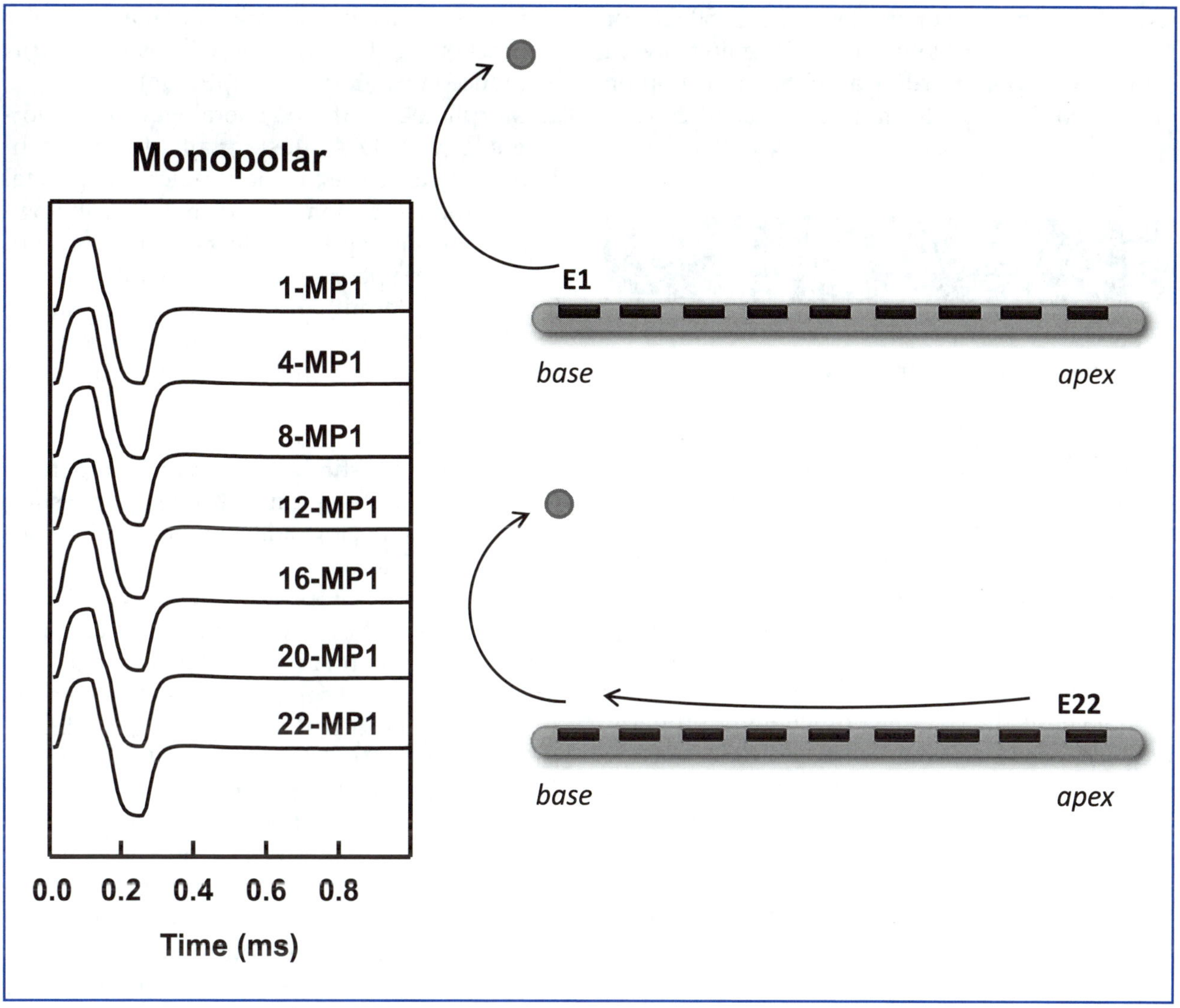


**FIGURE 5–5. Left:** Normal AEV patterns for a Nucleus 24M recipient with monopolar stimulation. **Right:** Corresponding schematics illustrating the path of current flow (*arrows*) for active electrodes 1 and 22. Adapted with permission from Figure 3, Hughes et al. (2004), "Sensitivity and specificity of averaged electrode voltage measures in cochlear implant recipients," *Ear and Hearing*, *25*, 431–446, Lippincott, Williams & Wilkins.

current path illustrations (right). Data are from a Nucleus 24M recipient (adapted from Hughes et al., 2004, Figure 3). With monopolar stimulation, each intracochlear electrode is used as the active, and an extracochlear ground (MP1 in this example) is used for the return (see Chapter 2). If we consider the cochlea as a closed tube encased in insulating bone with an open end at the base, then the return current path is likely basalward for all intracochlear electrodes. As a result, the normal AEV pattern is a positive-leading biphasic waveform for all electrodes. AEV amplitudes are relatively large (on the order of 10 times larger than for common ground; Hughes et al., 2004) because the distance between each intracochlear electrode and the monopolar return is relatively large (that is, compared with the distance between intracochlear active-return electrode pairs). Monopolar AEV amplitudes are also generally uniform across the array because the amplitude decrements (from base to apex) that are typically observed in other modes are negligible given the relatively large amplitudes overall. When using monopolar stimulation for AEV testing, care should be taken to use relatively low current levels (e.g., 50 CL for Nucleus devices) or lower amplifier gain to avoid saturation of the recording amplifier and clipping of the recorded waveforms (Hughes et al., 2004).

## ATYPICAL PATTERNS

Abnormally functioning electrodes are typically identified by comparing the AEV amplitude, polarity, and morphology with that of the expected pattern and the rest of the electrodes in the array. Abnormally functioning electrodes typically yield abnormal AEVs in more than one coupling mode, which is why it is important to measure AEVs in multiple modes. It is also important to keep in mind that abnormal cochlear anatomy (such as ossification or cochlear malformations) can produce AEV patterns that deviate from the norm even if the device is functioning properly. In those cases, decisions about electrode function may be based more on relative changes across the array and less on comparisons to the normal or expected patterns. The following criteria are used as a guideline for identifying abnormally functioning electrodes. These rules apply to any electrode coupling mode:

1. Amplitude differences—If the AEV peak-to-peak amplitude is significantly larger or smaller than that of the adjacent electrodes, it may indicate abnormal electrode function. Mens et al. (1994a) suggested that AEV amplitudes differing by more than 20% of the mean amplitude for adjacent electrodes should be considered abnormal.
2. Polarity inversion—Any waveform that is inverted in polarity relative to the expected pattern may be considered abnormal. Polarity inversion indicates a reversal in the direction of current flow, which is only expected near the middle of the array with common ground stimulation.
3. Monophasic waveforms—Because the stimulus is a biphasic pulse, the recorded AEV should also be biphasic. A monophasic waveform is typically indicative of an abnormally functioning electrode (and will also present as reduced peak-to-peak amplitude).
4. Morphology—If the general waveform morphology differs substantially from neighboring electrodes, it may indicate abnormal electrode function. Abnormal morphology may include spiky artifacts on one or both phases, or a poor signal-to-noise ratio.
5. Absent/intermittent—AEVs that are absent (flat) or intermittently present over repeated test intervals may indicate electrode or device malfunction.
6. Lack of growth—AEV amplitudes should increase with stimulus level. It is important to use a range of current levels for testing that are well below a level that might induce amplifier saturation.

Figure 5–6 shows an example of common ground (left column), BP+1 (middle column), and variable mode (right column) AEVs characterized by inverted polarity and abnormal amplitudes for electrodes 12 and 16. These AEVs, obtained from a Nucleus 22 recipient who was 14 years old at the time of testing, represent one of the more common types of abnormal patterns. The top row of graphs shows AEV waveforms for the region surrounding electrode 12 (for brevity, results for electrode 16 are not illustrated). The bottom row plots peak-to-peak AEV amplitudes as a function of active electrode, with the thick gray lines representing the normal range of amplitudes for a large group of pediatric Nucleus 22 users (University of Iowa Cochlear Implant Electrophysiology Laboratory, unpublished data).

In common ground, the AEV recorded for electrode 12 was much larger and reversed in polarity relative to the AEVs for adjacent electrodes. For BP+1, abnormally large AEVs were obtained when electrode 12 was used as either the active (pair 12–14) or return electrode (pair 10–12, which also demonstrated a polarity reversal). For variable mode, the AEV for pair 1–12 was abnormally small and reversed in polarity relative to the AEVs for adjacent electrodes. Behaviorally, stimulation of electrode 12 resulted in an abnormal percept and was therefore disabled in the recipient's map as both an active and return electrode.

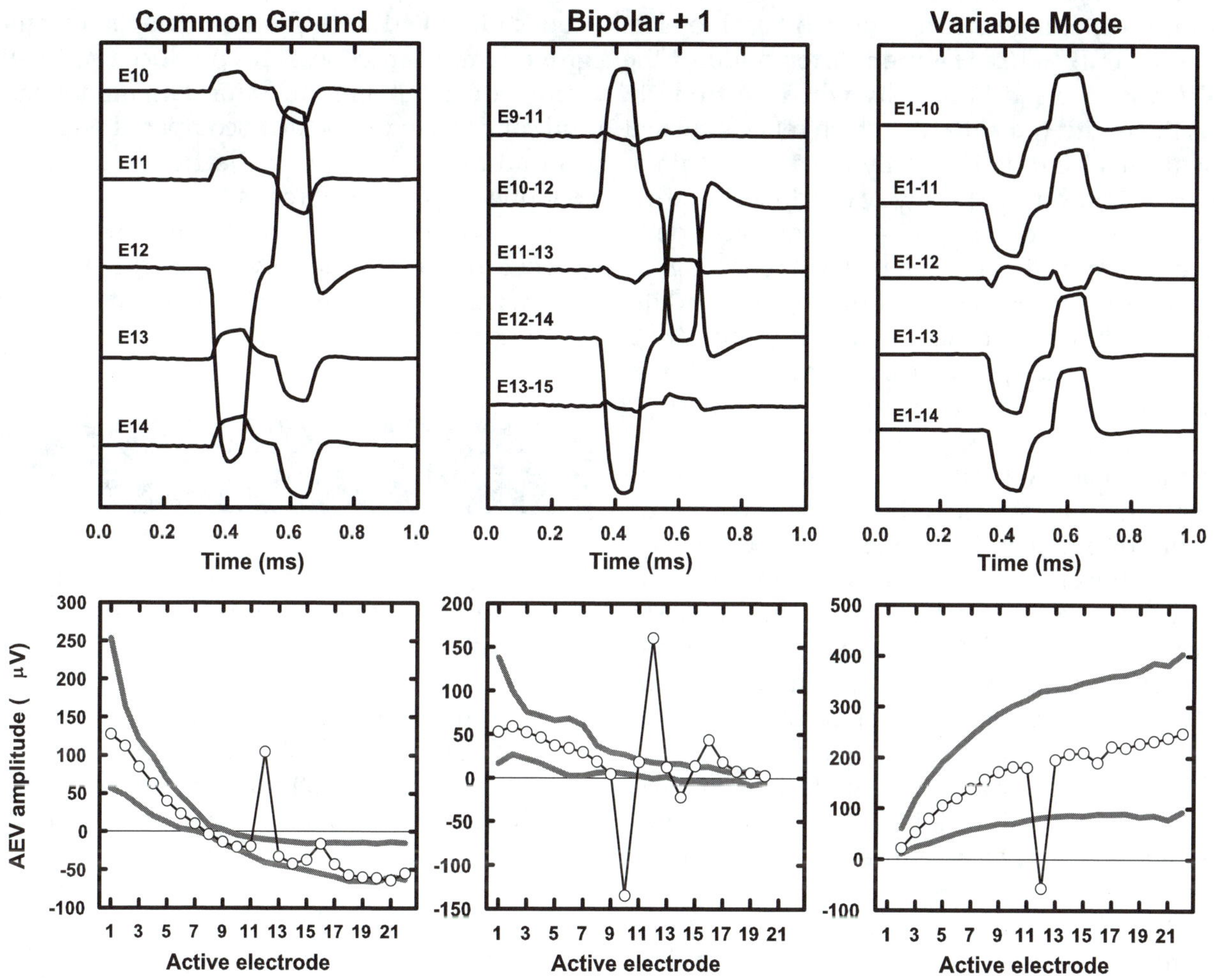


**FIGURE 5–6.** Example of abnormal AEVs for electrodes 12 and 16, obtained from a pediatric Nucleus 22 recipient. Common ground (*left column*), BP+1 (*middle column*), and variable mode (*right column*) AEVs are shown. **Top row:** AEV waveforms for selected electrodes surrounding electrode 12. **Bottom row:** Peak-to-peak amplitudes as a function of all active electrodes, where positive amplitudes represent a negative-leading potential. Thick solid lines represent normative data from a large group of pediatric Nucleus 22 recipients. (Unpublished data courtesy of the University of Iowa Cochlear Implant Electrophysiology Laboratory.)

Collectively, these results suggest that electrode 12 may have been shorted to one of the stiffening rings, which are located basal to electrode 1. Stiffening rings are inactive electrodes used to help guide surgical insertion (see Chapter 1). Recall that normal common ground AEVs are largest for the most basal active electrode because: (1) it is closest in proximity to the recording electrodes, and (2) all of the current is flowing in one direction because all remaining electrodes used for the common ground are located apical to the active electrode. The polarity is also negative-leading, which reflects an apical direction of current flow. If electrode 12 was shorted to a stiffening ring, and the stiffening ring provided the path of least resistance, then current would flow apically from the stiffening ring toward all intracochlear electrodes for common ground mode, resulting in the negative-leading polarity seen in the top left panel of Figure 5–6. The AEV for electrode 12 would also be larger than for the most basal electrode (E1) because stiffening rings are located basal to electrode 1. For BP+1 (see Figure 5–6, top middle), the AEV was reversed in polarity when electrode 12 was the return (pair 10–12), which reflects current flow from electrode 10 basally toward the stiffening ring instead of apically toward electrode 12. The amplitudes of the BP+1 AEVs for electrode 12 were also much larger than normal, reflecting the larger spacing between the stiffening ring and the normally functioning active (E10) or return (E14) electrodes. Finally, for variable mode (see Figure 5–6, top right), the reversed polarity reflects current flow from the active electrode (E1) toward the more basally located stiffening ring, instead of apically toward electrode 12. The smaller AEV amplitude for pair 1–12 reflects the shorter distance between electrode 1 (active) and the stiffening ring (return) versus the distance between electrodes 1 and 12 if 12 were functioning normally. The relative location of the stiffening ring (i.e., within the extreme basal end of the cochlea) would also account for unpleasant or aversive percepts.

Aberrant peak-to-peak amplitudes and polarity reversals for this recipient are illustrated in the bottom three graphs of Figure 5–6. As mentioned previously, electrode 16 also yielded abnormally small AEV amplitudes (re: the 20% rule) for both common ground and variable mode. When BP+1 was used, abnormally large AEVs were recorded when electrode 16 was used either as the active or return electrode. AEVs were also reversed in polarity relative to adjacent electrodes when electrode 16 was used as the return electrode with BP+1 coupling. Overall, the patterns for electrode 16 across the three coupling modes are similar to the patterns for electrode 12, although less pronounced. This suggests a lower-impedance path linked to electrode 16 that was shunting current somewhere toward the base of the cochlea (such as a partial short circuit; see Chapter 3). Stimulation of electrode 16 in a BP+1 mode (used for the recipient's map), however, did not result in unusual percepts and the electrode was therefore not disabled in the recipient's map.

Now that all newer devices are equipped with telemetry capabilities for measuring electrode impedance, some insight can be gained regarding how abnormal AEV patterns relate to impedance measures. Hughes et al. (2004) found that electrodes identified with short circuits via common ground impedance measures produced AEVs that were reduced in amplitude (or flat), monophasic, and/or reversed in polarity compared with adjacent normally functioning electrodes. Electrodes identified with open circuits via impedance measures produced AEVs with abnormal morphology (specifically, a large negative polarity spike at the end of the second phase), with either asymmetric or monophasic waveforms.

## CLINICAL USES FOR AEVS

Clinically, AEVs are used to assess device function when the following issues are suspected, reported, or observed:

1. Intermittent device function
2. Lack of stimulation/sound (nonfunctioning internal receiver/stimulator)
3. Decreased performance, or poorer performance than expected
4. Abnormal changes in programming levels
5. Changes in sound quality
6. Abnormal pitch or loudness percepts in the presence of normal impedance
7. Pitch reversals or abnormal pitch order
8. Nonauditory percepts (dizziness, facial nerve stimulation, pain)
9. Intermittent overstimulation
10. Short or open circuits for devices without telemetry capabilities

Although all newer devices have telemetry capabilities for reporting impedances, abnormal electrode function can persist in the presence of normal impedance (Hughes et al., 2004; examples are given below). Postlingually deafened/experienced CI users can typically provide reliable feedback regarding changes in sound quality, loudness, nonauditory percepts, and so forth. For very young CI users or those without prior auditory experience or adequate language abilities to describe abnormal percepts, AEVs can provide additional information regarding device function.

Thus, it is necessary to understand how AEV measures relate to impedances and subjective perceptions for each electrode.

Hughes et al. (2004) compared common ground impedances to AEVs obtained with both common ground and monopolar stimulation to assess the sensitivity and specificity of AEVs for a group of Nucleus 24M and 24R(CS) recipients. The sensitivity of a test is how often the test accurately identifies an anomaly as present, whereas the specificity is how often the test accurately identifies an anomaly as not being present. Results showed good sensitivity for common ground AEVs (91.7%), but poor sensitivity for monopolar AEVs (7.7%). Both common ground and monopolar AEVs had excellent specificity (97.9%, common ground; 99.8% for monopolar). In general, open circuits were accurately identified with both common ground and monopolar AEVs. Short circuits were accurately identified with common ground AEVs but were missed with monopolar AEVs. In sum, AEV results are generally consistent with impedance results for both monopolar and common ground coupling: open circuits can be identified using any electrode coupling mode (monopolar, any bipolar mode, common ground, pseudomonopolar), and short circuits can be identified with any mode except monopolar.

Figures 5–7 and 5–8 show examples of abnormal electrode function in the presence of normal impedance, and how AEVs were used to objectively confirm abnormal perceptions. Figure 5–7 shows common ground impedances (left column), common ground AEVs (middle), and monopolar AEVs (right) for three adult Nucleus 24M recipients. Each recipient presented with a single electrode that yielded an abnormal percept described as sounding unpleasant or aversive (E11 for M45b, E7 for M17, and E14 for M5). In each case, impedances were within the normal range, common ground AEVs were abnormal for the electrodes with abnormal percepts (bolded waveforms), and monopolar AEVs were normal. For subjects M45b (top row) and M5 (bottom row), impedances for the electrode producing the unpleasant/aversive percept and abnormal common ground AEV (indicated by an arrow in the left column) were not markedly different from that of the adjacent electrodes. For subject M17, the impedance difference for electrode 7 was more noticeable, although still well within the normal range. For all three subjects, the offending electrode presented with negative-leading polarity and abnormally large amplitudes (exceeding the 20% rule proposed by Mens et al., 1994a) in common ground mode. It was hypothesized that the lead wires of these three electrodes may have been shorted to one of the basal stiffening rings, similar to the example shown in Figure 5–6 (electrode 12). Because the stiffening rings are inactive electrodes, they are not shorted with the intracochlear electrodes to create the common ground return path. Thus, a short circuit of this type will not be identified using common ground impedance testing.

Figure 5–8 shows another example of abnormal electrode function in the presence of normal impedance. Results are from the initial stimulation of a child implanted with a Nucleus 24M at the age of 5 years 7 months. A full insertion was achieved, including all 10 stiffening rings. Panel A shows common ground impedance, indicating short circuits on electrodes 12 and 22. These two electrodes were immediately disabled at the initial programming visit. Note that the impedance for electrode 15 was substantially lower than for the adjacent electrodes, although still within normal limits. Panel B shows the initial map levels, obtained with reliable behavioral responses. Because the behavioral levels for electrode 15 were significantly elevated relative to those for the rest of the array, AEV testing was immediately performed. Panel C shows common ground AEVs for electrodes 12 through 22. AEVs for the two electrodes with a known short circuit (12 and 22) were abnormal, as expected. The AEV for electrode 15, which presented with normal impedance, was abnormally large and reversed in polarity compared with those for the adjacent electrodes. Panel D shows the peak-to-peak amplitudes for AEVs obtained with common ground (filled circles) and monopolar (open squares) stimulation. Note that the AEV amplitudes for the two short-circuit electrodes are abnormal in common ground but not in monopolar mode. Finally, the AEV amplitudes for electrode 15 were abnormally large for common ground stimulation and abnormally small for monopolar stimulation (following the 20% rule of Mens et al., 1994a). As with the examples shown in

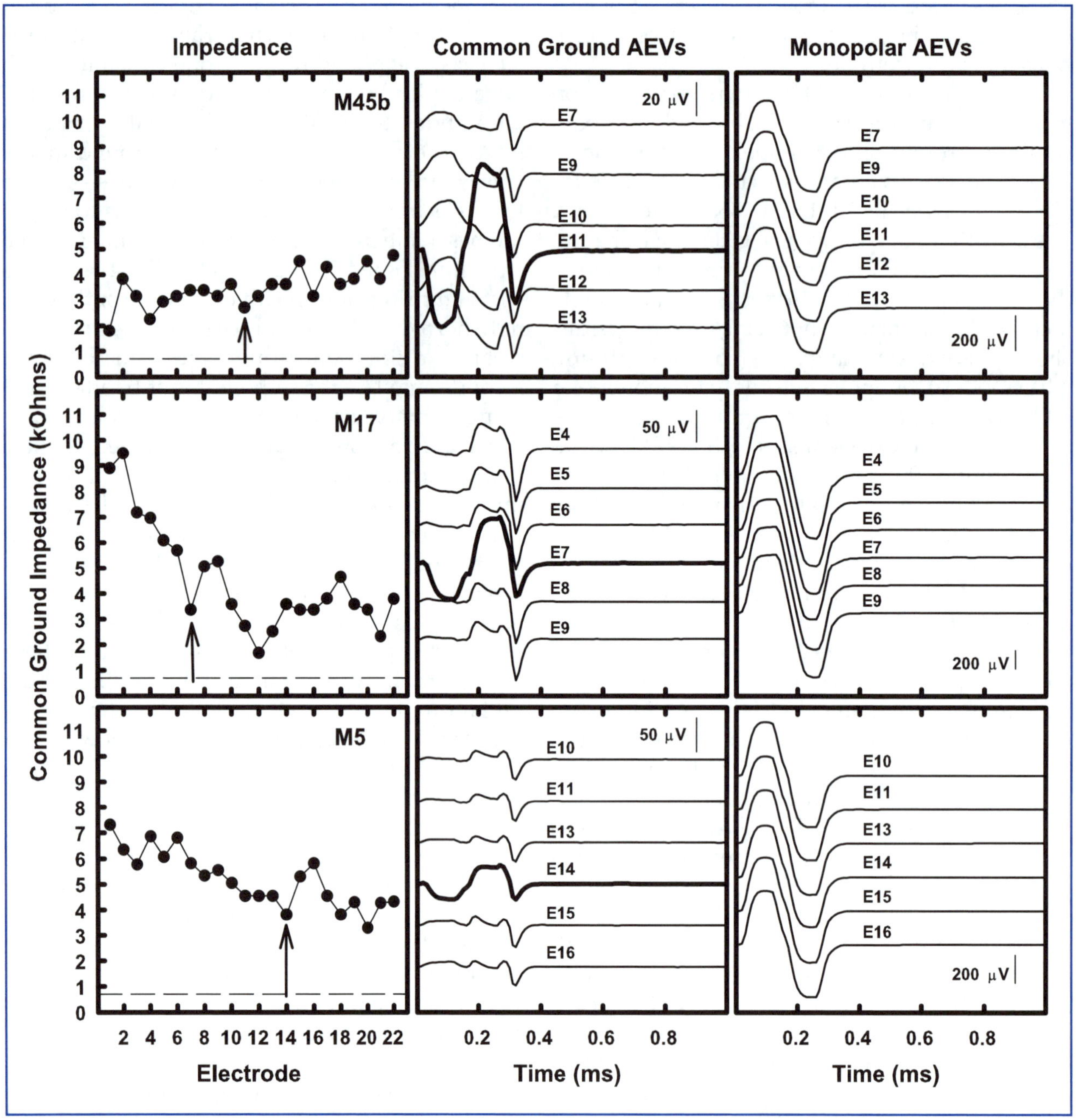


**FIGURE 5–7.** Examples from three adult Nucleus 24M recipients (subject number indicated on each row), each presenting with an electrode with common ground impedances in the normal range (*left column*), abnormal common ground AEVs (*middle*), and normal monopolar AEVs (*right*). Arrows in the left column of graphs indicate the electrode that produced abnormal perceptions. The horizontal dashed lines on the impedance graphs indicate the manufacturer's cutoff for a short circuit. Electrode numbers are indicated on each AEV waveform in the middle and right columns. Republished with permission from Figure 8, Hughes et al. (2004), "Sensitivity and specificity of averaged electrode voltage measures in cochlear implant recipients," *Ear and Hearing, 25*, 431–446, Lippincott, Williams & Wilkins.

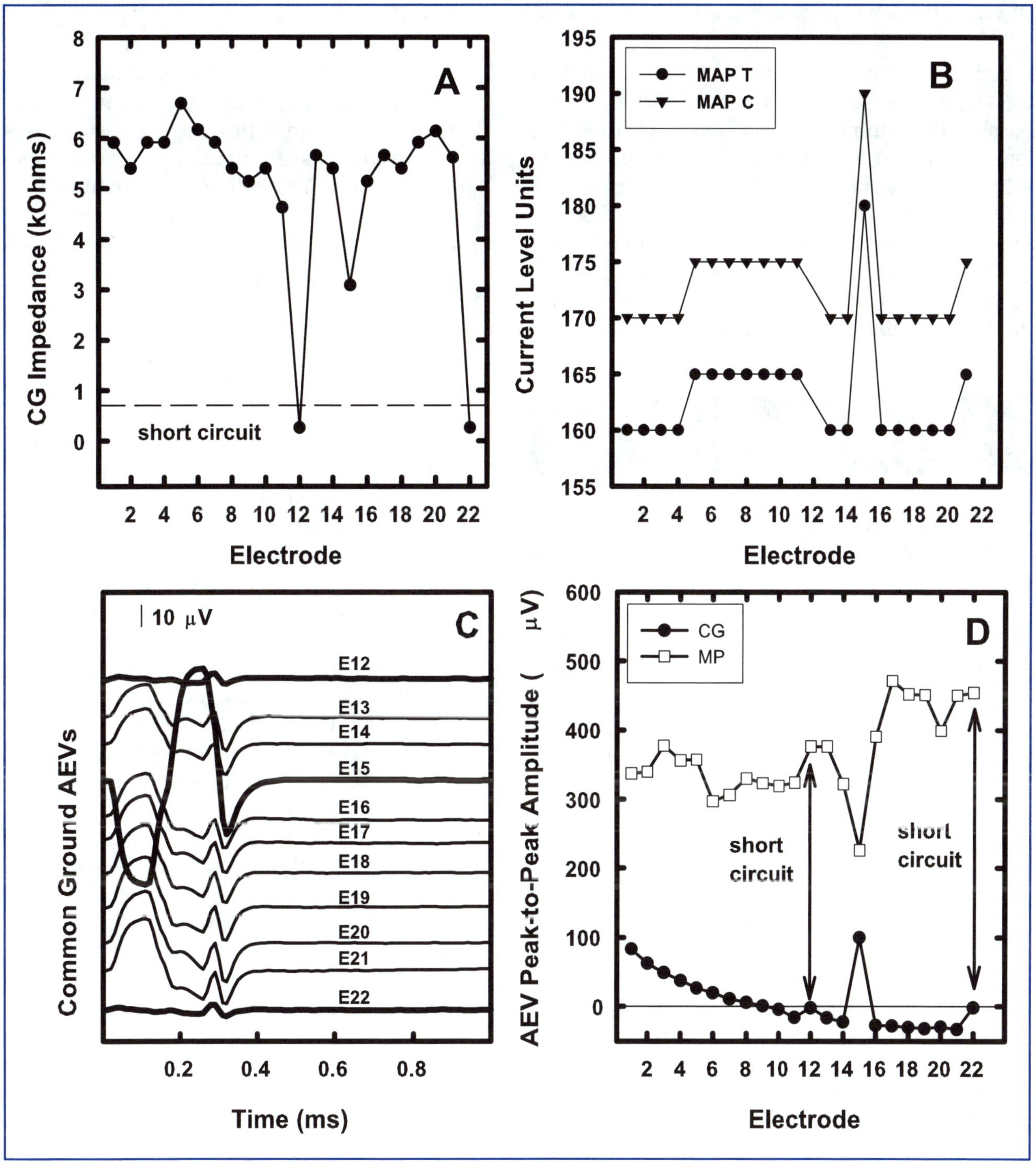


**FIGURE 5–8.** Test results from a pediatric Nucleus 24M recipient at the initial stimulation. **A.** Common ground impedances as a function of electrode number. The horizontal dashed line indicates the manufacturer's cutoff for a short circuit. Electrodes 12 and 22 presented with short circuits. Electrode 15 was within the normal range, but the impedance was substantially lower than for the adjacent electrodes. **B.** Map levels (T = threshold, C = upper comfort levels) as a function of electrode number. **C.** Common ground AEVs for electrodes 12 to 22. Abnormal responses can be seen for the two known short circuits (E12 and E22), as well as for E15 (*bolded waveforms*). **D.** AEV peak-to-peak amplitudes for common ground (*filled symbols*) and monopolar (*open symbols*) stimulation. Amplitudes for the two known short-circuit electrodes (E12 and E22) are indicated with arrows. Republished with permission from Figure 9, Hughes et al. (2004), "Sensitivity and specificity of averaged electrode voltage measures in cochlear implant recipients," *Ear and Hearing, 25*, 431–446, Lippincott, Williams & Wilkins.

Figures 5–6 and 5–7, it was hypothesized that electrode 15 was shorted to a basal stiffening ring because the common ground AEV amplitude was larger than that for electrode 1 (see Figure 5–8D), with the same negative-leading polarity as the AEVs obtained for the most basal electrodes. It is worthwhile to note that this type of anomaly will not be seen for the newer Nucleus Contour arrays or for other manufacturers' devices because those do not have platinum stiffening rings.

## SUMMARY

This chapter has described the basics of averaged electrode voltages. Key concepts are summarized below:

1. AEVs are far-field measurements of the artifact associated with stimulating an intracochlear electrode, and are measured with surface recording electrodes.
2. AEV amplitudes increase with increased stimulus current level, distance between active and return electrodes, and more basal location of the active electrode.
3. AEV polarity reflects the direction of current flow. For a negative-leading biphasic stimulus pulse, a negative-leading AEV represents current flow in an apical direction between the active and return electrodes.
4. The typical AEV pattern for common ground stimulation is a relatively large negative-leading biphasic waveform that progressively decreases in amplitude, reverses polarity, and then increases slightly in amplitude as stimulation progresses from base to apex. The disadvantages of common ground stimulation for AEVs is that the phases may be asymmetric (i.e., falsely identified as abnormal), and responses for electrodes near the middle of the array are typically in the noise floor and thus difficult to evaluate.
5. The typical AEV pattern for BP+1 stimulation is a relatively large negative-leading biphasic waveform that progressively decreases in amplitude as stimulation progresses from base to apex. The primary disadvantage of BP+1 stimulation is that responses for electrodes in the apical portion of the array may fall within the noise floor and be difficult to evaluate.
6. The normal AEV pattern for variable bipolar mode is a small, negative-leading AEV for the most basal electrode pair, which gets progressively larger in amplitude as the bipolar spacing is increased. The primary disadvantage of variable mode is that loudness percepts increase as the bipolar spacing widens, which increases the possibility of overstimulation.
7. The normal AEV pattern for monopolar stimulation is a very large, positive-leading waveform that is fairly uniform in amplitude across the array. The primary disadvantages of monopolar stimulation for AEVs are that: (a) lower current levels and/or lower amplifier gains must be used to avoid saturation of the recording amplifier and clipping of the recorded waveforms, and (b) they do not accurately identify short-circuit electrodes.
8. Abnormal AEVs may be characterized by one or more of the following: amplitude difference of 20% or more relative to adjacent electrodes, polarity inversion, monophasic waveforms, abnormal morphology, absent/intermittent waveforms, and lack of amplitude growth with increased current level.
9. AEVs can be used to assess device function for the following issues: intermittent device function, lack of stimulation/sound, decreased performance or performance poorer than expected, abnormal changes in programming levels, changes in sound quality, abnormal pitch or loudness percepts in the presence of normal impedance, pitch reversals, nonauditory percepts, intermittent overstimulation, or suspected short/open circuits in devices without telemetry capabilities.

# Part III

## Physiological Objective Measures

# 6

# Electrically Evoked Stapedial Reflexes

## INTRODUCTION TO PHYSIOLOGICAL OBJECTIVE MEASURES

The final five chapters of this book each describe physiological measures from different levels of the auditory system in response to electrical stimulation through a cochlear implant. Electrically evoked stapedial reflexes (ESRs) are described in Chapter 6, electrically evoked compound action potentials (ECAPs) in Chapter 7, electrically evoked auditory brainstem responses (EABRs) in Chapter 8, electrically evoked auditory middle latency responses (EAMLRs) in Chapter 9, and electrically evoked auditory cortical potentials in Chapter 10. These assessment tools are designed to measure various aspects of auditory responses through an implant, which can provide information regarding behavioral thresholds and comfort levels, spread of excitation within the cochlea, channel interaction, binaural interaction, neural maturation, and objective measures of stimulus discrimination.

This chapter begins with a basic description of ESRs, and then describes how ESR thresholds (ESRTs) are measured. The last section describes how ESRTs are used clinically, and includes a relevant summary of the literature. ESRTs have been referred to in the literature by various other names and acronyms, including the electrically evoked auditory reflex thresholds (EART), electrically evoked middle ear muscle response (eMEMR), and eSRT.

## BASIC DESCRIPTION

Electrically evoked stapedial reflexes are the same as their acoustic counterparts, except that the stimulus consists of electrical current delivered via the cochlear implant. The stapedial reflex is a muscular contraction within the middle ear in response to loud sounds, and involves both sensory and motor neurons in an afferent/efferent arc. The stimulus (loud acoustic sound or electrical current) elicits a response in the afferent auditory nerve fibers (eighth cranial nerve), which travels to the ipsilateral cochlear nucleus, then to motor nuclei of the facial nerve (seventh cranial nerve) on both the ipsilateral and contralateral sides (Hall, 1992). The reflex arc is completed via the efferent path from the motor nuclei to the facial nerve, which innervates the stapedius muscles on both the ipsilateral and contralateral sides. The stapedius muscle, which attaches to the stapes, contracts bilaterally. This contraction stiffens the ossicular chain, resulting in decreased compliance of the middle ear system. The decreased compliance is measured with a hermetically sealed probe integrated with a clinical impedance bridge.

## MEASUREMENT

ESRs can be measured clinically using a standard impedance bridge and cochlear implant programming equipment. Figure 6–1 illustrates the equipment configuration. The stimulus that is used to elicit the ESR is typically the same stimulus used to measure map levels in the clinical programming software. This is usually a 500-ms duration pulse train of the same per-channel rate and pulse width used in the recipient's map. The stimulus parameters are specified in the programming software, and the stimulus is delivered via the recipient's speech processor, which is connected to the programming computer via a standard manufacturer-specific programming interface.

For recording, the probe tube of the impedance bridge should be placed in the ear contralateral to the implant and then pressurized to attain a hermetic seal. Hodges, Butts, Dolan-Ash, and Balkany (1999) reported greater success with obtaining ESRTs in the contralateral ear versus the ipsilateral ear for unilateral implant recipients. However, because the stapedial reflex occurs bilaterally, regardless of which ear is stimulated, either ear can theoretically be used for measurement. It is important to note that the ear used for measurement should have normal middle ear function, so it is necessary to always obtain a tympanogram before attempting ESR measurements.

Once the ear canal has been pressurized and a normal tympanogram obtained, the impedance bridge should be set to the "Reflex Decay" setting to allow for an ample time window to record the response. Note that the contralateral stimulus probe of the impedance bridge is not needed, because the stimulus is provided by the cochlear implant. Once the decay setting is initiated, the stimulus is presented via the programming software, typically in a group of 3 to 5 pulse trains (Hodges et al., 1999). The ESR appears as a single downward deflection and should be time-locked to each stimulus presentation. An example

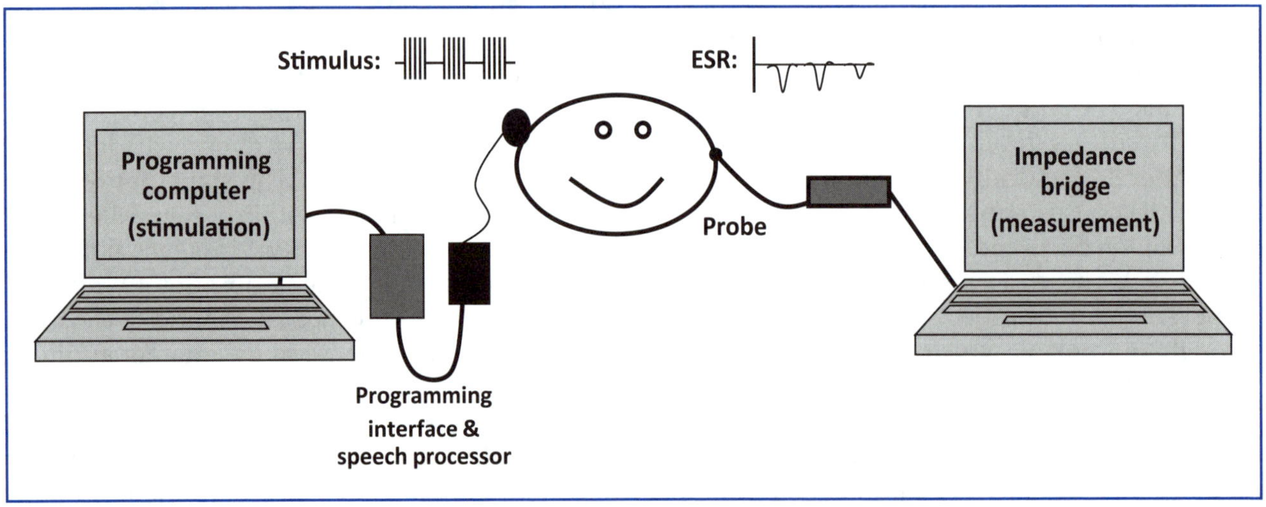


**FIGURE 6–1.** Stimulus and recording setup for electrically evoked stapedial reflexes. **Left:** The stimulus is a pulse train delivered via the implant using standard programming software and equipment. The same stimulus used to program the speech processor is typically used to elicit the ESR. In this example, a series of three pulse trains is illustrated. **Right:** A standard clinical impedance bridge is used to record the stapedial reflex. The probe is inserted into the contralateral ear (ipsilateral ear can also be used if not contraindicated by middle ear dysfunction) and a hermetic seal is obtained. The impedance bridge should be set to the reflex decay setting and then the stimulus is presented via the programming software. Three ESRs are illustrated; one in response to each of the three pulse trains.

of an ESR is shown in Figure 6–2 for a series of five stimulus presentations; thus, five downward deflections are observed.

To obtain a threshold (ESRT), an initial ascending approach for the stimulus level should be used because ESRTs tend to occur near the upper comfort levels (e.g., Hodges et al., 1997; Hodges et al., 1999; Jerger, Oliver, & Chmiel, 1988; Stephan & Welzl-Müller, 2000), so it is important to avoid potential overstimulation. Hodges et al. (1999) recommended beginning with a relatively low stimulus level, and then slowly increasing the current until an ESR is visualized. When a clear response is obtained, the stimulus level should be reduced using smaller current step sizes until the response is no longer present. The lowest visible repeatable response on the descending run is taken as threshold. Figure 6–3 shows an ascending series of ESRs obtained from a Nucleus CI512 recipient. In this example, no responses were visualized for stimulus levels of 189 CL and 192 CL, but clear responses were present for 194 CL and 196 CL. For this electrode, 194 CL would be considered the ESRT if the responses were repeatable on a descending run (not shown).

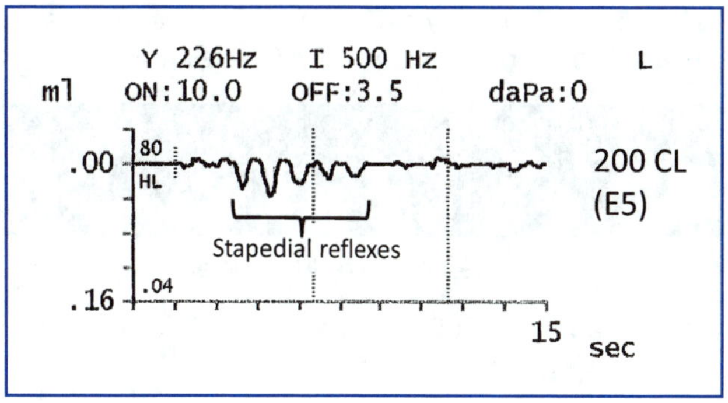


**FIGURE 6–2.** Example of an electrically evoked stapedial reflex measured contralaterally from a Nucleus CI512 recipient by stimulating electrode 5 at 200 CL with a 900-pps pulse train. The reflex presents as a series of downward deflections, time-locked to the stimulus presentation. In this example, a series of five pulse trains were presented, each one eliciting a reflex.

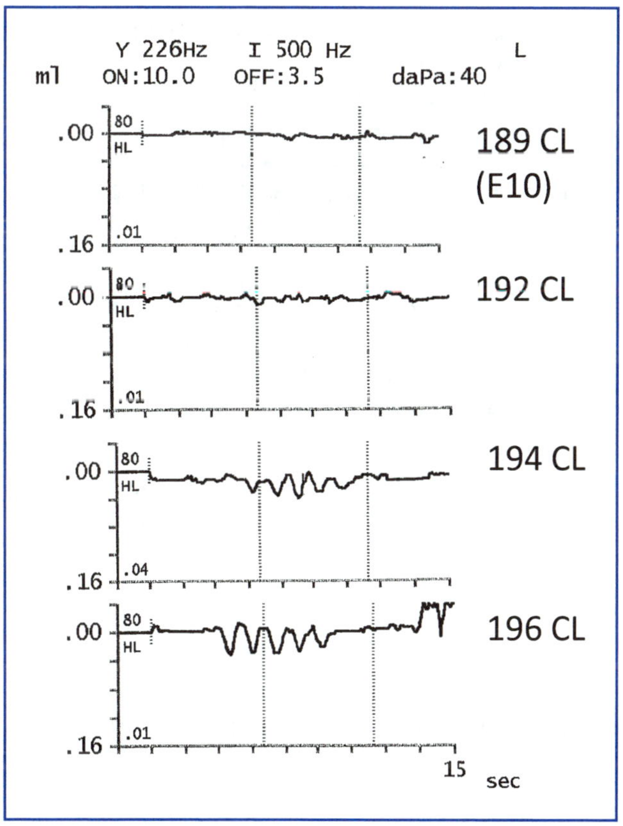


**FIGURE 6–3.** Examples of electrically evoked stapedial reflexes for a series of stimulus levels, obtained from electrode 10 in a Nucleus CI512 recipient. The stimulus was a 900-pps pulse train. No responses were seen for 189 CL and 192 CL; clear responses were seen for 194 CL and 196 CL. In this example, 194 CL would be considered threshold.

## CLINICAL USES FOR ESRTS

Clinically, ESRTs can be used to confirm device function, and confirm that the auditory pathway (at least to the level of the brainstem) is functioning in response to electrical stimulation from the implant. ESRTs have also been used to assist with speech processor programming. Table 6–1 summarizes key findings from a number of research studies that have examined the relation between ESRTs and map upper comfort levels. Several studies (e.g., Han et al., 2005; Hodges et al., 1997; Lorens, Walkowiak, Piotrowska, Skarzynski, & Anderson, 2004; Spivak & Chute, 1994; Stephan & Welzl-Müller, 2000) have shown strong correlations between ESRTs and map upper comfort levels (i.e., C- or M-levels). This finding is important because it can be difficult to obtain accurate estimates of upper comfort levels for young children, especially those who are congenitally deafened. This population typically lacks the concepts of

**Table 6–1.** Summary of Research Studies Assessing the Relation Between Electrically Evoked Stapedial Reflex Threshold (ESRT) and C/M-Levels

| Study | Recipients/Device | Stim Mode | # Subjs with Measurable ESRTs | ESRT vs. C/M-Levels |
|---|---|---|---|---|
| Battmer et al. (1990) | Adult Nucleus 22 | BP+1 | 19/25 (76%) | ESRT @ 66-78% map DR |
| Bresnihan et al. (2001) | Pediatric Nucleus 22/24 | [N/R] | 20/26 (77%) | ESRT ~20 CL below C-level |
| Caner et al. (2007) | Pediatric AB CII/90K | MP | 48/60 (80%)* | 1-year M-levels @ 76% of intraop ESRT |
| Gordon et al. (2004) | Nucleus 24M | MP | 13/35 (37%)† <br> 32/43 (74%)‡ | [N/R] |
| Han et al. (2005) | Pediatric AB CII | [N/R] | 7/9 (78%) | *r* = 0.71 |
| Hodges et al. (1997) | Adult Nucleus 22 <br> Pediatric Nucleus 22 | BP+1 <br> [N/R] | 17/25 (68%) <br> 31/40 (78%) | *r* = 0.91 <br> [N/R] |
| Hodges et al. (1999) | Pediatric AB Clarion | [N/R] | 11/17 (65%) | [N/R] |
| Jerger et al. (1988) | Adult Nucleus 22 | BP+1 | 7** | *r* = 0.09*** |
| Lorens et al. (2004) | Pediatric MED-EL C40 | MP | 7/10 (70%) | *r* = 0.89 |
| Opie et al. (1997) | Adult & pediatric <br> Nucleus 22, AB Clarion EBP, MED-EL C40 | CG, MP | 8/10 (80%) | ESRT near or above C/M-level |
| Spivak & Chute (1994) | Adult Nucleus 22 <br> Pediatric Nucleus 22 | BP+1 | 12/16 (75%) <br> 12/19 (63%) | ESRT near, above, or below C-level |
| Stephan & Welzl-Müller (2000) | Adult MED-EL C40, C40+ | MP | 6^ | *r* = 0.44 to 0.99 across subjs; *r* = 0.92 for group |

*Note:* DR = dynamic range; N/R = not reported; AB = Advanced Bionics; EBP = enhanced bipolar; C40 = Combi 40; CG = common ground; MP = monopolar.

*Number of measurements, not subjects.

†At 1 month post.

‡At 3 months post.

**Unclear how many subjects were initially screened.

***Calculated from their Table 1 data.

^Measurable ESRT was part of the inclusion criteria.

soft and loud, and often will tolerate stimulus levels much higher than what postlingually deafened children or adults indicate as maximum comfort levels. As a result, those patients may be at higher risk for the implant operating out of voltage compliance limits, poorer battery life, and potentially further degraded spectral resolution due to broad current spread from high stimulus levels. It is therefore valuable to have an objective measure that can be used to estimate upper comfort levels.

For children with Nucleus devices, Hodges et al. (1997) recommended setting C-levels to 15%

below ESRT at the initial programming visit, and then gradually working up to the ESRT levels over time. For pediatric Advanced Bionics (AB) recipients, Hodges et al. (1999) recommended setting M-levels to 70%, 80%, and 90% of the ESRT levels for the different program slots in the processor. They recommended using the 70% map at the initial visit, and then gradually working up to the 90% map over a period of several weeks. It should be noted that these recommendations were made based on older technology and older processing strategies; more work is needed to assess ESRT and map C/M-level relationships for newer devices and strategies.

Other studies have shown weaker agreements between ESRTs and upper comfort levels (e.g., Battmer, Laszig, & Lehnhardt, 1990; Bresnihan, Norman, Scott, & Viani, 2001; Caner, Olgun, Gültekin, & Balaban, 2007; Jerger et al., 1988; Spivak & Chute, 1994). Battmer et al. (1990) reported that ESRTs fell at approximately 66 to 78% of the map (behavioral) dynamic range for a group of adult Nucleus 22 recipients, which suggests that ESRTs underestimated the C-levels. Similarly, Bresnihan et al. (2001) found that ESRTs were an average of 20 CL below behavioral C-levels for a group of children with Nucleus 22 and 24 devices. Conversely, Caner et al. (2007) reported that M-levels obtained at the initial stimulation and at one year post were 63% and 76%, respectively, of the ESRT obtained intraoperatively for a group of pediatric AB recipients, suggesting that ESRTs overestimated M-levels. Similarly, Spivak, and Chute (1994) reported ESRTs that were up to 40 to 50 CL above map C-levels for a group of adults with the Nucleus 22 device. However, they noted that none of the subjects reported that the ESR stimulus was uncomfortably loud, and postulated that perhaps those subjects' C-levels had not been set using an appropriate loudness criterion. In that same study, another group of adult subjects presented with ESRTs that were up to 40 to 50 CL below map C-levels, primarily for mid-to-apical electrodes, suggesting that ESRTs underestimated C-levels.

Figure 6–4 shows the relation between ESRTs and map C-levels for four electrodes measured for the Nucleus CI512 recipient whose responses are shown in Figures 6–2 and 6–3. The stimulus in this example was a 900-pps pulse train. Although the correlation between the two measures is very strong ($r$ = 0.99), ESRTs were consistently above this recipient's map C-levels. Using a loudness rating scale, the loudness estimates for the levels corresponding to the ESRT were either at or just below the uncomfortable level (UCL). ESRTs were attempted for two additional electrodes (E1 and E3), but loudness comfort levels were exceeded before an ESR could be measured. These results are consistent with those of Caner et al. (2007) and Spivak and Chute (1994), which suggested that ESRTs can overestimate upper comfort levels for some recipients.

One factor that may account for the different findings across studies is the location of the electrodes that were tested. The correlation between ESRT and upper comfort levels has been shown to vary across the electrode array. Caner et al. (2007) showed a stronger correlation between AB M-levels and ESRTs for basal electrodes than for

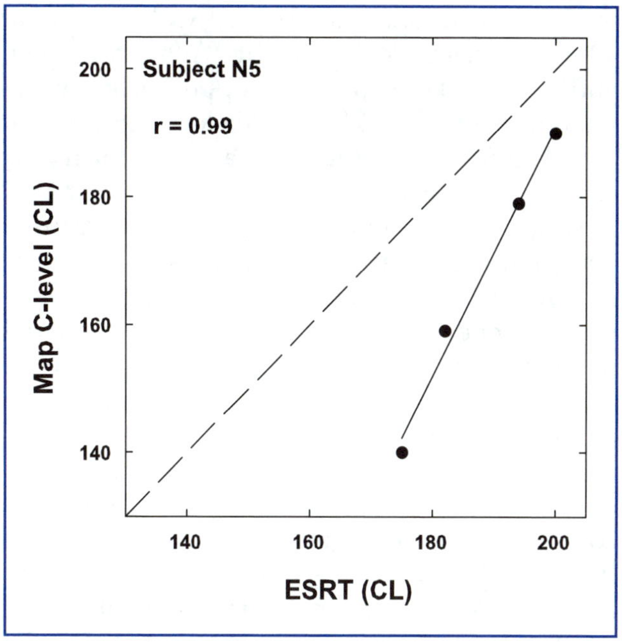


**FIGURE 6–4.** Correlation between ESRTs and map C-levels for electrodes 5, 10, 16, and 22 measured for the Nucleus CI512 recipient whose data are shown in Figures 6–2 and 6–3. The stimulus was a 900-pps pulse train. The solid line is the linear regression line, and the diagonal dashed line represents the point at which C-level and ESRT would be equal.

apical electrodes. For a group of MED-EL Combi 40+ and Nucleus 24M recipients, Allum, Greisiger, and Probst (2002) showed the opposite; better correlations were found for apical electrodes.

Another factor that may account for different outcomes across studies is the time interval at which ESRTs and C/M-levels were measured. Some studies compared ESRTs obtained intraoperatively to C/M-levels obtained postoperatively (e.g., Caner et al., 2007), whereas others compared measures made at the same visit (e.g., Hodges et al., 1997; Stephan & Welzl-Müller, 2000). This is a particularly critical detail, as C/M-levels have been shown to change over time (e.g., Gordon et al., 2004; Hughes et al., 2001), and this time course differs from changes observed in ESRT over time (Gordon et al., 2004). Both measures tend to increase over time, but not at the same rate.

One final issue to keep in mind is that the upper comfort levels are defined differently across manufacturers. For Cochlear (Nucleus) devices, C-level is loud but comfortable; for MED-EL devices, M-level is loud (maximum comfortable level), and for AB devices, M-level is most comfortable. Because the upper comfort level (M-level) for AB devices is, by definition, lower than that for the other two manufacturers, ESRTs for AB recipients will likely overestimate M-levels (Caner et al., 2007). Despite the large variability across studies, the data suggest that ESRTs represent a level that should be audible, but should not exceed uncomfortable levels (UCLs) for many cochlear implant recipients.

One of the disadvantages of ESRTs is that they cannot be measured in all cochlear implant recipients. Previous research has reported that ESRTs were measured in 37 to 80% of subjects tested (e.g., Gordon et al., 2004; Opie, Allum, & Probst, 1997; see Table 6–1). As mentioned, this result is dependent on the time interval at which the measures are obtained. As indicated in Table 6–1, Gordon et al. (2004) were able to measure ESRTs in 37% of their pediatric subjects at the 1-month postoperative visit, but measurements were successful for 74% of subjects at the 3-month visit. Factors that can preclude ESRT measurement include pressure equalization tubes in the tympanic membrane, middle ear effusion or other dysfunction, surgically altered middle ear, inability to maintain a pressurized seal, excessive movement or stiffness of the tympanic membrane, facial nerve dysfunction, or loudness discomfort of the stimulus. In sum, ESRTs may not be possible for a significant number of patients. Furthermore, because ESR measurements require cooperation on the part of the patient (i.e., sit still, no talking or swallowing), it can be more difficult to obtain ESRs for young children or otherwise uncooperative patients.

Finally, several researchers have examined outcomes with behaviorally measured map levels versus maps with C/M-levels set according to ESRTs (Bresnihan et al., 2001; Hodges et al., 1997; Lorens et al., 2004; Spivak, Chute, Popp, & Parisier, 1994). Spivak et al. (1994) measured speech perception performance for the two types of maps in a group of seven adults with the Nucleus 22 device. Two subjects performed better with the measured C-level map, two performed better with the ESRT map, and the remaining three showed no significant difference. Using a similar study design, Hodges et al. (1997) measured speech perception performance for the two types of maps for five adults with the Nucleus 22 device. All five subjects showed similar or slightly improved performance with the ESRT-based map. In general, results across studies suggest that performance and/or preference is similar for the two methods.

## SUMMARY

This chapter has described the basics of ESRs. Key concepts are summarized below:

1. Normal middle ear function is necessary for measurement of the ESR.
2. Either the ipsilateral or contralateral ear (re: the cochlear implant) can be used to measure the ESR; however, the contralateral ear appears to yield a slightly higher probability of obtaining a response.
3. An ascending-descending approach should be used to obtain the ESRT. The lowest level

that yields a repeatable visible response on the descending run is taken as threshold.

4. ESRs are useful for confirming device function, assessment of the auditory pathway to the level of the brainstem, and assisting with estimating map upper comfort levels.
5. ESRTs have been shown to correlate strongly with upper comfort map levels (C/M-levels) in some studies.
6. One disadvantage of ESRTs is that they are not measurable in a significant percentage of cochlear implant recipients.

# 7

# Electrically Evoked Compound Action Potential

Of all the physiological potentials covered in this book, the electrically evoked compound action potential (ECAP) is probably the most widely used in the clinical setting. Reverse telemetry, which allows for ECAPs to be recorded quickly and easily without the need for surface/scalp electrodes, was first commercially available in the United States in 1998 when the Nucleus CI24M was introduced. Since that time, all cochlear implant manufacturers with FDA approval in the United States have introduced devices that are equipped with reverse telemetry systems. This chapter begins with a basic description of what ECAPs are and how they are measured. Common artifact reduction methods are explained, and a discussion of the different types of measurements that can be made with ECAPs is included. Finally, some of the challenges associated with measuring ECAPs are discussed, and a summary of the clinical uses for ECAPs is provided.

## BASIC DESCRIPTION

The ECAP is a synchronous physiological response from an aggregate population of auditory nerve fibers in response to electrical stimulation. It is characterized by a negative deflection, N1, followed by a positive peak or plateau, P2 (Figure 7–1). The ECAP is measured using the intracochlear electrodes of the implant, so it is the near-field version of wave I of the electrically evoked auditory brainstem response (EABR; Miller, Brown, Abbas, & Chi, 2008). The latencies of N1 and P2 are on the order of approximately 0.2 to 0.4 msec and 0.6 to 0.8 msec, respectively (Abbas et al., 1999; Brown, Abbas, & Gantz, 1998; Cullington, 2000). As with most physiological potentials, ECAP amplitudes increase with increased stimulus levels. The peak-to-peak amplitudes can be as large as 1 mV, but are typically between tens and hundreds of microvolts (μV), depending on the recipient's loudness tolerance levels. Because the ECAP is elicited by stimulation through the cochlear implant, a measurable ECAP response can be used to verify device and electrode function. ECAPs can also be used to verify the function of the auditory nerve, monitor physiological responses over time, and can be used to some extent to assist with programming the sound processor. In contrast to the electrically evoked stapedial reflex threshold (ESRT), which can only be measured in 37 to 80% of recipients (Gordon et al., 2004; Opie et al., 1997; see Chapter 6), the ECAP can be measured in approximately 95 to 96% of cases (Cafarelli Dees et al., 2005; van Dijk et al., 2007).

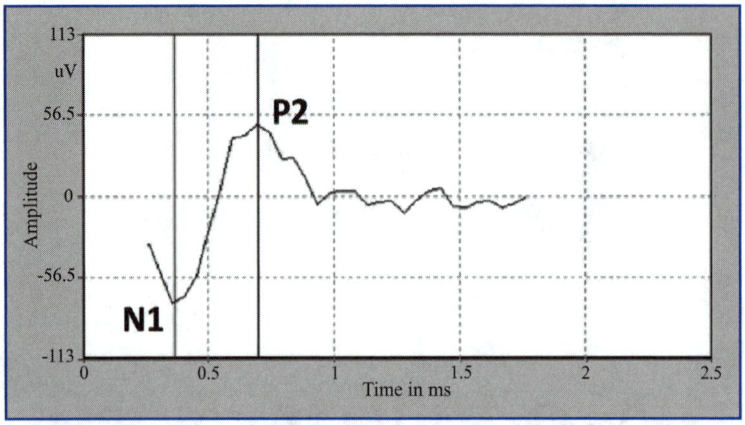


**FIGURE 7–1.** Example of a single electrically evoked compound action potential (ECAP) response. The ECAP is characterized by a leading negative trough, N1, followed by a positive peak or plateau (P2). N1 and P2 are indicated by solid vertical lines.

## MEASUREMENT

### Stimulus

ECAPs can be measured clinically using standard programming software and hardware. Figure 7–2A illustrates the stimulating and recording equipment configuration. The stimulus that is used to elicit the ECAP is typically a single biphasic current pulse delivered using monopolar coupling (Figure 7–2B). Other electrode coupling modes can be used as the device allows (e.g., bipolar, BP+1); however, monopolar is the standard mode for both stimulating and recording, and tends to yield the best results. The stimulus and recording parameters are specified in the clinical software, and the effects of these parameters are detailed in the following sections. The stimulus is delivered by the implanted array via a speech processor that is connected to the programming computer with a standard manufacturer-specific processor interface.

### Recording

The ECAP is recorded using the cochlear implant electrodes, also typically in a monopolar configuration. The measured ECAP is the voltage change (as a function of time) produced by depolarization of auditory nerve fibers. This voltage change is measured across an intracochlear recording electrode (typically located two positions apical to the stimulating electrode) and an extracochlear monopolar ground electrode (see Figure 7–2B).

ECAPs offer several advantages over more central auditory physiological responses. First, they are relatively immune to anesthesia effects, so they can be used for intraoperative assessments. Second, contamination by myogenic activity (muscle artifact) is not an issue because the responses are measured using the intracochlear electrodes instead of surface/scalp electrodes. As a result, patients do not need to lie still, sleep, or be sedated during ECAP measurements. Third, because the ECAP is measured within the cochlea (i.e., closer to the neural generator site), the responses are much larger than those obtained far-field with surface/scalp electrodes. Fewer averages are therefore needed for ECAP measures (about 10 to 100) than for more central measures obtained with scalp electrodes (several repetitions of about 1000 sweeps). As a result, the test time for ECAPs is substantially shorter than for brainstem or cortical measures. Finally, ECAPs are present within the first year of life, so they are much less influenced by maturational effects, as compared to cortical potentials.

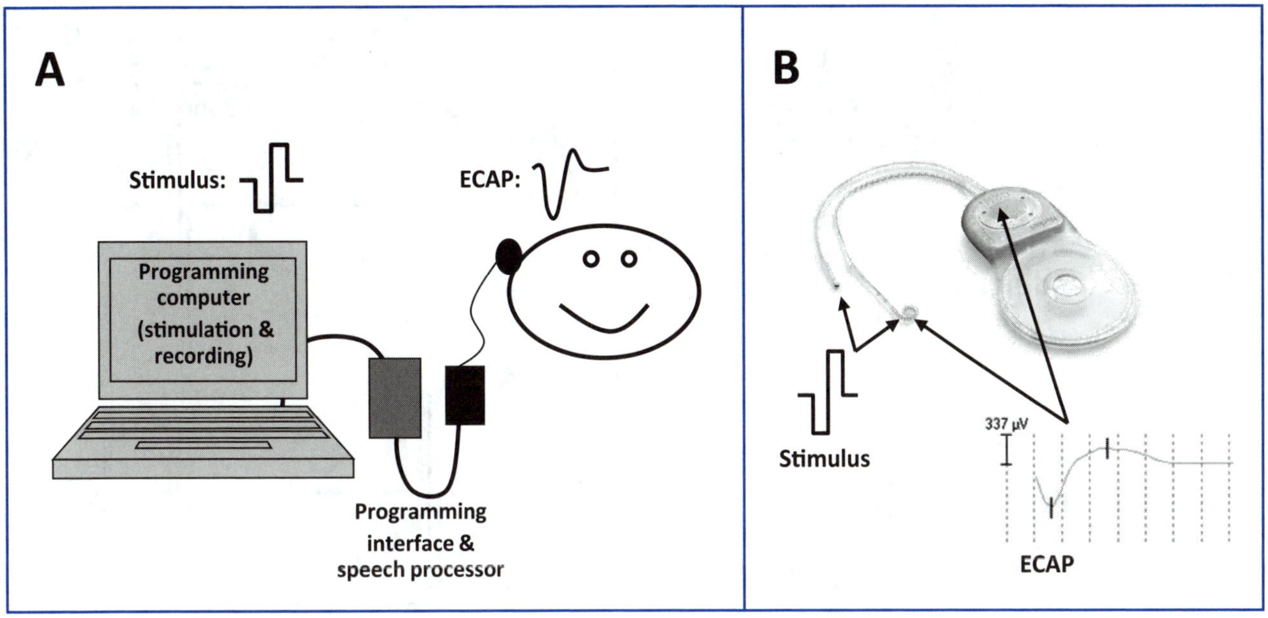


**FIGURE 7–2. A.** Stimulus and recording setup for electrically evoked compound action potentials (ECAPs). **B.** The stimulus is a biphasic current pulse delivered to an intracochlear electrode and extracochlear monopolar ground (MP1 ball electrode, in this example). The ECAP is recorded as the voltage difference across another intracochlear electrode relative to the other extracochlear monopolar ground (MP2 case electrode, in this example). Photo of the Nucleus CI24R(CS) provided courtesy of Cochlear™ Americas, ©2011 Cochlear Americas.

## Artifact Reduction Methods

One of the disadvantages to recording from an intracochlear electrode is that the artifact, like the ECAP, is also larger than when measured with scalp electrodes. Because the ECAP is an early-latency response and the artifact is typically several orders of magnitude larger than the physiological potential, it is more difficult to separate the stimulus artifact from the neural response. Several methods can be used to isolate the ECAP. Three of these methods are outlined in the following sections.

### *Alternating Polarity*

Alternating the stimulus polarity is a method that is commonly used with acoustic auditory brainstem and EABR measurements. This method is illustrated in Figure 7–3. Alternating polarity is the only method currently used in Advanced Bionics' Neural Response Imaging (NRI), is the default method in MED-EL's Auditory Nerve Response Telemetry (ART) software, and is an optional method in Cochlear's Neural Response Telemetry (NRT) software. When the polarity of the stimulus current pulse is reversed, the artifact also reverses in polarity but the physiological response does not. When the response to a cathodic-leading pulse is averaged with the response to an anodic-leading pulse, the artifact primarily cancels out, leaving the neural response. This process can be expressed mathematically as ([C+A]/2), where C is the response to the cathodic-leading pulse and A is the response to the anodic-leading pulse.

The primary disadvantage to this method is that the amplitude and latency of the ECAP can differ slightly for anodic- versus cathodic-leading pulses (Miller et al., 1998). The averaged waveform will therefore have slightly different amplitude and/or morphology compared with the response to either polarity alone. As a result, thresholds obtained with alternating polarity can be slightly elevated relative to those obtained with other methods, such as the forward-masking subtraction method described in the following section (Frijns et al., 2002; Hughes et al., 2003).

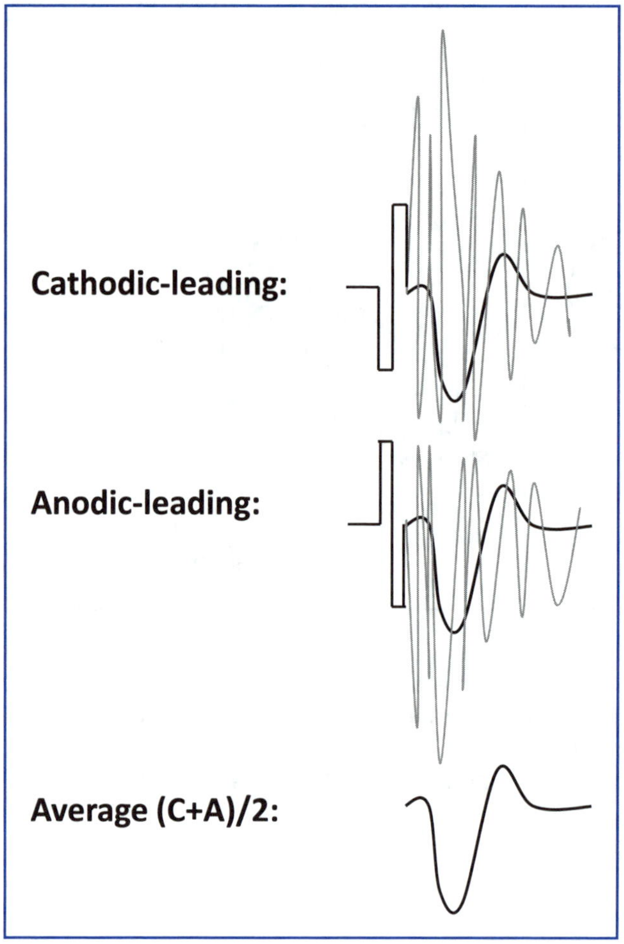


**FIGURE 7–3.** Schematic illustration of the alternating polarity method of artifact reduction. The response for the cathodic-leading current pulse (C) is averaged with the response for the anodic-leading pulse (A). When the stimulus polarity is inverted, the artifact inverts but the neural response does not.

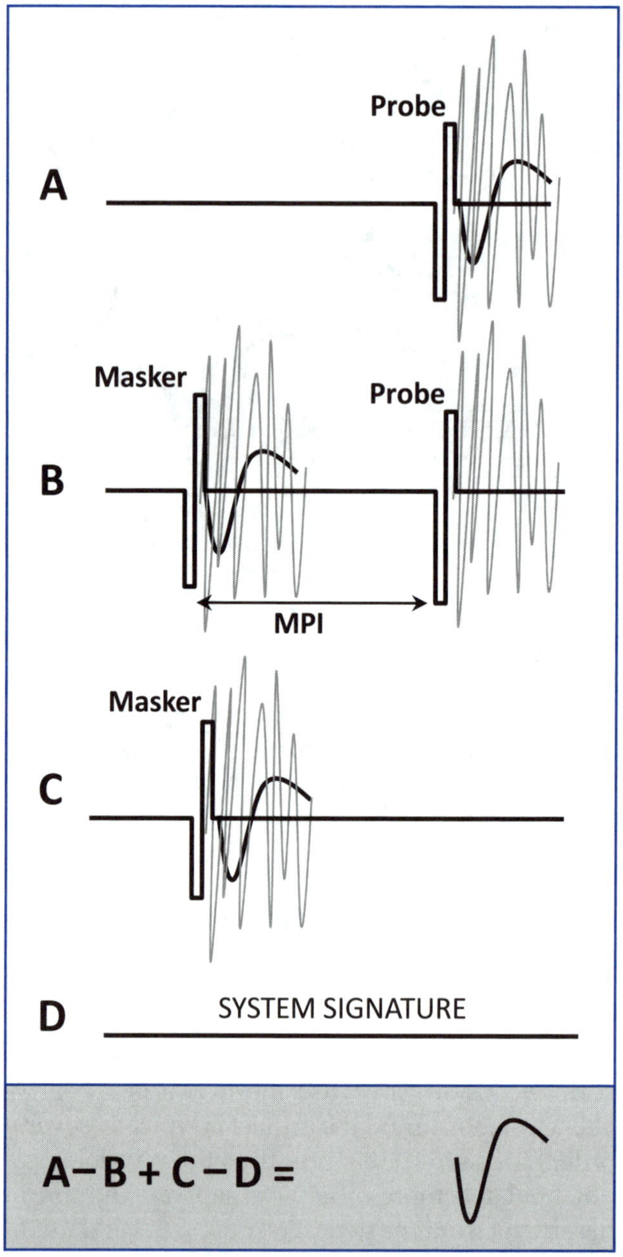


**FIGURE 7–4.** Schematic illustration of the forward-masking subtraction method of artifact reduction. Trace A is the probe alone, trace B is the masker followed by the probe, trace C is the masker alone, and trace D is a zero-amplitude pulse to obtain the system signature (artifact). MPI is the masker-probe interval. All traces are aligned in time (x-axis). The formula A − B + C − D is applied to resolve the neural response to the probe in trace A.

### *Forward-Masking Subtraction Method*

The forward-masking subtraction method takes advantage of neural refractory properties to separate the ECAP from the stimulus artifact (e.g., Abbas et al., 1999; Brown et al., 1998; Dillier et al., 2002). This method is illustrated in Figure 7–4. The forward-masking subtraction method is the default method used in Cochlear's NRT software; it is not used with either Advanced Bionics' or MED-EL's ECAP telemetry systems.

The forward-masking subtraction method uses a four-frame stimulus paradigm. The first frame consists of a single pulse called the probe, which elicits a neural response as well as stimulus artifact (see Figure 7–4A). The second frame (see Figure 7–4B) consists of a pair of pulses (masker and probe) separated by a short time interval called the masker-probe interval, or MPI. The first pulse in the pair (masker) elicits a neural response and stimulus artifact. When the MPI is sufficiently short, the second pulse (probe) occurs during the absolute refractory period for the neurons that discharged in response to the masker. The current NRT software default MPI is 400 µsec, but the optimal MPI can vary between 300 and 500 µsec (Miller et al., 2000; Morsnowski, Charasse, Collet, Killian, & Muller-Deile, 2006). In this frame, the probe pulse only generates artifact, with no embedded neural response. When the artifact response to the probe in frame B is subtracted from the response in frame A, the neural response to the probe alone in frame A is resolved. The last two frames are used to remove the artifact and neural response from the masker in frame B. The third frame (see Figure 7–4C) consists of the masker pulse alone, which elicits a neural response and stimulus artifact. The final frame is a zero-amplitude current pulse, which represents the artifact associated with switching on the current source. The formula applied to the four frames in Figure 7–4 is A – B + C – D. Figure 7–5 shows this process expressed mathematically.

### *Artifact Template Subtraction Method*

The template subtraction method uses a subthreshold current pulse to obtain a template of the stimulus artifact (Miller, Abbas, & Brown, 2000; Miller, Abbas, Nourski, Hu, & Robinson, 2003; Miller, Robinson, Rubinstein, Abbas, & Runge-Samuelson, 2001). This method is illustrated in Figure 7–6. First, a reduced-amplitude version of the target stimulus is delivered. With this method, it is critical that the stimulus level be sufficiently below the physiological threshold to ensure that no neural response is embedded in the trace (i.e., 10 µA). As a result, only the stimulus artifact is recorded. In the second step, the artifact obtained in the first step is scaled up by the same amount as the target stimulus. This step produces the template of the stimulus artifact. In the third step, the target stimulus is delivered, resulting in a neural response and stimulus artifact. In the fourth step, the template of the artifact obtained in step

**Formula for the forward-masking subtraction method:**

$$A = A_p + N_p + S$$

$$B = A_m + N_m + A_p + S$$

$$C = A_m + N_m + S$$

$$D = S$$

$$\begin{aligned} A - B + C - D &= (A_p + N_p + S) - (A_m + N_m + A_p + S) + (A_m + N_m + S) - S \\ &= A_p + N_p + S - A_m - N_m - A_p - S + A_m + N_m + S - S \\ &= N_p \end{aligned}$$

**FIGURE 7–5.** Mathematical expression of the forward-masking subtraction method shown in Figure 7–4. Trace A is the probe alone, trace B is the masker and probe, trace C is the masker alone, and trace D is the zero-amplitude pulse. $A_p$ is the artifact in response to the probe, $N_p$ is the neural response to the probe, S is the system signature (switching artifact), $A_m$ is the artifact in response to the masker, and $N_m$ is the neural response to the masker.

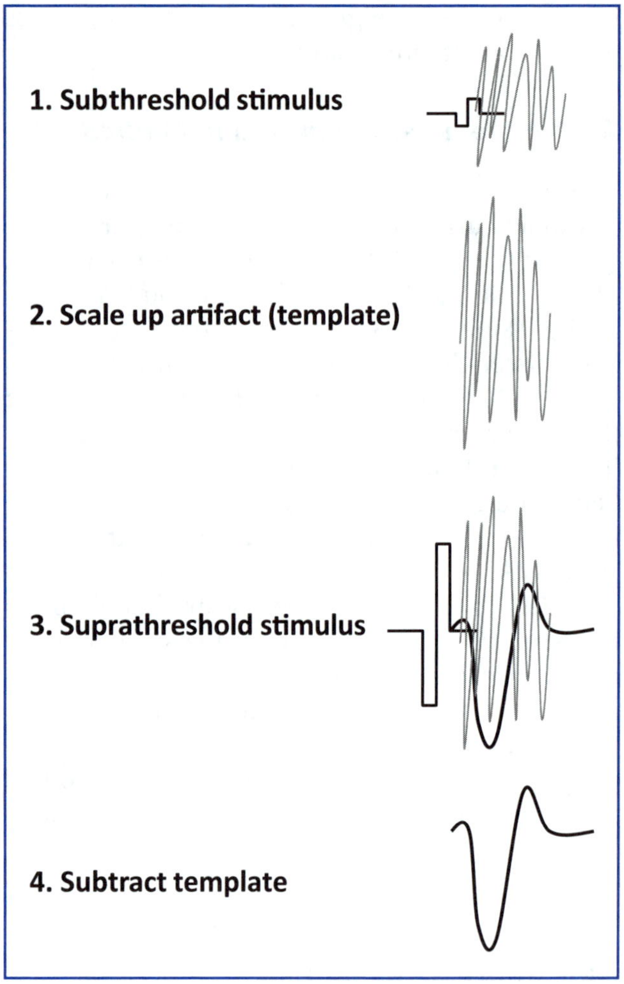


**FIGURE 7–6.** Schematic illustration of the artifact template subtraction method. In trace 1, a subthreshold pulse is presented, which elicits only artifact. In trace 2, the artifact from trace 1 is scaled up by the same proportion as the stimulus in trace 3. In trace 3, the suprathreshold stimulus elicits artifact and a neural response. In trace 4, the template artifact from trace 2 is subtracted, yielding the neural response.

two is subtracted from the response in step three to resolve the ECAP. This method is an optional method in Cochlear's Neural Response Telemetry (NRT) software, and is a method that is commonly used in animal ECAP experiments (e.g., Miller et al., 2000, 2001, 2003).

## Types of Measurements

Stimulus and/or recording parameters can be manipulated to measure different aspects of auditory nerve response properties with a cochlear implant. Some of these parameter manipulations or measurements are only possible with certain types of artifact reduction methods. The following subsections focus on parameter changes that are used to measure ECAP threshold and growth of response with level, refractory recovery, and neural spread of excitation.

### *Threshold and Growth of Response with Level*

As with most physiological responses, the magnitude of the ECAP increases with greater stimulus levels. When the peak-to-peak amplitude is plotted as a function of stimulus level, the result is an input-output (I/O) function, or amplitude growth function (AGF). The AGF can be obtained using any of the artifact reduction techniques described above. An example of an AGF using the forward-masking subtraction method is shown in the upper right panel of Figure 7–7 (data are from a Nucleus 24RE recipient).

Two primary measures are derived from the AGF: slope and threshold. The slope represents the rate of ECAP response growth as a function of stimulus level, and the threshold represents the minimum amount of current needed to elicit a measurable neural response. ECAP thresholds have been used clinically to estimate behavioral levels used to program the sound processor (discussed further at the end of this chapter). Slope and threshold can be affected by a number of variables including the electrode coupling mode used for stimulation (e.g., monopolar, bipolar), the distance between the electrode and neurons, and the density and specific characteristics (e.g. fiber-threshold distribution) of the surviving neural population. Specifically, the rate of response growth tends to be steeper for broader stimulation modes (e.g., Frijns, de Snoo, & Schoonhoven, 1995; Miller, Woodruff, & Pfingst, 1995; Miller et al. 2003) and greater degrees of nerve survival (Hall, 1990; Miller, Abbas, & Robinson, 1994; Smith & Simmons, 1983). Electrode-nerve distance, however, has not been shown to affect the slope of the ECAP growth function (Eisen & Franck, 2004; Van Weert, Stokroos, Rikers, & Van Dijk, 2005). Physiological thresholds tend to be lower for broader stimulation modes (e.g., Miller et al., 1995, 2003),

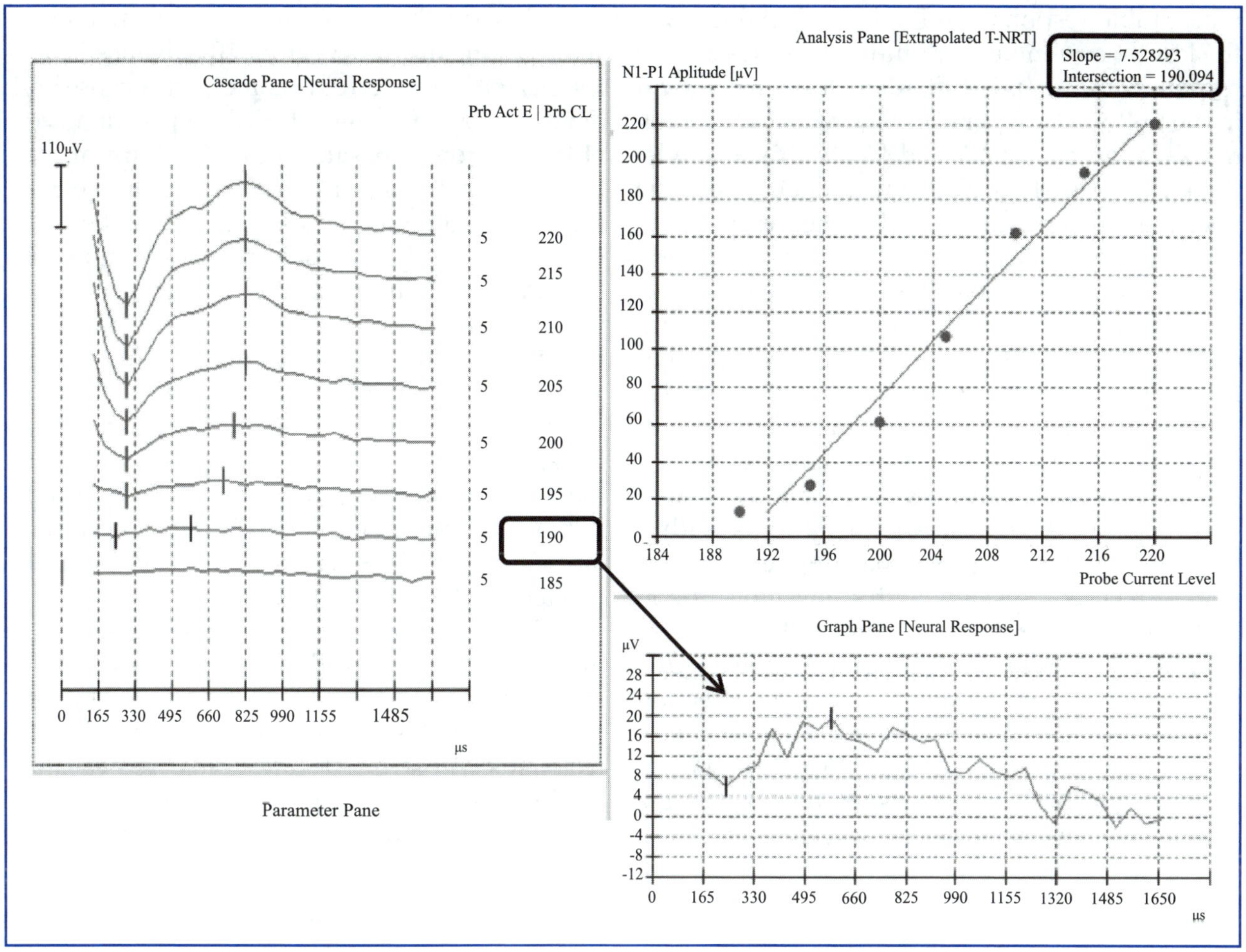


**FIGURE 7–7.** Screen shot of an amplitude growth function in Cochlear's Custom Sound EP software for electrode 5 in a Nucleus 24RE recipient. **Left:** Cascade view of individual waveforms from high (220 CL) to low (185 CL) current level. N1 and P2 peaks are indicated by small vertical hash marks on each waveform with a measurable response (220 CL to 190 CL). **Upper right:** Peak-to-peak amplitudes plotted as a function of stimulus current. Slope (7.5 μV/CL) and linear regression threshold (190 CL) are indicated above the graph in the outlined box. **Bottom right:** Larger view of the threshold waveform (190 CL) that is highlighted in the left panel.

closer electrode-nerve distances (Eisen & Franck, 2004; Gordin, Papsin, James, & Gordon, 2009; Seidman, Vivek, & Dickinson, 2005), and greater neural density or broader fiber-threshold distributions (Miller, Abbas, & Rubinstein, 1999).

The slope is calculated by applying a linear regression to the data points in the AGF. For the example shown in Figure 7–7, the AGF is plotted in the upper right panel, along with the regression line. The slope value, 7.528 μV/CL, is indicated above the graph.

With the commercially available software, threshold can be determined using one of two methods. The first method is to use the AGF linear regression line to extrapolate to the stimulus current level that yields an ECAP amplitude of zero. This "linear regression method" is used in the clinical software by all three manufacturers. For Cochlear devices, the linear regression threshold is referred to in the software as T-NRT; for AB devices, it is called t-NRI; MED-EL does not have a specific name for the regression-based ECAP threshold. In the example shown in Figure 7–7, the T-NRT is given above the top right graph (indicated as "intersection"), which is 190.094 CL.

The second method of threshold determination is called visual detection. With this method, threshold is the lowest current level that yields a measurable response. In Figure 7–7, 190 CL was the lowest current level resulting in a measurable response (13.7 µV). The ECAP for 190 CL is shown in the bottom right panel of Figure 7–7, with peak markers indicating N1 and P2. In this example, there was a nearly perfect agreement between the linear regression and visual detection methods.

Typically, linear regression thresholds are lower than visual detection thresholds because of the criteria used to define each method. Linear regression threshold is defined as the current for a zero-amplitude ECAP, whereas visual detection necessitates a measurable (larger than zero) amplitude. The advantage of the linear regression method is that it can provide a better approximation of ECAP threshold for systems with a high noise floor (Hughes, 2006; Hughes & Glassman, 2011). For systems with a low noise floor, both methods are strongly correlated (Hughes & Glassman, 2011). Figure 7–8 illustrates the relation between linear regression and visual detection methods for two manufacturers. The left graph shows data from six Nucleus 24RE subjects and four Nucleus 24R(CS) subjects (plotted as separate symbols because the devices have different internal chips and thus different noise floors), and the right graph shows data from 10 Advanced Bionics CII/90K subjects (data combined because both devices use the same internal chip). Data were obtained from a basal, middle, and apical electrode for each subject. For the Nucleus devices, there was generally good agreement between the two methods (i.e., data points fall along the diagonal unity line). For AB devices, thresholds were almost always higher with the visual detection method; this was consistent with findings by Han et al. (2005), who reported visual detection thresholds were an average of 32 CU higher than linear regression thresholds. It should be noted that the noise floors for the older Nucleus 24R(CS) and Advanced Bionics CII/90K devices are similar (~20 to 40 µV), whereas the noise floor for the Nucleus 24RE is around 2 to 4 µV.

One disadvantage of the linear regression method is that at least three suprathreshold measures are necessary to reasonably perform the regression analysis. This may not be possible for recipients whose ECAP thresholds are near their loudness tolerance levels. Another disadvantage of the linear regression method is that the AGF

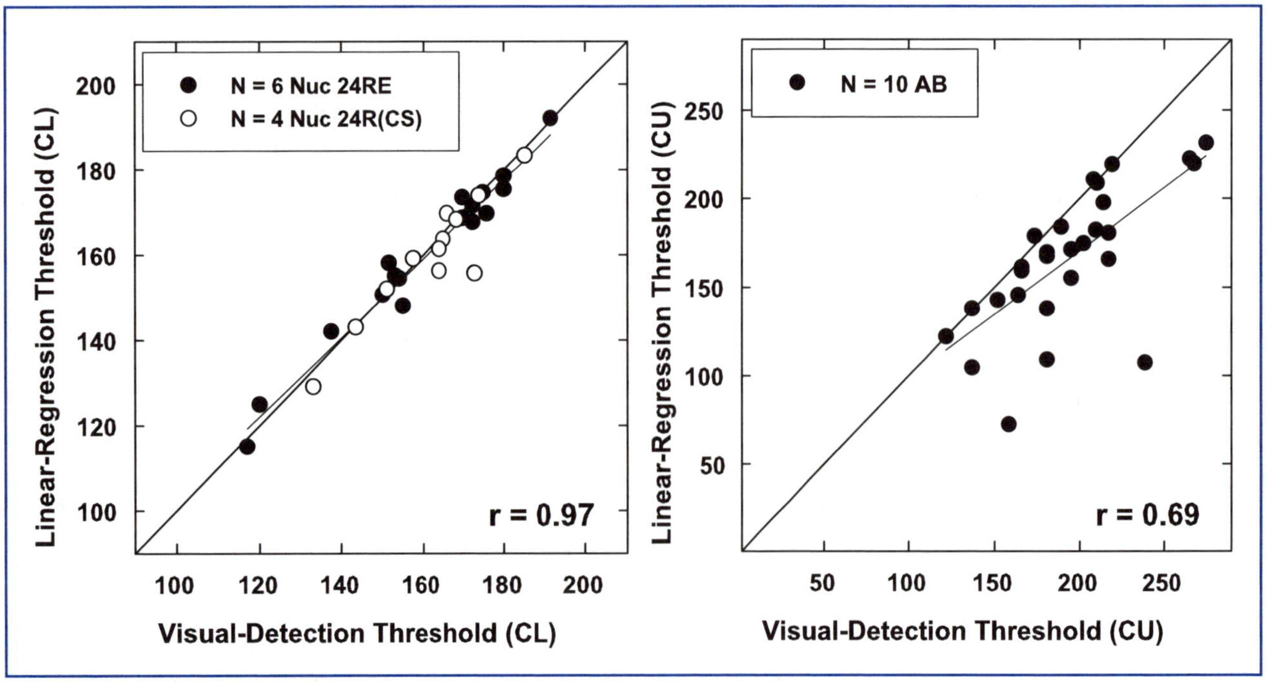


**FIGURE 7–8.** Comparison of linear regression and visual detection methods of threshold determination. **Left:** Nucleus. **Right:** Advanced Bionics. The diagonal solid line represents unity.

can flatten or roll over at the top of the function, or present with a long, shallow tail at the bottom of the function. The result is an AGF that is nonlinear, sigmoidal, or nonmonotonic, which makes a linear regression analysis inappropriate (Botros, van Dijk, & Killian, 2007; Lai & Dillier, 2007). Three examples are shown in Figure 7–9. In panel A, the function plateaus and rolls over slightly at the top. This phenomenon can be due to amplifier saturation or insufficient masking (forward-masking method only). In this example from a Nucleus 24RE recipient, the visual detection threshold was 167 CL and the regression threshold was 164.8 CL. In panel B, the function presents with a tail at the

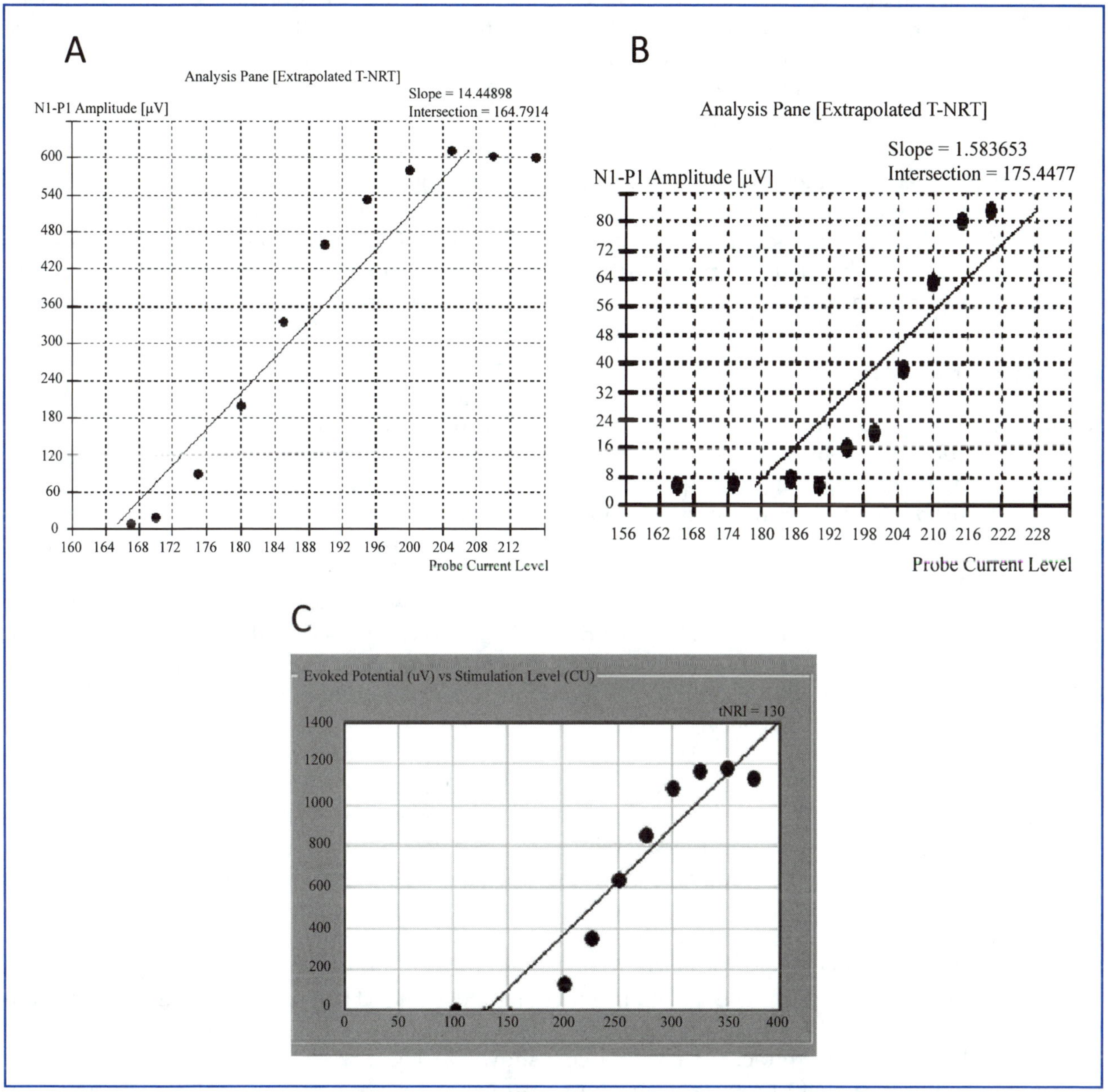


**FIGURE 7–9.** Individual examples of nonlinear amplitude growth functions with linear regression (*diagonal solid line*) applied to each function. **A.** Nucleus 24RE recipient exhibiting plateau and rollover at high stimulus levels. **B.** Nucleus 24RE recipient exhibiting a "tail" at low stimulus levels. **C.** HiRes 90K recipient exhibiting both rollover and tail.

bottom. The visual detection threshold for this Nucleus 24RE recipient was 165 CL and the regression threshold was 175.4 CL. Panel C shows an example of both a rollover at the top and tail at the bottom. In this Advanced Bionics HiRes 90K recipient, the visual detection threshold was 202 CU and the regression threshold was 130 CU.

In sum, it is important to carefully examine the data points that are included in the AGF when using the linear regression method for threshold determination. Most software algorithms allow users to deselect points in the function (such as those that roll over at the top of the function), and the linear regression threshold is automatically adjusted. Because there can be differences between visual detection and linear regression methods, it is important that clinicians be aware of these differences when using (and reporting) ECAP measures clinically.

### Refractory Recovery

Refractory recovery is assessed by measuring the ECAP amplitude in response to a masked probe as a function of varying the time between the masker and probe. Refractory-recovery functions have been shown to reflect the size of the underlying neural population, where slower recovery is associated with larger neural populations (Botros & Psarros, 2010b). Of the three artifact-reduction techniques described above, the forward-masking subtraction method is the only one that can be used to measure the auditory nerve's ability to recover from the refractory period. This is because it is the only method that utilizes a preceding masker pulse.

Figure 7–10 illustrates a simplified version of how the forward-masking technique is used to measure refractory recovery (only frames A and B are shown). Frame A (top) represents the neural response to the probe alone (for clarity, artifact is not shown in this figure). The second frame ($B_1$) represents a short MPI, where all fibers that respond to the masker are refractory and unable to respond to the subsequent probe (i.e., absolute refractory period). The result is no measurable response to the probe pulse, and is the ideal MPI for the standard forward-masking subtraction method. The third frame ($B_2$) represents a slightly longer MPI, where some fibers that respond to the masker are recovered from the refractory period and able to respond to the subsequent probe. The result is a reduced-amplitude ECAP in response to the probe. The bottom frame ($B_3$) represents an MPI that is longer than the absolute and relative refractory periods, where all fibers that respond to the masker are recovered and respond fully to the subsequent probe. Finally, the subtraction method must be applied to eliminate the stimulus artifact. As indicated within the dashed box, each of the responses in the forward-masked probe condition (bottom three frames, $B_n$) is subtracted from the probe-alone condition (top frame, A). The masker-alone (see Figure 7–4, frame C) and system signature (Figure 7–4, frame D) traces are applied as described in Figure 7–4 (for brevity, these two traces are not shown in Figure 7–10). The resulting ECAP waveforms, shown in the right column of Figure 7–10, represent the population of neurons that were still in a refractory state when the probe was presented.

Figure 7–11 shows ECAP amplitudes, obtained using the method described above, plotted as a function of MPI. Data are from a Nucleus 24RE recipient; each curve represents a different stimulating electrode. The top panel shows the raw ECAP amplitudes, and the bottom panel shows the amplitudes normalized to (i.e., divided by) the response obtained with MPI = 500 μsec, which typically yielded the largest response for this recipient. Because ECAP refractory recovery functions are highly dependent on stimulus level (Finley et al., 1997), it is useful to normalize the data to examine the time course of recovery across individuals and electrodes, independent of level.

Miller et al. (2000) proposed an alternative method to eliminate stimulus artifact and circumvent possible distortions introduced by the traditional forward-masking subtraction method for refractory recovery measures. The problem with the traditional forward-masking subtraction method is that it operates under the assumption that a partially masked response (such as that shown in Figure 7–10, probe response in frame $B_2$) has the same morphology and latency as an unmasked response (i.e., probe alone). Miller et al. (2000) illustrated the flaw with this assumption; partially masked single-fiber responses demonstrated slightly longer latencies and reduced amplitudes relative to unmasked responses. When

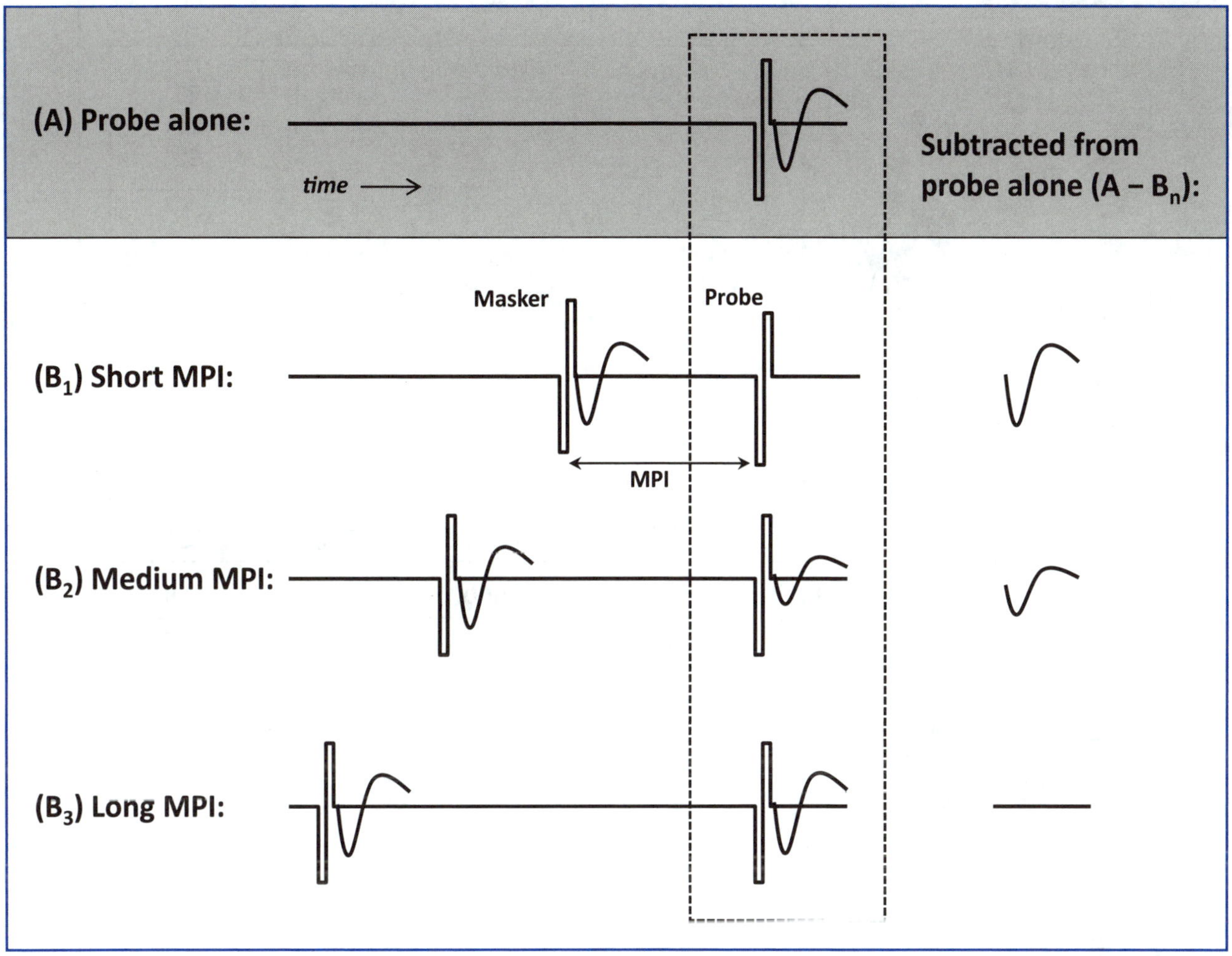


**FIGURE 7–10.** Simplified schematic illustration of the standard forward-masking subtraction method used to measure the refractory recovery function (artifacts, masker-alone, and system signature frames are not shown). **A.** Probe-alone trace. The bottom three frames ($B_1$–$B_3$) represent gradual increases in the masker-probe interval, yielding progressively larger neural responses to the probe. Traces in the far right column represent the difference between the probe-alone (*A*) and the response to the probe in the masked condition ($B_1$–$B_3$) for each corresponding frame outlined in the dashed box.

the standard subtraction method is applied in this case, the resulting difference waveform (unmasked response minus partially masked response) can have a distorted morphology.

With the alternative method proposed by Miller et al. (termed "masked response extraction" in the NRT software), four different frames are used. This method is illustrated in Figure 7–12. Frame A represents the masked condition with the MPI of interest. In the example shown in Figure 7–12, the MPI falls within the relative refractory period. The masker elicits a neural response and artifact, whereas the probe elicits a response from a subset of recovered fibers (partially masked response) as well as artifact. Frame B consists of the masker and probe with a sufficiently short MPI (software default is 400 μsec) to ensure no neural response to the probe, resulting in a template of the probe artifact. When trace B is subtracted from trace A, the artifact is removed from the probe response in trace A. Trace C (masker alone) removes the neural response and artifact generated by the masker in Trace A, and Trace C′ removes the time-shifted neural response and artifact generated by the masker in Trace B. The formula to resolve the probe response in trace A

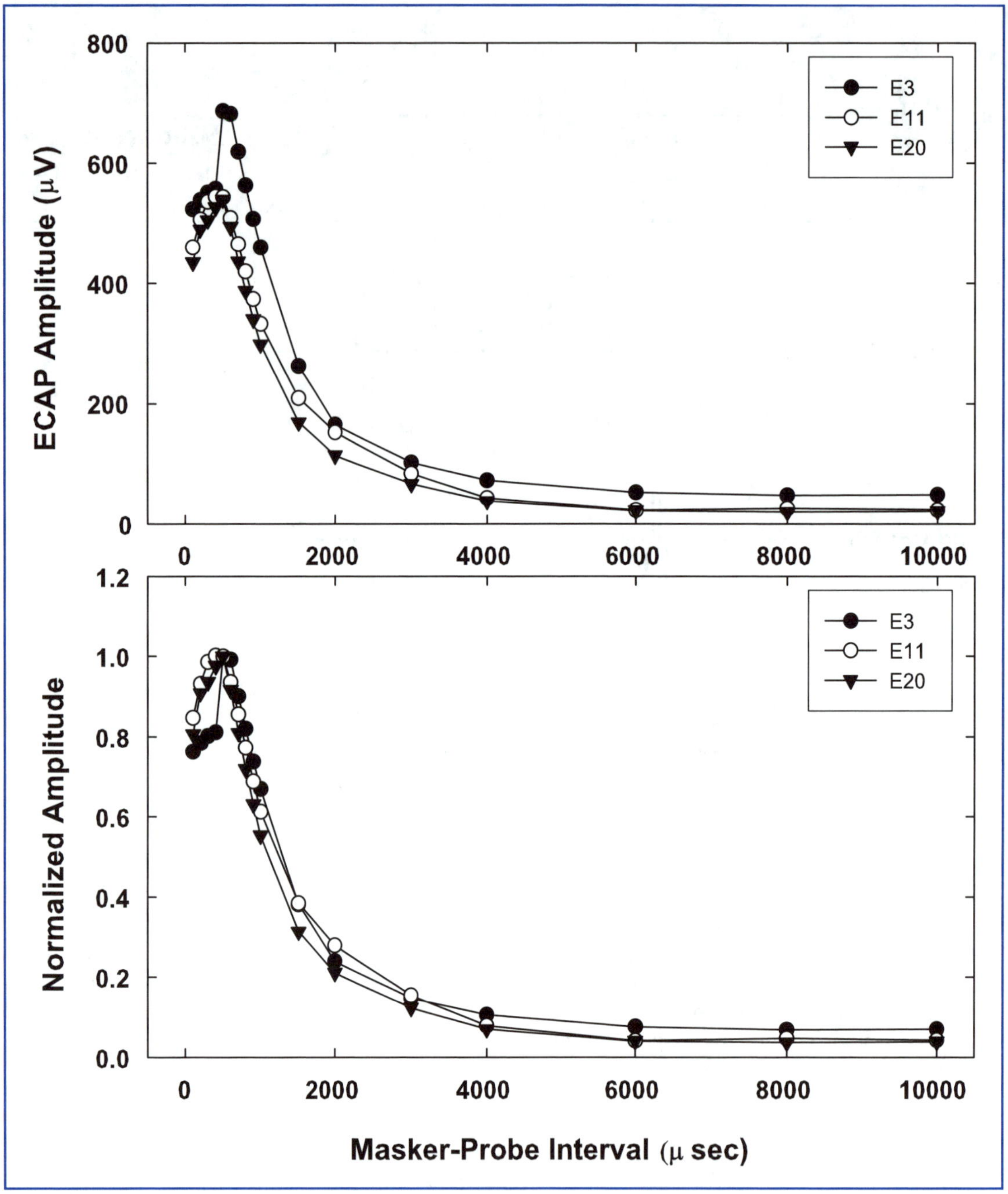


**FIGURE 7–11.** Example of refractory recovery functions from three different electrodes for a Nucleus 24RE recipient. **Top:** Raw ECAP amplitudes plotted as a function of masker-probe interval. **Bottom:** Data from the top panel normalized to (divided by) the amplitude obtained for a masker-probe interval of 500 μsec.

is A − B − C + C′. There is no separate system signature trace (D, from Figure 7–4) because the system signature is present in all four frames, and is thus eliminated with the subtraction formula described here.

Because this method simply removes the artifact from the probe in the masked condition, the ECAP amplitude will increase as the MPI increases, reflecting less influence of the masker for longer MPIs. This is the inverse of the refractory recovery function generated by the standard subtraction method, which represents the difference between the unmasked and masked conditions. Figure 7–13 shows examples of refractory recovery functions obtained with the standard forward-masking subtraction method (filled circles) and the masked response extraction method described by Miller et al. (2000; open circles). Each panel represents data from a different electrode; data are from a Nucleus 24RE recipient.

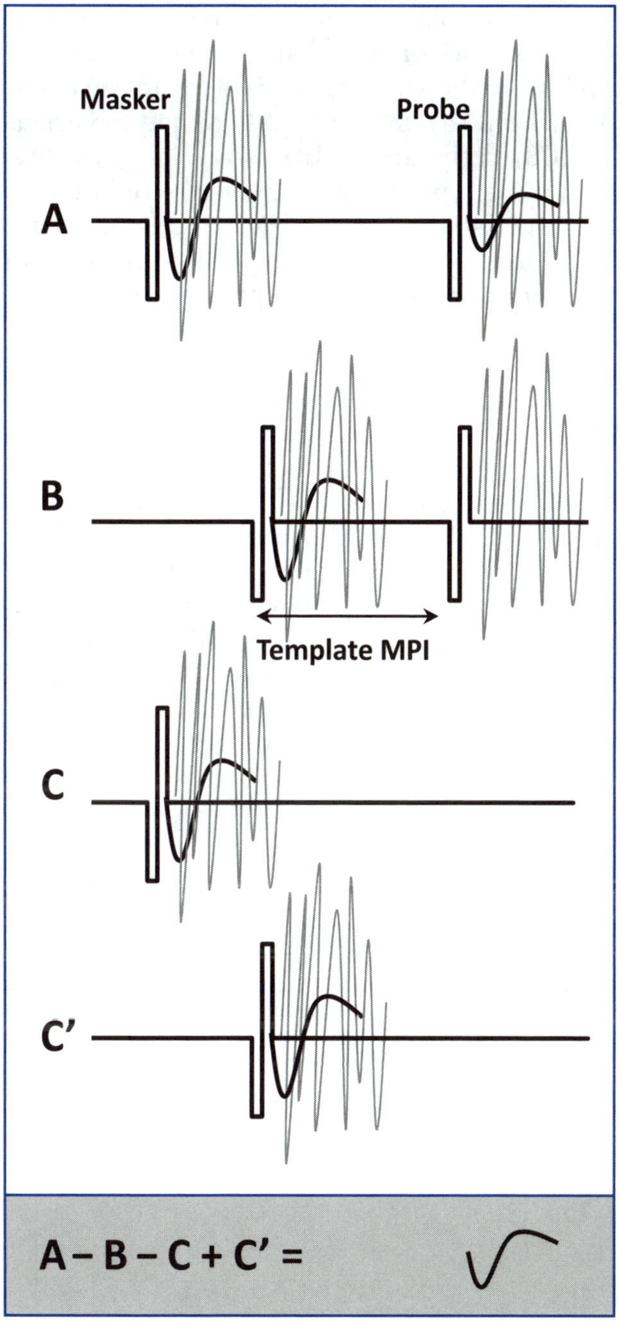


**FIGURE 7–12.** Schematic illustration of the modified forward-masking subtraction method described by Miller et al. (2000). Trace A is the masked condition with the masker-probe interval (MPI) of interest. Trace B is the masked condition with a short MPI to ensure no neural response to the probe; this generates a template of the probe artifact. Traces C and C′ are the masker alone, respectively lined up in time with the maskers in traces A and B. The formula A – B – C + C′ is applied to resolve the neural response to the probe in trace A.

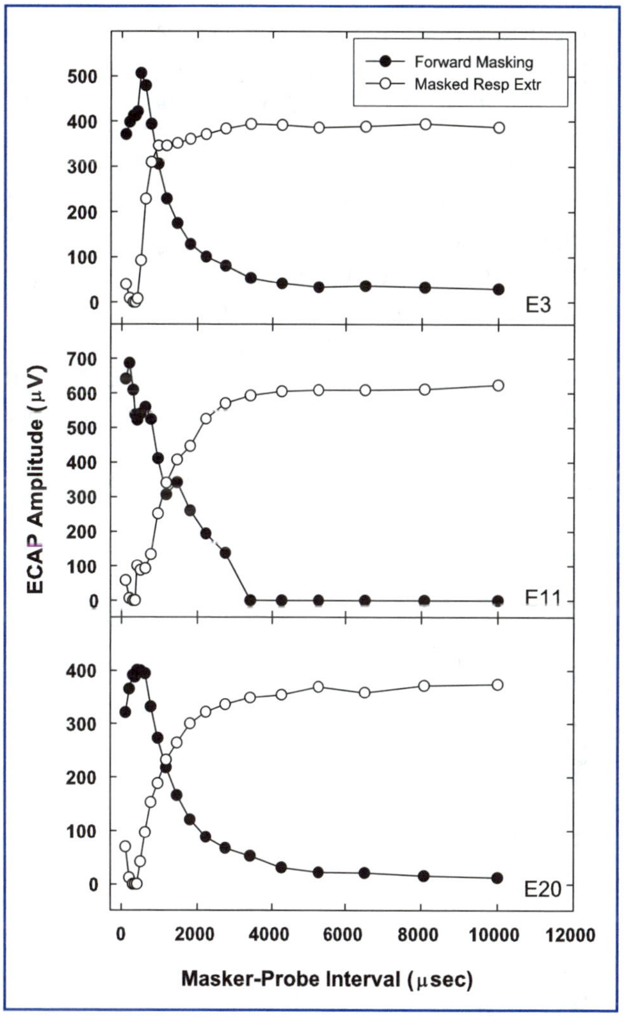


**FIGURE 7–13.** Comparison of refractory recovery functions obtained with the standard forward-masking technique illustrated in Figure 7–4 and 7–10 (*filled circles*) and the modified forward-masking technique (also called "masked response extraction") described by Miller et al. (2000) illustrated in Figure 7–12 (*open circles*). Each graph represents data from a different electrode, indicated in the bottom right corner of each panel.

### Spread of Excitation

Because the ECAP is recorded from within the cochlea, it can be useful in estimating the amount of current spread from a stimulated electrode, as well as the spread of neural excitation. The degree to which excitation fields overlap across electrodes has been shown to correlate with recipients' ability to discriminate electrodes on the basis of pitch (Hughes, 2008). There are two basic types of spatially related measures that can be generated through different manipulations of stimulus or recording parameters. The first measure, spatial spread, is obtained by fixing the location of the stimulating electrode and varying the location of the recording electrode across the array (e.g., Cohen et al., 2004; Hughes & Stille, 2010). This method represents a coarse measure of spatial spread because it encompasses both the neural excitation pattern resulting from current spread throughout the cochlea, as well as the conduction of the voltage change generated by the ECAP response along the fluid-filled cochlea. Because spatial spread involves only changing the location of the recording electrode, it can be measured using any artifact reduction technique with any of the manufacturers' devices that allow for reverse telemetry. Two examples of spatial spread measures (filled circles) are shown in Figure 7–14 for an Advanced Bionics HiRes 90K recipient (left) and a Nucleus 24R(CS) recipient (right). With this measure, ECAPs are typically largest when recording near the stimulating electrode. Amplitudes decrease as the recording electrode is located farther from the stimulating electrode, representing the decay in the measured ECAP response along the length of the cochlea (Hughes & Stille, 2010).

The second measure, called spatial masking or spread of excitation (SOE), is obtained using the standard forward-masking subtraction technique described earlier (Busby et al., 2008; Cohen et al., 2003; Hughes & Abbas, 2006; Hughes & Stille, 2010). As a result, this measure can only be made clinically with the Nucleus 24- or CI512-generation devices. (Specialized experimental research software can be used to implement the forward-masking technique with other manufacturers' devices.) With this method, the probe and recording electrodes are fixed, whereas the masker electrode is roved across the array. Figure 7–15 shows a simplified version of how this method works (reproduced from Hughes & Abbas, 2006,

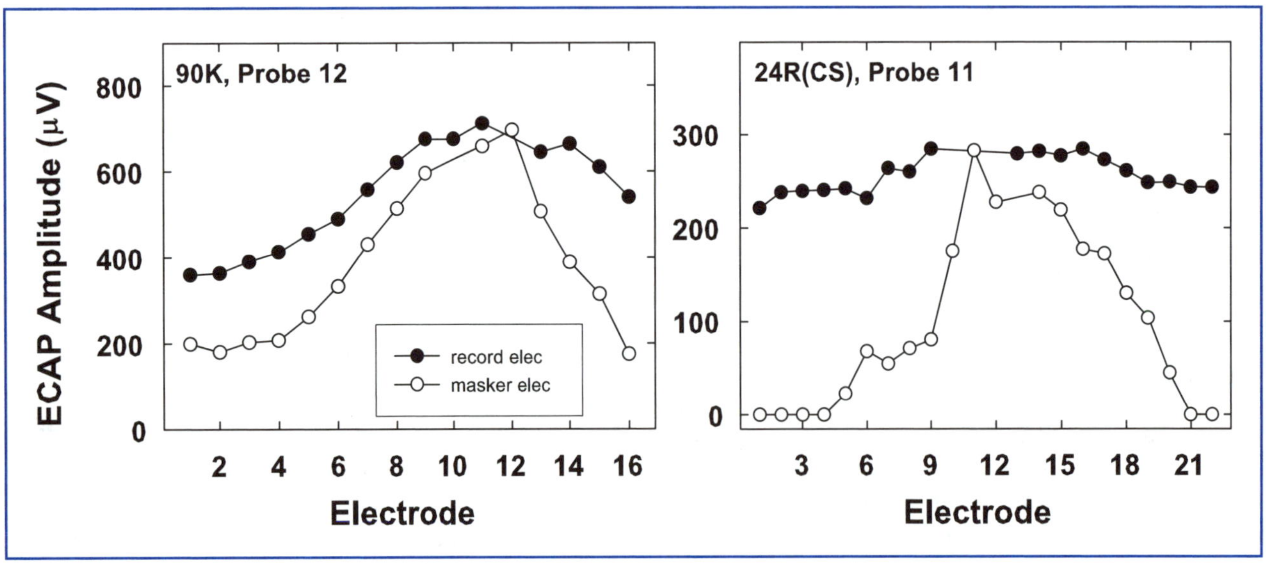


**FIGURE 7–14.** Comparison of spatial spread functions (*filled circles*) obtained by changing the location of the recording electrode, and spatial spread-of-excitation functions (*open circles*) obtained by changing the location of the masker with the standard forward-masking subtraction technique. **Left:** Data from a HiRes 90K recipient. **Right:** Data from a Nucleus 24R(CS) recipient.

Fig. 1). In the top panel, the masker and probe are delivered to the same electrode, recruiting the fibers shown in bold. The probe in the masked condition yields only artifact (B), which is subtracted from the probe alone (A). This maximal ECAP response represents a maximum overlap between the masker and probe. In the middle panel, the masker and probe are delivered to different electrodes that recruit independent (bold lines) and overlapping (bold dotted lines) regions of neurons. The partially masked response in B is subtracted from A, resulting in an ECAP that represents the region of overlap between masker and probe (bold dotted lines). In the bottom panel, the masker and probe are delivered to widely spaced electrodes with independent regions of excitation.

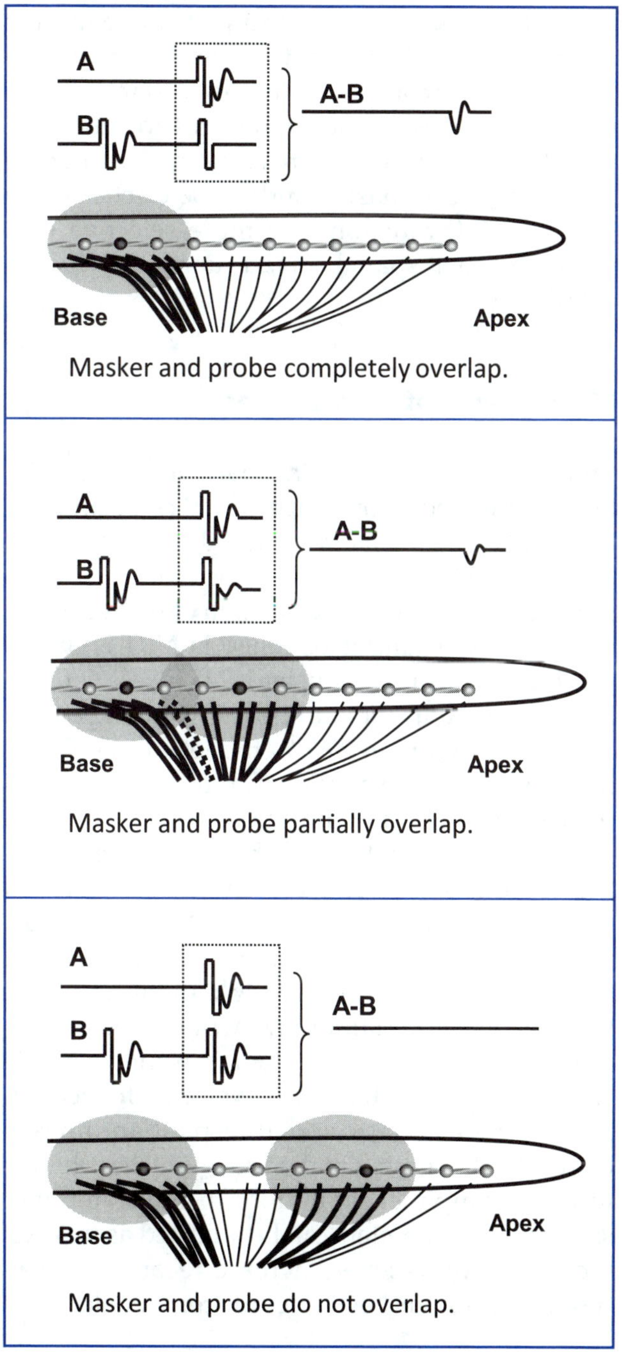


**FIGURE 7–15.** Simplified schematic illustrating how the forward-masking subtraction method is used to obtain spread-of-excitation patterns with the electrically evoked compound action potential (ECAP). **Top:** Masker and probe are delivered to the same electrode (*recruited fibers in bold*). The response to the probe in the masked condition generates only artifact (*B*), which is subtracted from the probe alone (*A*), yielding a maximal ECAP response (maximum overlap of masker and probe). **Middle:** Masker and probe are delivered to spatially separated electrodes that excite independent (*bold lines*) and overlapping (*bold dotted lines*) regions of neurons. The subtraction yields an ECAP generated by the region of overlap between masker and probe (*bold dotted lines*). **Bottom:** Masker and probe are delivered to widely spaced electrodes yielding independent regions of excitation. Subtraction of the maximal response to the probe in both A and B yields zero amplitude (complete nonoverlap of masker and probe). Reproduced from Figure 1 of M. L. Hughes and P. J. Abbas (2006), "The relation between electrophysiologic channel interaction and electrode pitch ranking in cochlear implant recipients," *Journal of the Acoustical Society of America, 119*(3), 1527–1537.

The probe elicits a maximal response in both A and B, yielding zero amplitude (complete nonoverlap) when subtracted. ECAP amplitudes are then plotted as a function of masker electrode to yield the SOE function, which represents the relative amount of *overlap* between populations recruited by the masker and probe. Two examples are shown in Figure 7–14 (open circles) for the same subjects and electrodes for which the spatial spread functions were obtained. For SOE functions, the peak typically occurs when the masker and probe are delivered to the same electrode, representing the greatest amount of overlap between electrodes. As with the spatial spread functions, the ECAP amplitude decreases for greater separations between masker and probe electrodes. In general, SOE functions are more selective (i.e., narrower) than spatial spread functions (Hughes & Stille, 2010).

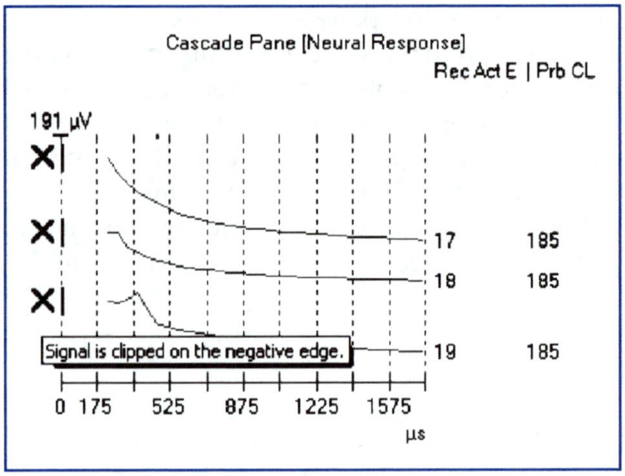


**FIGURE 7–16.** Sample waveforms from Cochlear's Custom Sound EP software showing an upward drift at the beginning of the trace, indicative of amplifier saturation. The stimulus was delivered to electrode 16 at 185 CL; recording electrode number (17, 18, and 19) is indicated to the right of each trace.

## Measurement Challenges

Stimulus and/or recording parameters can also be manipulated to optimize ECAP recordings for a given type of measurement (Abbas et al., 1999; Hughes, 2006). One of the most common measurement challenges is saturation of the recording amplifier. An example obtained in NRT is shown in Figure 7–16 for a Nucleus 24RE recipient. In NRT, traces that violate the software algorithm are marked with an "X" to the left of the waveform with an explanation for the violation. In most cases, amplifier saturation is due to stimulus amplitudes that are too high, beginning the recording too quickly after the stimulus is presented (i.e., short "delay" parameter in NRT and ART), recording too close to the stimulating electrode, or gain settings that are too high. In this example, the masker/probe stimuli were presented to electrode 16 at 185 CL, while the recording electrode was varied. Note that the waveforms for recording electrodes 17, 18, and 19 exhibit an upward drift at the beginning of the trace, which is characteristic of amplifier saturation. To avoid amplifier saturation, parameters can be adjusted as follows: reduce stimulus level, increase recording delay (not an option in NRI), record from an electrode one to two positions farther apically, record from an electrode one to two positions basal to the stimulating electrode (software defaults are apical), or reduce the amplifier gain. Reducing the amplifier gain is typically the last choice because it results in noisier responses and thus requires at least a doubling of the number of averages.

## What Constitutes a Measurable Response?

Learning how to identify physiological responses and differentiate them from artifact or the noise floor might be considered an art that is learned with practice. Differentiating responses from the noise floor is primarily an issue when attempting to determine threshold. All cochlear implant manufacturers have algorithms that automatically mark peaks on the waveforms and calculate threshold using linear regression. However, it is important to make sure the peak markers have been placed in accordance with what you as the clinician would deem appropriate. This section presents several guidelines that can help with identifying what constitutes a measurable response, and provides rules that can be applied to other physiological potentials beyond the ECAP.

1. Morphology and latency — Compare the morphology and latency of the waveform in question to that of waveforms obtained at higher stimulus levels. The response amplitude should grow with increased stimulus level and the latency should decrease slightly. It is important to realize that artifact can also grow with stimulus level, although usually at a faster rate than physiological potentials. Also, latency does not tend to shift as much with electrical stimulation as compared with acoustic stimulation. Figure 7–17B shows an example of an ECAP AGF obtained from electrode 17 in a Nucleus 24RE recipient. Panel A shows the respective waveforms from high to low stimulus level (top to bottom). Panels C and D show a larger view of the waveforms at 200 CL and 195 CL, respectively. The waveform in panel C exhibits similar morphology to those at higher levels, with slightly longer N1 latency. The waveform in panel D exhibits no distinguishable peaks (thus, assessing latency is not possible). In this example, the

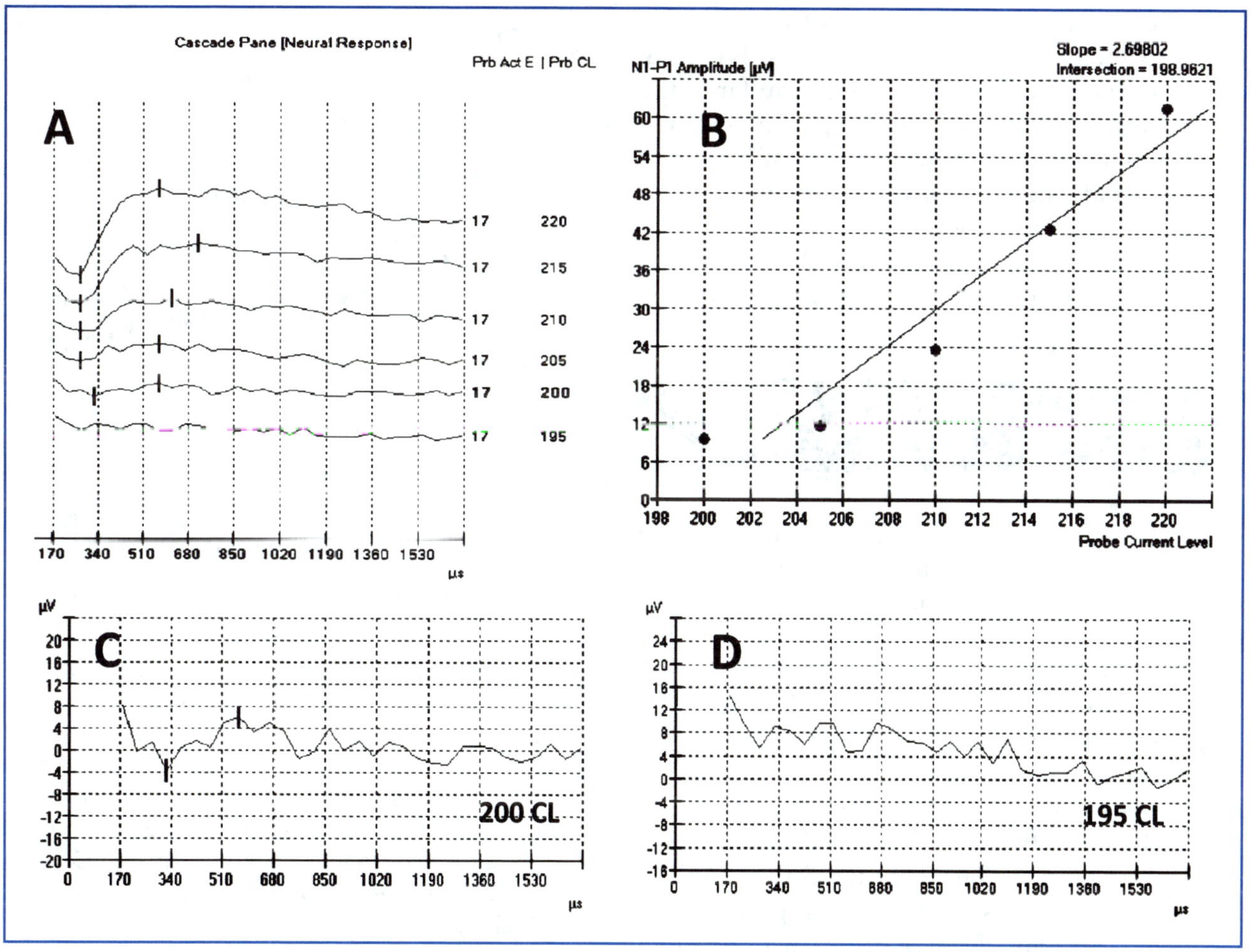


**FIGURE 7–17.** Sample amplitude growth function and selected waveforms from a Nucleus 24RE recipient. **A.** Cascade panel showing individual waveforms for stimulation of electrode 17 at 220 CL (*top*) down to 195 CL (*bottom*). **B.** Peak-to-peak amplitudes from A, plotted as a function of stimulus level. **C.** Larger view of the waveform for 200 CL. **D.** Larger view of the waveform for 195 CL, which shows no measurable ECAP response. Visual detection threshold in this case was 200 CL, and the regression threshold was 198.96 CL (see upper right corner of panel B).

waveform for 200 CL would represent the visual detection threshold.

2. Scaling—Because all three manufacturers' software show a cascade view of the waveforms, large-amplitude responses at high levels can make low-level responses difficult to resolve visually because the amplitude scale is so large. Clinical software typically allows for the amplitude scale to be changed, or a specific waveform to be selected and displayed in a separate window for better viewing of low-level responses (i.e., Figures 7–17C and 7–17D).
3. Noise floor—When using visual detection methods, the ECAP should always be larger than the noise floor. One way to decide whether a "response" is an actual response is to measure the negative-to-positive peak amplitude obtained at latencies similar to the N1 and P2 of a higher-level response, and then compare with a negative-to-positive peak amplitude measured at any other later latency in the trace (this would be the noise). If the "response" and the noise are the same size, then the "response" is probably just noise.

## CLINICAL USES FOR ECAPS

Clinically, ECAPs can be used to confirm device function, and confirm that the peripheral auditory neurons are functioning in response to electrical stimulation from the implant. ECAPs have also been used to assist with sound processor programming and verify questionable behavioral responses. A number of investigators have proposed different ways in which ECAP thresholds can be used to assist with setting map T- and/or C/M-levels (Botros & Psarros, 2010a; Brown et al., 2000; Franck, 2002; Hughes, Brown, Abbas, Wolaver, & Gervais, 2000; Smoorenburg, Willeboer, & van Dijk, 2002). Figure 7–18 shows an example of the method described by Brown et al. (2000) and Hughes et al. (2000). With this method, ECAP thresholds are measured on all electrodes (see Figure 7–18, Step 1). Next, behavioral threshold and maximum comfort (C-level, in this case) are measured on a single electrode in the middle of the array (see Figure 7–18, Step 2). Last, the ECAP threshold function is shifted up (for C/M-levels) or down (for T-levels) by the difference between the ECAP threshold and the measured T-level and C/M-level (see Figure 7–18, Step 3).

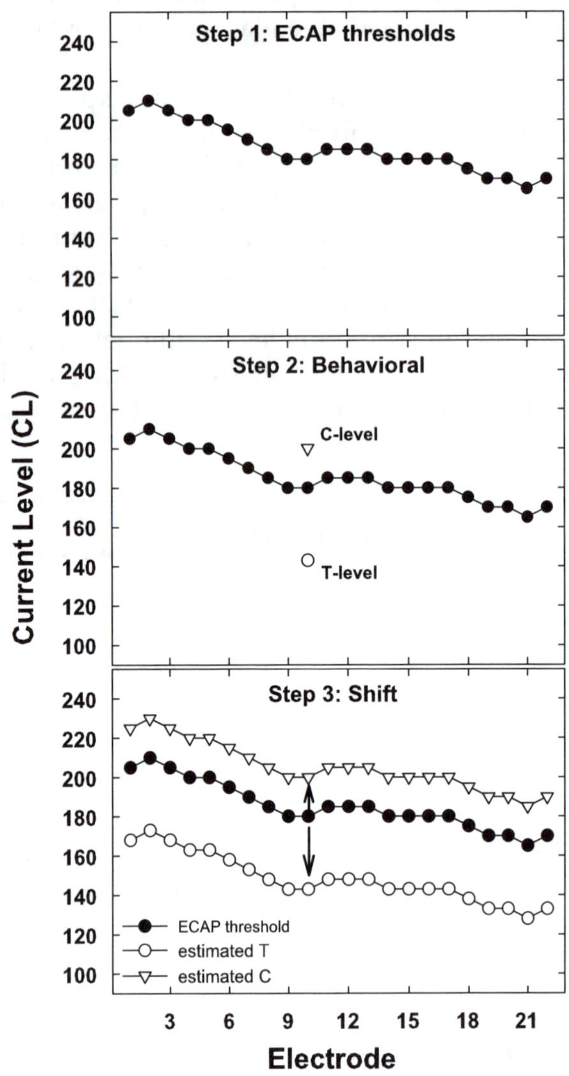


**FIGURE 7–18.** Example illustrating the ECAP-based method of estimating map levels described by Brown et al. (2000) and Hughes et al. (2000). **Step 1:** ECAP thresholds are obtained on all electrodes. **Step 2:** Behavioral threshold (T-level) and upper comfort levels (C-level) are obtained for a single electrode in the middle of the array (in this case, electrode 10). **Step 3:** The ECAP threshold profile is shifted up (for estimated C-level) or down (for estimated T-level) to match the behavioral level obtained for electrode 10.

Figure 7–19 shows an example of the method described by Smoorenburg et al. (2002). With this method, ECAP thresholds are obtained on all electrodes (see Figure 7–19, Step 1). Next, both the T- and C/M-levels are set to equal the ECAP threshold profile (i.e., offset of 0 CL between T and C/M), and levels are globally reduced to a range well below behavioral threshold (see Figure 7–19, Step 2). Live speech mode is turned on, and the T-levels (linked with C/M-levels) are globally raised until a behavioral threshold response is obtained (see Figure 7–19, Step 3). The C/M-levels are globally raised further until a behavioral response of upper loudness comfort is reached (see Figure 7–19, Step 4).

The methods described above rely on only a single behavioral threshold response and a single behavioral upper comfort response, in addition to objective ECAP measures across all electrodes. These methods can therefore be useful for estimating individual electrode map levels for populations who can only provide limited behavioral responses. However, research comparing the estimated map levels to those obtained from reliable behavioral measures has shown only moderate correlations (e.g., Brown et al., 2000; Franck 2002;

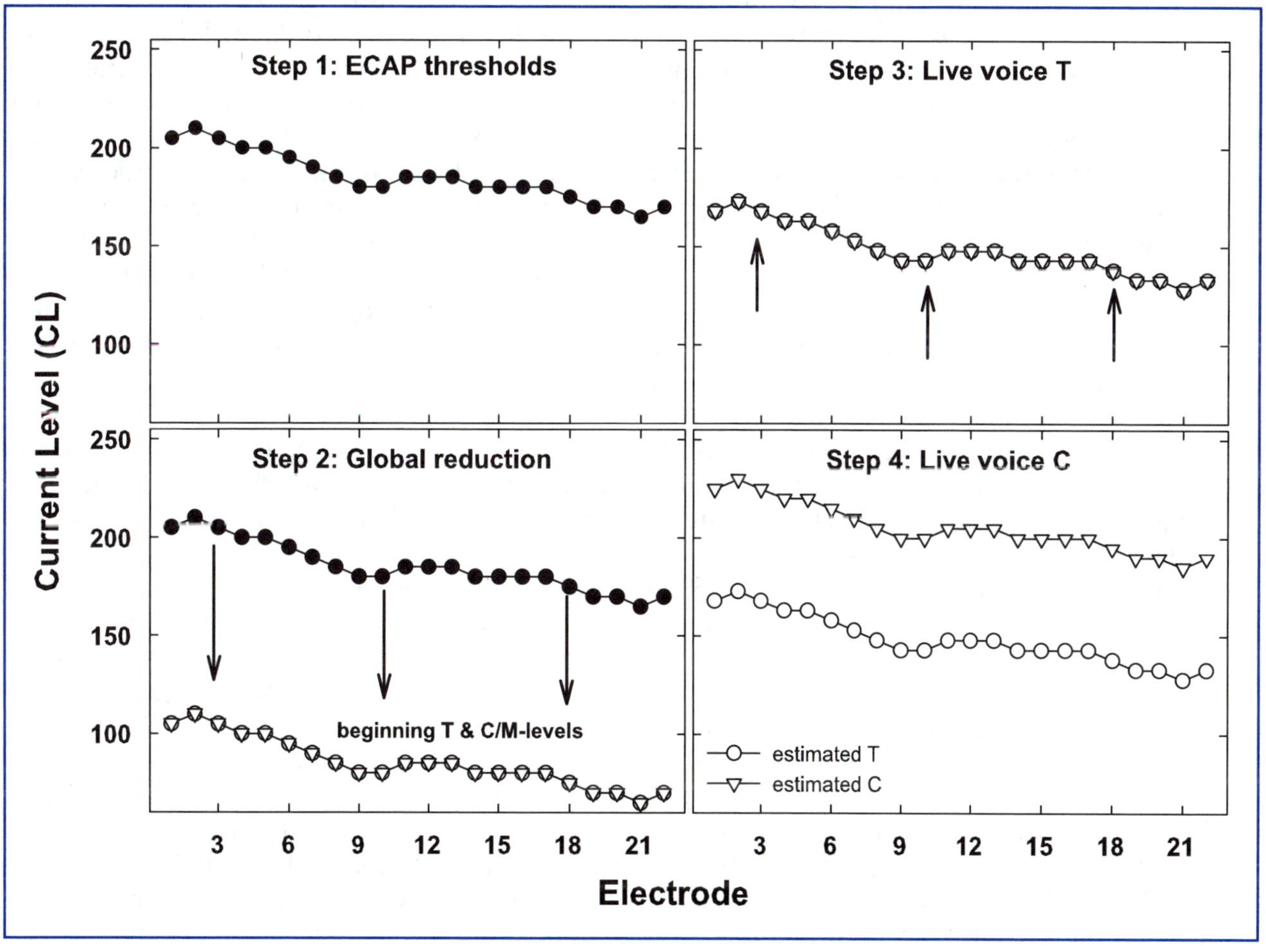


**FIGURE 7–19.** Example illustrating the ECAP-based method of estimating map levels described by Smoorenburg et al. (2002). **Step 1:** ECAP thresholds are obtained on all electrodes. **Step 2:** Map T- and C-levels are set to equal the ECAP threshold profile, which is then reduced to a subthreshold level. **Step 3:** Live voice is turned on and the T/C levels are globally increased until they are audible. The ECAP threshold profile is set at this level for the estimated T-levels. **Step 4:** For estimated C-levels, the profile is further increased until loudness comfort is reached.

Hughes et al., 2000; Smoorenburg et al., 2002). For a group of postlingually deafened adults, Seyle and Brown (2002) compared speech perception with a traditional behavioral map, an ECAP-based map, and a map using a combination of ECAP and limited behavioral information (following Brown et al., 2000 and Hughes et al., 2000). Subjects exhibited only slightly poorer performance for the two ECAP-based maps, with a very limited acclimatization period. Similar findings were also reported by Smoorenburg et al. (2002) for traditional versus ECAP-based maps. The authors concluded that, although the ECAP-based maps were not necessarily ideal, listeners were still able to achieve relatively high levels of performance. Thus, ECAP-based maps may be sufficient for providing adequate audibility for the development of speech and language while young children mature and develop the skills needed to provide more reliable behavioral responses.

Other key findings from research assessing the relation between ECAP thresholds and map levels are summarized below (see also Hughes, 2010):

1. ECAP thresholds are obtained with a single pulse presented at a slow repetition rate (for signal averaging). As with any other physiological response, using a faster stimulation rate for ECAP measures will result in a degraded neural response (i.e., higher thresholds). Map levels, on the other hand, are obtained with a fast-rate pulse train (~250 to 5000 pps) of 300 to 500 ms in duration. Temporal integration across the stimulus will make the longer-duration, fast-rate pulse train more easily detected by the brain, thus resulting in lower behavioral thresholds. As a result, the relation between ECAP thresholds and behavioral map levels will change with different map stimulation rates (Botros & Psarros, 2010a; McKay, Fewster, & Dawson, 2005; Potts, Skinner, Gotter, Strube, & Brenner, 2007; Zimmerling & Hochmair, 2002). The correlation between ECAP thresholds and map levels tends to worsen for faster rates.
2. ECAP thresholds almost always occur above behavioral threshold (T-level), regardless of the strategy rate (e.g., Cafarelli Dees et al., 2005; Di Nardo, Ippolito, Quaranta, Cadoni, & Galli, 2003; Jeon et al., 2010; Potts et al., 2007; Seyle & Brown, 2002). Thus, ECAP thresholds should indicate a level that is audible, and may be useful for indicating a level to begin conditioning a child to respond behaviorally.
3. ECAP thresholds tend to occur in the upper portion of the behavioral dynamic range, and will be more likely to exceed C/M-levels for faster stimulation rates (Akin et al., 2006; Brown et al., 2000; Cullington, 2000; Eisen & Franck, 2004; Franck & Norton, 2001; Han et al., 2005; Holstad et al., 2009; Hughes et al., 2000; Jeon et al., 2010; McKay et al., 2005; Potts et al., 2007; Smoorenburg et al., 2002).
4. The ECAP threshold profile may be similar to the profile of T- or C/M-levels across the array. If the T and C/M profiles differ from each other, the ECAP profile is more likely to follow that of the T-level (Franck & Norton, 2001; Hughes et al., 2001; Smoorenburg et al., 2002). However, there are cases where the ECAP profile does not follow that of either the T- or C/M-levels (Miller et al., 2008; Potts et al., 2007). Also, C-level profiles tend to flatten at higher stimulation levels (Botros & Psarros, 2010a).

In sum, ECAPs are quick and easy to obtain in the clinical setting, which makes them ideal for use with pediatric or other difficult-to-test populations. However, ECAPs can only be used to predict map levels with modest accuracy, and should not be used as a substitute for behavioral responses. When ECAP thresholds are combined with a few behavioral measures, significant correlations are found between predicted and measured map levels (Brown et al., 2000; Franck, 2002; Hughes et al., 2000; Smoorenburg et al., 2002). In addition, combining ECAP measures with other objective measures such as the ESRT (see Chapter 6) can improve the accuracy of estimating map levels (Gordon et al., 2004; Polak, Hodges, & Balkany, 2005; Wolfe & Kasulis, 2008). Given the large variability across subjects regarding the relation between ECAP thresholds and map levels, more sophisticated models are needed to improve the accuracy with which ECAPs can be used to assist with sound processor programming.

## SUMMARY

Key concepts for ECAP measures are summarized below:

1. The ECAP is a synchronous response from an aggregate population of auditory nerve fibers in response to electrical stimulation, and is characterized by a negative peak (N1) at a latency of approximately 0.2 to 0.4 msec, followed by a positive peak or plateau (P2) at approximately 0.6 to 0.8 msec. It is the near-field version of wave I of the EABR.
2. Because ECAPs are recorded using the intracochlear electrode array (near-field) instead of surface (far-field) electrodes, responses are not subject to contamination from muscle artifact; thus, recipients do not need to be still, asleep, or sedated during testing. Furthermore, ECAPs are roughly an order of magnitude larger than EABRs, so fewer averages and shorter test times are needed.
3. ECAPs are not strongly influenced by maturational or anesthesia effects.
4. The types of ECAP measurements that can be made depend on the type of artifact reduction technique that is used (alternating polarity, forward-masking subtraction, or artifact template).
5. Common ECAP measurements include the amplitude growth function (which yields threshold and slope measures), refractory recovery, and spread of excitation.
6. Amplifier saturation is a common problem that can interfere with ECAP measurements. Various manipulations of stimulus and/or recording parameters can be made to avoid amplifier saturation. These may include reducing the stimulus level, increasing the recording delay, recording farther from the stimulating electrode, or reducing the amplifier gain.
7. To differentiate questionable ECAP responses from the noise floor, compare the morphology and latency of the waveform in question to that of more robust waveforms obtained at higher stimulus levels, change the amplitude scale for better viewing, and compare the peak-to-peak amplitude of the questionable response to the peak-to-peak amplitude of the noise in the same waveform.
8. Clinically, ECAPs can be used to confirm device function, confirm auditory nerve function, assist with sound processor programming, and verify questionable behavioral responses.
9. The correlation between ECAP thresholds and map levels tends to worsen with increased map stimulation rates.
10. ECAP thresholds almost always occur above behavioral thresholds, and more likely approximate or exceed upper comfort levels.
11. ECAP measures alone cannot predict map levels with adequate accuracy, and thus should not be used as a substitute for behavioral responses. However, when combined with limited behavioral information and/or other objective measures such as the ESRT, ECAP thresholds can be very useful for predicting map levels that correlate strongly with those measured behaviorally.

# 8

# Electrically Evoked Auditory Brainstem Response

Although the clinical use of the electrically evoked auditory brainstem response (EABR) has waned with the advent of telemetry systems for measuring the electrically evoked compound action potential (ECAP), the EABR offers several advantages over the ECAP (Miller et al., 2008). First, EABRs can be obtained in a wider population of implant users because the measures are not dependent on the implant having telemetry capabilities. Second, EABRs can provide information about the auditory pathway up to the level of the brainstem. Third, EABRs can often be recorded in cases when excessive stimulus artifact precludes successful acquisition of ECAPs, such as in ossified cochleae. Finally, the primary wave of interest of the EABR, wave V, occurs at a later latency than the ECAP, and is therefore easier to isolate from the stimulus artifact. This chapter begins with a basic description of what EABRs are and how they are measured. Next, challenges associated with measuring EABRs are discussed, and different types of measurements with the EABR are described. Finally, a summary of the clinical uses for the EABR is provided.

## BASIC DESCRIPTION

The EABR is a synchronous physiological response from the auditory nerve to structures in the brainstem. As with its acoustic counterpart, the EABR is characterized by waves I through V (Figure 8–1), although wave I (and sometimes wave II) can be obscured by stimulus artifact. Each wave represents a different synapse point or structure within the auditory pathway. Waves I and II presumably arise from the distal and proximal portions of the auditory nerve, respectively; wave III from the cochlear nucleus; wave IV from the superior olivary complex; and wave V from the lateral lemniscus and inferior colliculus (Hall, 1992).

The absolute latencies of the EABR are approximately 1 to 1.5 ms earlier than those of the acoustic ABR because direct electrical stimulation from the cochlear implant eliminates the latency from sound traveling down the ear canal, through the middle ear, generation of the traveling wave, and synaptic activity at the level of the

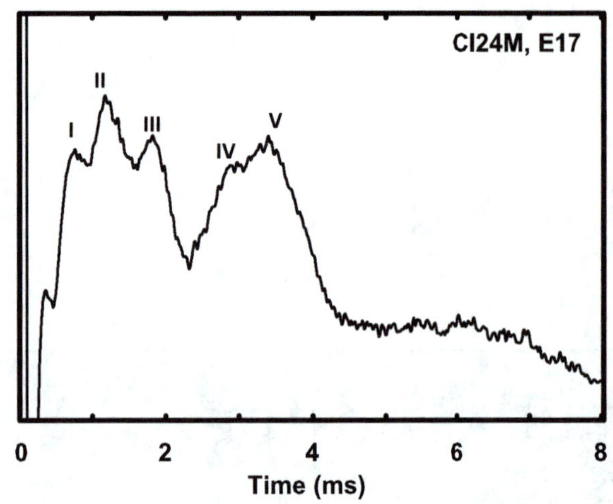


**FIGURE 8–1.** Electrically evoked auditory brainstem (EABR) waveform obtained near upper comfort level for an adult Nucleus CI24M recipient. Waves I through V are indicated on the trace. Data courtesy of Paul Abbas and Carolyn Brown, the University of Iowa Cochlear Implant Electrophysiology Laboratory.

hair cells (e.g., Shallop, Beiter, Goin, & Mischke, 1990; Starr & Brackmann, 1979; van den Honert & Stypulkowski, 1986). The interpeak latencies have been shown to be similar to those of the acoustic ABR (~1.0 ms; van den Honert & Stypulkowski, 1986) or slightly shorter than those of the acoustic ABR (~0.8 ms; Firszt, Chambers, Kraus, & Reeder, 2002; Gardi, 1985). The latencies of waves I through V of the EABR generally occur within the first 4 to 5 ms following stimulus onset (Brown, Abbas, Fryauf-Bertschy, Kelsay, & Gantz, 1994; Kileny, Zwolan, Boerst, & Telian, 1997; Kileny, Zwolan, Zimmerman-Phillips, & Telian, 1994; Shallop, VanDyke, Goin, & Mischke, 1991; van den Honert & Stypulkowski, 1986). On average, the latency of wave V is approximately 3.7 to 4.0 ms at high levels and 4.1 to 4.7 ms near threshold (Firszt, Chambers, Kraus, & Reeder, 2002; Kileny et al., 1997; van den Honert & Stypulkowski, 1986). Firszt, Chambers, Kraus, and Reeder (2002) reported an average latency shift of 0.4 msec between upper comfort level and wave V threshold. EABR latencies increase slightly with decreased stimulus levels, but are much less affected by level than the acoustic ABR (Abbas & Brown, 1991a; Gordon, Papsin, & Harrison, 2003; van den Honert & Stypulkowski, 1986). Additionally, wave V latencies tend to be shorter for apical electrodes and longer for basal electrodes (Firszt, Chambers, Kraus, & Reeder, 2002; Shallop et al., 1990).

As with most physiological potentials, EABR amplitudes decrease with stimulus level. Wave V is typically the most robust, and is usually the only wave of the EABR that remains visible at the lowest levels. Maximum peak-to-peak amplitudes of wave V are typically around 1 to 2 microvolts (μV), depending on the recipient's loudness tolerance levels (Firszt, Chambers, Kraus, & Reeder, 2002; Miller et al., 2008; Shallop et al., 1990). This is several orders of magnitude smaller than the ECAP, which can be several hundred microvolts to one millivolt at upper comfort levels. Threshold amplitudes for wave V are typically around 0.25 μV (Firszt, Chambers, Kraus, & Reeder, 2002). EABR wave V is often larger than the acoustic wave V for comparable loudness levels because electrical stimulation excites a larger portion of the cochlea than an acoustic click, and produces greater neural synchrony (Kiang & Moxon, 1972). As with the ECAP (see Chapter 7), the EABR can be used to verify device and electrode function, verify the function of the peripheral auditory pathway to the level of the brainstem, monitor physiological responses over time, and can be used to some extent to assist with programming the sound processor.

## MEASUREMENT

### Stimulus

EABRs can be measured clinically using standard programming software and hardware to provide the stimulus, a standard clinical evoked potentials system for recording, and a trigger pulse output from the programming interface to synchronize the recording system. Figure 8–2 illustrates the stimulating and recording equipment configuration for EABRs. The stimulus that is used to elicit the EABR is typically a single biphasic current pulse delivered

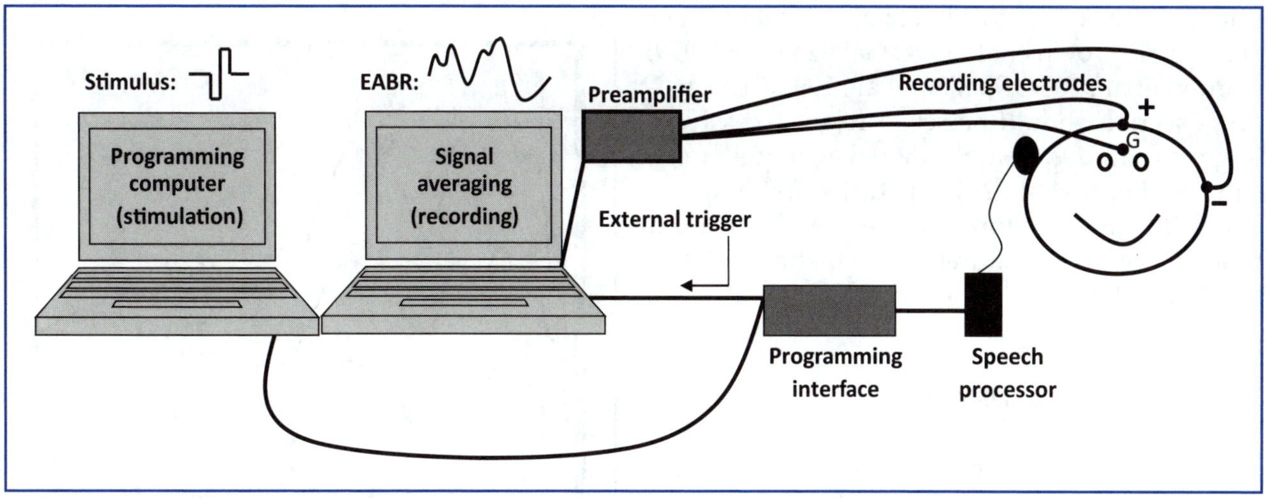


**FIGURE 8–2.** Stimulus and recording setup for electrically evoked auditory brainstem (EABR) responses. The recording electrode montage in this example is vertex positive (+), contralateral mastoid negative (−) and forehead ground (G). The recording electrodes are input to a preamplifier, which in turn provides input to the signal averaging equipment. The stimulus is defined within the clinical cochlear implant software, and is sent to the internal implant via the programming interface and speech processor. A trigger pulse from the programming interface synchronizes the signal averaging equipment to begin recording.

at a relatively slow repetition rate (~10 to 50 Hz). As with the ECAP, electrode coupling modes can be used for stimulation based on the specific device capabilities (e.g., bipolar, monopolar).

## Recording

The EABR is a far-field response recorded using scalp electrodes that are attached to a preamplifier. The typical montage is vertex positive with the mastoid (or earlobe) contralateral to the stimulated implant as the negative, and forehead or ipsilateral mastoid as the ground (e.g., Bierer, Faulkner, & Tremblay, 2001; Brown et al., 1994, 2000; Brown, Hughes, Lopez, & Abbas, 1999; Shallop et al., 1991; Thai-Van et al., 2007). Because the EABR is recorded using scalp electrodes, responses can be easily contaminated by myogenic (muscle) activity. Therefore, patients must be still, asleep, or sedated for ease of recording. In contrast to the ECAP, which only requires 50 to 100 sweeps, the EABR is typically recorded using 1000 to 2000 sweeps and traces are replicated near threshold.

The recording time window is generally set to around 10 ms (Gallégo et al., 1999; Shallop et al., 1991). Although wave V has a longer latency than the ECAP, it is still affected by stimulus artifact, but to a lesser degree. The EABR can be resolved using the alternating polarity method (described in Chapter 7). For older Nucleus devices, this was previously only possible with bipolar stimulation because of limitations in the older versions of the clinical software (Brown et al., 1994, 2000). Newer software versions for Cochlear devices (Custom Sound EP v. 3.x) allow for the option of alternating the stimulus polarity for all stimulation modes. MED-EL's ART feature within the Maestro clinical software and Advanced Bionics' SCLIN software also allow for alternating stimulus polarity with a trigger output from the programming interface (DIB or CPI II, respectively). An EABR trigger is not available in Advanced Bionics' current version of SoundWave (2.1).

Filtering and artifact rejection can also be used to reduce stimulus artifact. The radio frequency from the transmitting coil tends to interfere with EABR recordings, so low-pass filtering at about 32 kHz (RF shielding) is necessary prior to the preamplifier (Brown et al., 1994, 1999; Firszt, Chambers, Kraus, & Reeder, 2002; Gordon et al., 2004). The recorded waveform is generally band-pass filtered between 10 to 150 Hz and 3 kHz (Bierer et al., 2011; Brown et al., 1994; Gallégo et al., 1999; Gordon et al., 2004; Shallop et al., 1991). The artifact rejection should be set to reject excessively large amplitudes from the signal averaging (e.g., ±15 µV, Bierer et al., 2011), and the first millisecond following the stimulus onset can be blocked to avoid amplifier saturation from stimulus artifacts (e.g., Bierer et al., 2011; Brown et al., 1994).

## Types of Measurements

As with the ECAP, stimulus and/or recording parameters can be manipulated to measure different aspects of neural response properties with a cochlear implant. The following subsections describe some useful measurements obtained with the EABR. Clinical implications for these measures are described further in the last section of this chapter.

### *Threshold and Growth of Response with Level*

As described in Chapter 7, the amplitude growth function (AGF) is obtained by plotting the response amplitude as a function of stimulus level. The peak-to-peak amplitude of wave V is typically used for an EABR growth function because wave V is the most robust. EABR thresholds are typically defined using visual detection (see Chapter 7). An alternative method described by Bierer et al. (2011) used an AGF of at least five points, which was subsequently interpolated to produce 100 points. Threshold in that study was defined as the lowest current level that yielded an EABR wave V amplitude of at least 0.1 µV.

Waveforms from an example EABR AGF are shown in Figure 8–3. Waveforms near threshold are typically replicated to ensure accurate detection of threshold (not shown). EABR and ECAP thresholds tend to occur at similar levels within the same subject (Brown et al., 2000; Gordon et al., 2004; Hay-McCutcheon, Brown, Clay, & Seyle, 2002). Some studies have reported slightly higher thresholds for EABR than for ECAP (Gordon et al., 2004; Lo, Chen, Horng, & Hsu, 2004), whereas others have reported slightly lower thresholds for the EABR (Brown et al., 2000; Hay-McCutcheon et al., 2002).

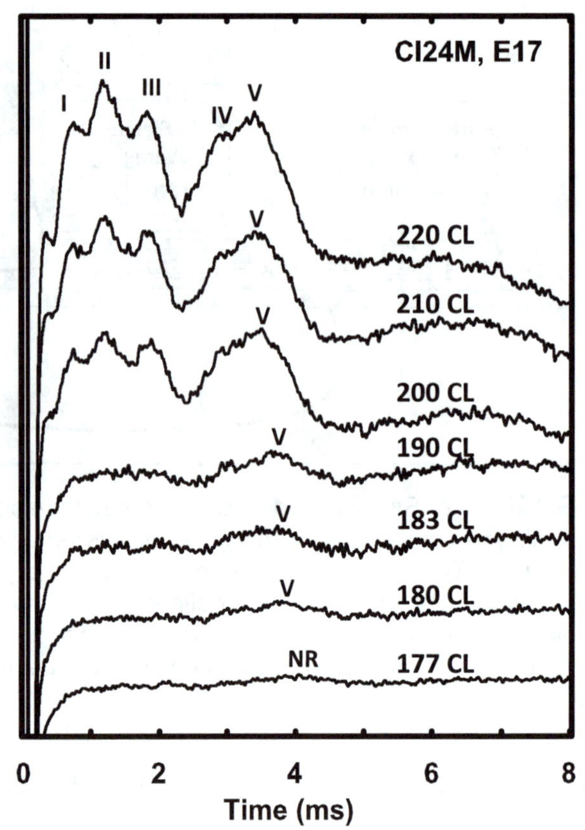


**FIGURE 8–3.** Example of a series of electrically evoked auditory brainstem (EABR) responses from an apical electrode in an adult Nucleus CI24M recipient. Responses represent a growth function from high to low stimulus levels (top to bottom, respectively). In this example, waves I–V are visible at the three highest stimulus levels (220–200 CL). Wave V is typically the most prominent and is the wave used to determine EABR threshold (180 CL in this example). NR = no response. Data courtesy of Paul Abbas and Carolyn Brown, the University of Iowa Cochlear Implant Electrophysiology Laboratory.

Probably the most common clinical use of EABR thresholds has been to assist with programming the sound processor (discussed further in the last section of this chapter). EABR threshold and slope of the AGF have also been used to assess a number of research-based questions with potential clinical applications. The most relevant include spread of excitation, channel interaction, nerve survival, and electrode placement relative to the stimulated neurons. As with the ECAP, lower thresholds and steeper AGFs are obtained with broader stimulation modes (e.g., monopolar). This means that greater spread of current results in a larger number of recruited neurons (i.e., lower thresholds) and a faster rate of neuronal recruitment with increased stimulus level (Abbas & Brown, 1991a).

Several studies have used EABRs to assess channel interaction (Abbas & Brown, 1988; Gardi, 1985; White, Merzenich, & Gardi, 1984). EABR responses were obtained with simultaneous stimulation of two electrode pairs, where the stimulus delivered to one pair was the same as or opposite of the phase for the first electrode pair. Results showed lower EABR thresholds and larger amplitudes in the AGF for simultaneous stimulation of electrodes with the same phase due to summation of the respective current fields. Conversely, higher EABR thresholds and smaller amplitudes resulted when the stimulus phases were inverted relative to each other. The effects were more pronounced for closer spacing between electrode pairs, representing greater spatial overlap and thus more channel interaction.

Regarding electrode placement and nerve survival, Shepherd, Hatsushika, and Clark (1993) showed lower EABR thresholds and shallower AGF slopes for electrode placements near the modiolar wall as compared with the outer wall of the cochlea (cat data). Other studies have shown conflicting results regarding the reliability of the EABR for predicting spiral ganglion cell survival (Lusted, Shelton, & Simmons, 1984; Shepherd, Clark, & Black, 1983; Smith & Simmons, 1983). In human subjects, Bierer et al. (2011) showed higher EABR thresholds for electrodes with higher behavioral thresholds and broader psychophysical tuning when obtained with both broad (monopolar) and spatially restricted (partial tripolar; see Chapter 2) stimulation. For partial tripolar stimulation, channels with low behavioral thresholds had shallower AGF slopes, whereas steeper slopes resulted for channels with high behavioral thresholds. Taken together, these results suggest that the EABR reflects the collective influence of nerve survival and electrode proximity, where lower thresholds, shallower AGF slopes, and more selective psychophysical tuning represent more focused stimulation regions within the cochlea.

### Refractory Recovery

Refractory-recovery functions can be measured with the EABR using a forward-masking subtraction paradigm that is slightly different from that described in Chapter 7 for the ECAP (Abbas & Brown, 1991b). With this method, two sets of averaged traces are obtained: (1) a single masker pulse alone, and (2) two pulses (masker and probe) presented in succession. The averaged response in the masker-alone condition is subtracted from the averaged response in the masker-plus-probe condition, leaving the response to the forward-masked probe. Because the stimulus artifact has less effect on wave V (due to its longer latency) than the earlier waves, the necessary subtractions are not as complex as those for the ECAP (see Chapter 7). For EABR refractory recovery, stimulus artifact is removed by zeroing out the first 1 to 2 ms of the trace, then digitally filtering between about 150 Hz and 3 kHz (Abbas & Brown, 1991b). The EABR amplitude (in response to the probe) is plotted as a function of the masker-probe interval to evaluate refractory recovery. As with the ECAP, stimulus level affects the time course of recovery. For stimulus levels in the upper portion of the behavioral dynamic range, effects of forward masking were essentially diminished by 4 to 6 ms (Abbas & Brown, 1991b).

### Binaural Interaction Component

The EABR can be elicited with either monaural (each ear separately) or bilateral (both ears at the same time via a synchronized processor) stimulation. When the bilateral EABR is subtracted from the sum of the two monaural EABRs, the result is the binaural interaction component (BIC) of the EABR (Gordon, Valero, & Papsin, 2007; Gordon, Valero, van Hoesel, & Papsin, 2008; He, Brown & Abbas, 2010; Pelizzone, Kasper, & Montandon,

1990; Smith & Delgutte, 2007). Figure 8–4 shows an example of the left and right monaural responses (top two traces, respectively), the sum of the two monaural responses (third trace), the binaural response (fourth trace), and the BIC (bottom trace). The BIC consists of a small negative deflection at a latency of 3.3 to 3.6 ms followed by a larger positive peak at a latency of approximately 4 to 4.4 ms (He et al., 2010; Pelizzone et al., 1990). The BIC amplitude is measured as the voltage difference between the initial negative trough and the following positive peak. This is in contrast to wave V, which is measured from the peak to the following trough. BIC amplitudes obtained in humans vary from approximately 0.4 to 1.2 μV (He et al., 2010).

The amplitude of the BIC is larger when both monaural stimulating electrodes occupy similar positions within the cochlea; the amplitude decreases as the interaural electrode spacing is less aligned (He et al., 2010; Smith & Delgutte, 2007). He et al. (2010) showed that this trend held for low stimulation levels but not for high levels, presumably due to more global current spread across the

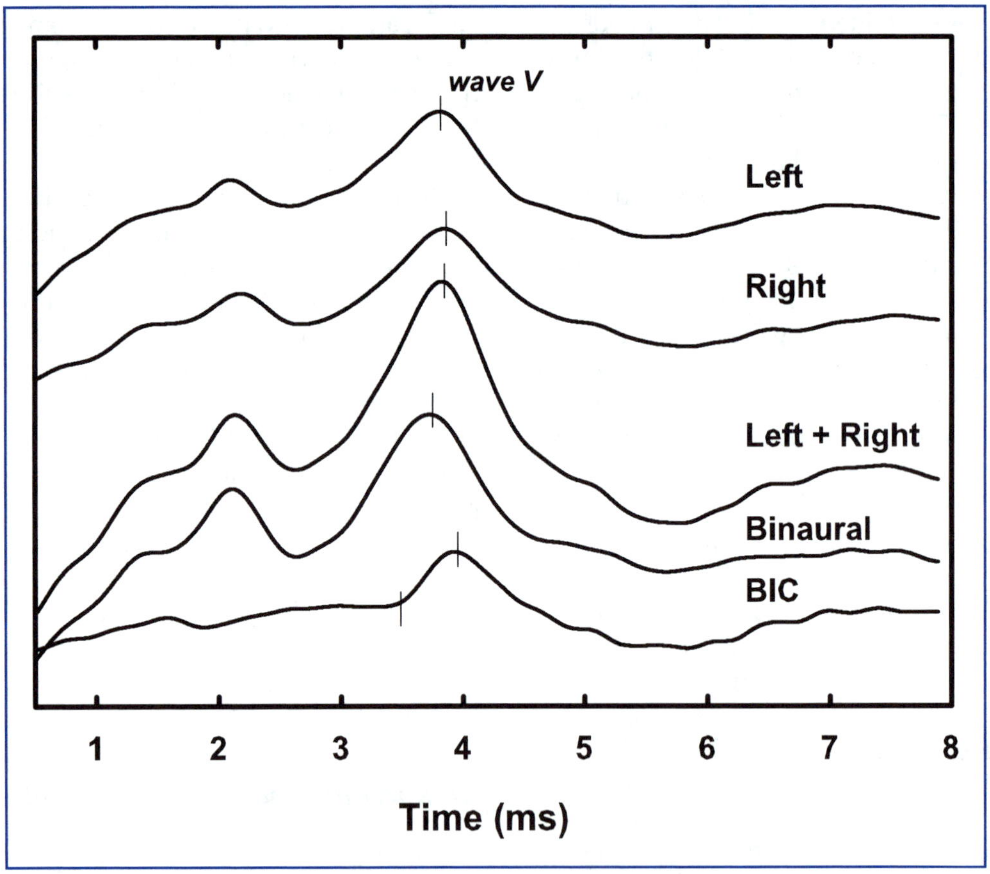


**FIGURE 8–4.** EABR waveforms for monaural and binaural stimulation, used to derive the binaural interaction component (BIC). **From top to bottom:** EABR elicited from the left ear, right ear, sum of the left and right monaural traces (left + right), both ears stimulated simultaneously (binaural), and BIC. The BIC is the difference between the summed monaural and binaural traces. Wave V is indicated on the top four traces. BIC amplitude is measured from the initial trough to the following peak, as indicated by hash marks on the bottom trace. Data are from an adult recipient of bilateral Nucleus 24M devices. Data courtesy of Shuman He, Paul Abbas, and Carolyn Brown, the University of Iowa Cochlear Implant Electrophysiology Laboratory.

cochlea at high levels. In cases where the duration of implant use is different between ears such that the EABR latencies differ, the latency of the BIC tends to be more similar to the longer latency of the more recently implanted ear (Gordon et al., 2007). Clinically, the BIC may be useful for adjusting sound processor programs between ears in bilaterally implanted recipients to optimize binaural advantages (Pelizzone et al., 1990).

### *Latency*

The human acoustic ABR is not fully developed until about 2 years of age. At birth, latencies are prolonged relative to those obtained in adults. Wave I latencies reach maturity at about 1 to 2 months of age and wave V at about 2 years (Ponton & Eggermont, 2007). EABR latency has been used to assess longitudinal changes in neural responsiveness to electrical stimulation. Gordon et al. (2003) showed significant decreases in ECAP, EABR wave III, and EABR wave V latencies within the first year of device use for a group of prelingually deafened children. Furthermore, interwave latencies (ECAP to EABR wave III and EABR waves III to V) also decreased within the first 6 months of implant use. Interestingly, there was no effect of age at implant on the time course of the latency change (Gordon et al., 2003; Gordon, Papsin, & Harrison, 2006; Thai-Van et al., 2007).

Gordon et al. (2007, 2008) also used the BIC response to assess auditory brainstem development in children who were bilaterally implanted either simultaneously, with a short time interval between ears (<1 year), or with a longer time interval between ears (>2 years). Results showed prolonged EABR and BIC latencies for the later-implanted ear for both groups of children implanted in sequential surgeries (short-delay and long-delay groups). Within the first 9 months of bilateral implant use, latencies for the short-delay group were similar to those for the simultaneous group. Although latencies decreased for the long-delay group over the first 9 months of implant use, delays were still evident. Assessments at longer postimplant intervals are necessary to fully characterize changes in physiological responsiveness over time, particularly for individuals with longer time intervals between sequentially placed implants.

## Measurement Challenges

In addition to the challenges described above for reducing stimulus artifact, EABR recordings can also be contaminated by unwanted physiological responses from the nearby facial and vestibular nerves. Reports indicate that EABRs can be measured in approximately 71 to 95% of cases (Gordon et al., 2004; Lo et al., 2004; Nikolopoulos, Mason, O'Donoghue, & Gibbin, 1997). Facial nerve stimulation can result in large myogenic or electromyographic (EMG) potentials that are easily recorded with scalp electrodes. EMG activity can be recorded in the absence of visible muscle twitches and/or in the absence of a physical percept by the recipient. EMG artifact presents as a very large, broad, positive-then-negative waveform at about the same latency as wave V, but can be several times larger and broader than the EABR wave V (see, for example, Figs. 4 and 12 in van den Honert & Stypulkowski, 1986). EMG activity is characterized by a very large magnitude response that grows quickly with increased stimulus level. Because EMG results from motor neurons, it is affected by paralytic agents (van den Honert & Stypulkowski, 1986).

Stimulation of the vestibular portion of the eighth nerve results in a smaller artifact than that recorded for myogenic activity. Vestibular responses present as a negative deflection near 2 ms with a smaller following positive peak or plateau around 3 ms (see, for example, Fig. 12 in van den Honert & Stypulkowski, 1986). Physiological vestibular responses can be recorded in the absence of a perceived vestibular disturbance by the recipient.

## What Constitutes a Measurable Response?

The following guidelines may be helpful for identifying EABR waveforms, determining whether physiological or stimulus artifacts are present, and differentiating near-threshold responses from the noise floor:

1. EABR waveform morphology should resemble that of the acoustic ABR. In many cases,

wave I (and sometimes even wave II) may be obscured by stimulus artifact.
2. EABR wave latencies should occur approximately 1 to 1.5 ms earlier than for acoustic ABR waveforms.
3. EABR amplitudes should increase with increased stimulus levels. Excessively large increases with stimulus level may indicate EMG activity.
4. Recordings should be repeatable. Obtain more averages or replications near threshold.
5. Stimulus levels that produce measurable EABR responses should be audible to the recipient (if able to provide reliable feedback).

## CLINICAL USES FOR EABRS

Clinically, EABRs can be used to confirm device function, and confirm that the peripheral auditory neurons up to the level of the brainstem are functioning in response to electrical stimulation from the implant. Like the ECAP, EABR wave V thresholds almost always occur above behavioral threshold, and in many cases, are more likely to approximate or even exceed upper comfort levels (e.g., Bierer et al., 2011; Brown et al., 1994, 1999, 2002; Firszt, Rotz, Chambers, & Novak, 1999; Gallégo et al., 1999; Gordon et al., 2004; Hay-McCutcheon et al., 2002; Miller et al., 2008; Shallop et al., 1990, 1991; van den Borne, Mens, Snik, Spies, & van den Broek, 1994; van den Honert & Stypulkowski, 1986). The same constraints regarding stimulation rates that were discussed in Chapter 7 for ECAPs also apply to EABRs. Namely, there is a mismatch between the stimulation rates used for EABRs (slow rate, on the order of 10 to 50 Hz) and the fast rates used for programming the sound processor (250 pps to >5000 pps). Therefore, for faster map rates, EABR thresholds are more likely to approximate or exceed upper comfort levels, and correlations between EABR and map levels are likely to be poorer (Brown et al., 1999; Miller et al., 2008). However, when the same slow-rate stimulus is used for both EABR and behavioral responses, both measures are highly correlated (Abbas & Brown, 1991a; Brown et al., 1994). In sum, EABR thresholds represent a level that should be audible, and can be useful for verifying questionable behavioral responses or estimating a stimulation level that can be used to begin conditioning young children for behavioral testing. As always, care should be taken to ensure that the stimulus is not too loud, particularly for map levels that use faster stimulation rates.

Several studies have examined correlations between EABR thresholds and map levels (e.g., Brown et al., 1994, 1999; Lo et al., 2004). Results have shown moderate correlations that are not strong enough to suggest that EABR thresholds can be used in isolation for setting map levels for recipients who cannot provide reliable behavioral feedback. However, when EABR thresholds are coupled with limited behavioral information (as described in Chapter 7 for the ECAP), correlations between predicted and measured map levels improves substantially (Brown et al., 2000).

A few studies have examined whether EABR measures can be used to predict speech perception with the implant (Abbas & Brown, 1991a; Gibson, Sanli, & Psarros, 2009; Kubo et al., 2001). Gibson et al. (2009) showed that children with more robust EABRs had better speech perception. Abbas and Brown (1991a) showed a moderate positive correlation between the slope of the EABR AGF and word/sentence recognition as well as a moderate negative correlation between EABR threshold and performance for a group of Ineraid subjects. These trends did not hold for a comparison group of Nucleus 22 subjects, however. Kubo et al. (2001) showed a significant positive correlation between the slope of the EABR AGF and performance on consonant recognition at the 1-month postoperative visit. Correlations at later time intervals, however, were not significant. The same study also reported a significant negative correlation between EABR AGF slope and behavioral T-levels, where steeper slopes were found for lower T-levels. In sum, better performance, more robust EABRs, steeper AGFs, lower T-levels, and lower EABR thresholds appear to be interrelated; however, these results are not always consistent across time intervals or device type.

## SUMMARY

Key concepts for EABR measures are summarized below:

1. The EABR is a far-field neural response from the auditory nerve up to the inferior colliculus.
2. EABR waveform morphology is similar to its acoustic counterpart, except absolute latencies are approximately 1 to 1.5 ms shorter, and wave I and/or wave II may be obscured by stimulus artifact.
3. EABR wave V is typically larger than its acoustic counterpart because electrical stimulation results in greater synchrony and broader spatial spread through the cochlea.
4. The EABR can be used to measure physiological threshold, growth of response with level, channel interaction, refractory recovery, binaural interaction, and maturational effects.
5. EABRs can be contaminated by other physiological responses, such as those induced by electrical stimulation of the facial or vestibular nerves.
6. Clinically, EABRs can be used to confirm device function, confirm auditory nerve function, assist with sound processor programming, and verify questionable behavioral responses.
7. The correlation between EABR thresholds and map levels tends to worsen with increased map stimulation rates.
8. EABR thresholds almost always occur above behavioral thresholds, and more likely approximate or exceed upper comfort levels. When a slow-rate stimulus is used for both measures, they are strongly correlated.
9. EABR measures alone cannot predict map levels with adequate accuracy. Therefore, like the ECAP, EABR thresholds should not be used as a substitute for behavioral responses. However, when combined with limited behavioral information, EABR thresholds can be useful for predicting map levels that correlate strongly with those measured behaviorally.

# 9

# Electrically Evoked Auditory Middle Latency Response

Although more central physiological responses are not used as widely in clinical applications with cochlear implant recipients, these potentials are useful for providing information about physiological maturation at higher levels of the auditory system. Compared to the ECAP (see Chapter 7), EABR (see Chapter 8), and cortical potentials (see Chapter 10), relatively little has been published on the use of the electrically evoked auditory middle latency response (EAMLR) in cochlear implant recipients. This chapter begins with a basic description of what EAMLRs are and how they are measured. Next, different types of measurements with the EAMLR are described, and challenges associated with measuring these potentials are discussed. Finally, a summary of the clinical uses for the EAMLR is provided.

## BASIC DESCRIPTION

The EAMLR is a synchronous physiological response from the upper brainstem, thalamus, and auditory cortex (Pratt, 2007). The morphology of the EAMLR is similar to that of its acoustic counterpart (Kileny, Kemink, & Miller, 1989). Like the acoustic AMLR, the EAMLR is characterized by the Na-Pa-Nb complex (Figure 9–1). The Na component presumably arises from the midbrain and thalamic regions (Pratt, 2007). The generators of the Pa component are less clear, but studies suggest responses arise from the primary auditory cortex with contributions from other ascending subcortical regions, such as the reticular formation and/or medial geniculate (Pratt, 2007). The generator for the Nb component has not been determined (Pratt, 2007). In contrast to the more peripheral auditory evoked potentials, the EAMLR can be affected by arousal state (e.g., certain stages of sleep or anesthesia; see Gordon, Papsin, & Harrison, 2005).

The latencies of Na and Pa occur at approximately 15 to 18 ms and 25 to 27 ms, respectively (Firszt, Chambers, Kraus, & Reeder, 2002; Shallop et al., 1990); Nb occurs at approximately 25 to 55 ms (Gordon et al., 2005). These latencies are similar to those reported for the acoustic AMLR, which occur at approximately 15 to 20 ms for Na, 22 to 36 ms for Pa, and 45 to 50 ms for Nb (Hall, 1992; Pratt, 2007). EAMLR latencies may increase slightly with decreased stimulus levels, but to a lesser degree than for the EABR. Firszt, Chambers,

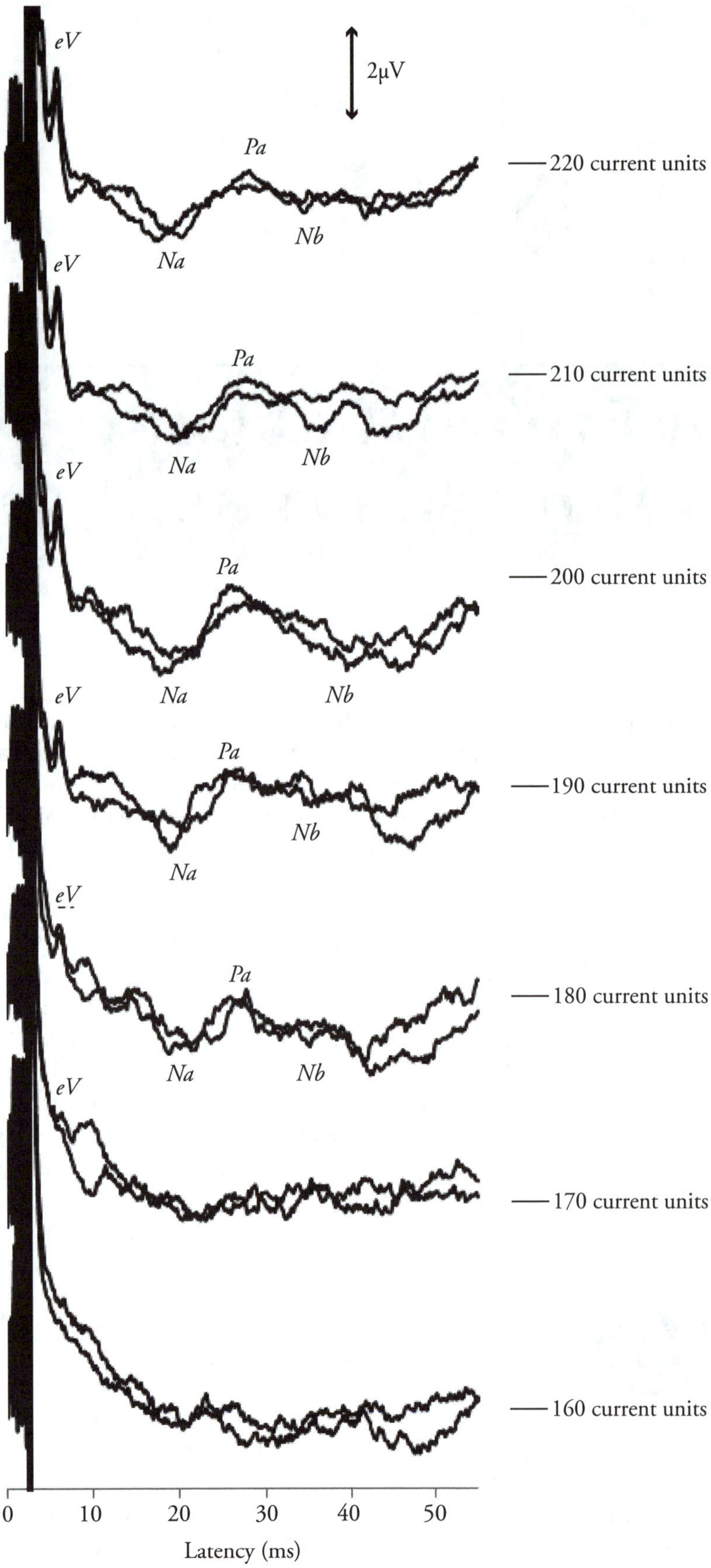


**FIGURE 9–1.** Example of a series of electrically evoked auditory middle latency responses (EAMLRs) from an apical electrode in a pediatric Nucleus 24RE(CA) recipient (age 8.7 years). Responses were obtained from the second-side implant (duration of device use, 2.6 years). Responses represent a growth function from high to low stimulus levels (top to bottom, respectively). In this example, waves Na, Pa, and Nb are visible at all but the two lowest stimulus levels (170 and 160 CL). Note that wave V of the EABR (eV) is also indicated near the beginning of each waveform. Figure courtesy of Karen Gordon and Salima Jiwani, Archie's Cochlear Implant Laboratory, The Hospital for Sick Children, Toronto, Canada.

Kraus, and Reeder (2002) reported average latency shifts of 1.1 ms and 0.7 ms for Na and Pa, respectively, when stimulus levels were reduced from upper comfort level to Na-Pa threshold; however, these differences were not statistically significant.

EAMLR amplitudes are calculated from the midpoint of the Na trough to the midpoint of the Pa peak. Maximum peak-to-peak amplitudes are typically around 2 to 3 microvolts (µV) at high (upper comfort) stimulus levels (Firszt, Chambers, Kraus, & Reeder, 2002). Threshold amplitudes for Na-Pa are typically around 1 µV (Firszt, Chambers, Kraus, & Reeder, 2002). Like other evoked potentials described in this book, Na-Pa amplitudes are larger with electrical stimulation than with acoustic stimulation (which are on the order of 0.5 to 1 µV at high levels; Pratt, 2007), presumably due to greater neural synchrony (Kileny et al., 1989). Also like the earlier potentials, the Na-Pa amplitude decreases with stimulus level. However, Firszt, Chambers, Kraus, and Reeder (2002) reported smaller amplitude decrements near threshold, consistent with trends seen for the acoustic AMLR (Özdamar & Kraus, 1983).

# MEASUREMENT

## Stimulus

EAMLRs can be elicited using the same stimulus configuration as for the EABR (see Chapter 8, Figure 8–2). The stimulus is delivered to the internal device via the sound processor and clinical programming interface. The stimulus parameters are defined within the clinical programming software in the same way as the EABR (see Chapter 8). A standard clinical evoked potentials system is used for recording, and a trigger pulse output from the programming interface is used to synchronize the recording system. The stimulus that is used to elicit the EAMLR is typically a single biphasic current pulse delivered at a slightly slower repetition rate (~11 Hz) than for the EABR (Firszt, Chambers, Kraus, & Reeder, 2002; Gordon et al., 2005).

## Recording

The EAMLR is a far-field response recorded using scalp electrodes that are attached to a preamplifier. As with the EABR, an RF filter (low-pass, ~32 kHz) is used to eliminate artifact from the transmitting coil. The typical montage is high forehead (Fz) or midline at the top of the head (Cz) for the positive (noninverting) electrode, with either the nape of the neck or ipsilateral earlobe or mastoid as the reference (inverting) electrode, and either the forehead or contralateral mastoid/earlobe as ground (Firszt, Chambers, Kraus, & Reeder, 2002; Gordon et al., 2005; Pratt, 2007). The recording time window is generally set to around 50 to 80 ms (Firszt, Chambers, Kraus, & Reeder, 2002; Gordon et al., 2005). Because the EAMLR has a longer latency than the EABR, responses are less affected by stimulus artifact. The EAMLR is usually resolved with band-pass filtering between approximately 5 to 10 Hz and 500 to 3000 Hz (Firszt, Chambers, Kraus, & Reeder, 2002; Gordon et al., 2005).

## Types of Measurements

### *Threshold and Growth of Response with Level*

EAMLR thresholds are typically defined using visual detection (see Chapter 7), where the lowest current level that yields a measurable, repeatable response is classified as threshold. To assist in determining the presence of a response, Firszt, Chambers, Kraus, and Reeder (2002) obtained a control condition using the lowest stimulus level possible for the device (3 clinical units for their group of Advanced Bionics Clarion 1.2 recipients). This condition served as a baseline of the individual subject's EEG activity that could be compared to responses obtained at higher stimulus levels. In general, waveform identification is made based on: (1) replication of the response, and (2) peaks occurring within the expected latency range (Gordon et al., 2005).

It is not clear how well EAMLR thresholds compare to EABR and/or ECAP thresholds. Shallop et al. (1990) reported that EAMLR thresholds were lower than EABR thresholds for some subjects; the opposite was found for other subjects. There are no comprehensive studies that have examined electrically evoked physiological thresholds at different levels of the auditory system for the same stimulus (i.e., ECAP, EABR, EAMLR).

EAMLR amplitudes can be affected by age at implant and duration of implant use. Gordon et al. (2005) examined EAMLR amplitudes longitudinally in two groups of children differing in age at implant (<5 years versus ≥5 years). In the first 2 months of implant use, amplitudes were larger for the older group. After approximately 6 months of device use, amplitudes for both groups were similar, and both increased with duration of implant use. This result suggests amplitude growth over time for both groups, with the rate of growth being faster for the younger group.

Finally, the slope of the EAMLR growth function is calculated by plotting the Na-Pa amplitude as a function of stimulus level. EAMLR slope is not a metric that has been widely assessed or reported in the literature. One study in guinea pigs (Jyung, Miller, & Cannon, 1989) reported that changes in the slope of the EAMLR growth function following ototoxic deafening was correlated with a reduction in spiral ganglion cell density; shallower slopes occurred with reduced cell density. Interestingly, EAMLR thresholds in that study did not change with reductions in slope and cell density.

### *Latency*

The human acoustic AMLR is not fully developed until about 8 to 10 years of age (Hall, 1992). EAMLR latency has been used to assess longitudinal changes in neural responsiveness to electrical stimulation (Gordon et al., 2005). After 6 months of device use, Gordon et al. (2005) showed longer EAMLR latencies for children implanted under the age of 5 versus those implanted over the age of 5. The difference between groups was no longer significant by the 1-year postimplant interval because latencies for the younger-implanted group decreased, whereas latencies for the older-implanted group showed little change. Further, when assessing EAMLR responses in subgroups of children that were the same age, Gordon et al. (2005) found that EAMLRs were more likely to be present for children who had at least 2 to 6 months of implant use. In sum, these results indicate that EAMLRs reflect some activity-dependent plasticity at the thalamocortical level in response to electrical stimulation.

### Measurement Challenges

As stated earlier, the EAMLR can be affected by sleep state, which makes these measures unsuitable for intraoperative assessments (Gordon et al., 2005). Furthermore, the EAMLR can be more difficult to detect in younger children, particularly with only limited durations of implant use (Gordon et al., 2005). As a result, the EAMLR has limited utility for verifying the function of the device and the auditory pathway in response to electrical stimulation, particularly for young children at intraoperative or early visits, when this information is most critical.

## CLINICAL USES FOR EAMLRS

Few studies have examined the relation between EAMLR and behavioral measures. EAMLR thresholds are similar to behavioral thresholds when the same stimulus is used for both measures (Kileny & Kemink, 1987; Miller, Arenberg, Middlebrooks, & Pfingst, 2001). No studies have systematically evaluated the use of EAMLR thresholds for predicting map levels for cochlear implant recipients. However, somewhat promising results have been found for speech perception. For adult implant users, Firszt, Chambers, and Kraus (2002) showed a significant correlation between speech perception in quiet and EAMLR amplitude and threshold. Better speech perception was correlated with larger amplitudes and lower EAMLR thresholds.

## SUMMARY

Key concepts for EAMLR measures are summarized below:

1. The EAMLR is a far-field neural response from the thalamocortical auditory pathway.

2. EAMLR waveform morphology is similar to its acoustic counterpart, except the amplitudes tend to be larger.
3. The primary measures of interest for the EAMLR are threshold, slope of the amplitude growth function, and latency.
4. EAMLR latencies tend to be prolonged for younger children and for shorter durations of implant use.
5. EAMLRs are difficult to measure intraoperatively because they can be affected by arousal state.
6. EAMLR thresholds correlate strongly with behavioral thresholds when the same stimulus is used for both measures. At this time, few studies have assessed clinical applications of the EAMLR for predicting map levels.

# 10

# Electrically Evoked Auditory Cortical Potentials

## INTRODUCTION

Central (cortical) physiological responses are useful for providing information about central auditory pathways, stimulus detection, perceptual discrimination, and/or physiological maturation at higher levels of the auditory system. One advantage that auditory cortical potentials have over more peripheral measures (ECAP, EABR) is that a wider range of stimuli can be used to elicit responses. The benefit is that it is possible to objectively evaluate the brain's ability to detect or discriminate different stimulus characteristics, such as loudness differences, temporal changes, or speech tokens (for example, differentiation of /ba/ versus /da/).

The term "cortical auditory evoked potentials" (CAEPs) is a relatively generic term that encompasses several specific types of auditory responses that differ based on how stimuli are presented and whether or not the listener attends to the stimuli. These potentials include the electrically evoked auditory late response (EALR), the electrically evoked acoustic change complex (EACC), the mismatch negativity (eMMN), and the P300. Auditory evoked potentials can be classified into two main groups: exogenous and endogenous potentials. Exogenous potentials do not require active participation on the part of the listener and are highly sensitive to stimulus characteristics used to evoke them (Hall, 1992; Martin, Tremblay, & Stapells, 2007). The ECAP, EABR, EAMLR, EALR, EACC, and eMMN can be considered exogenous responses in that they do not require the listener to actively attend to the stimulus. However, there are also endogenous aspects to some of these potentials in that attention and sleep can modulate middle and late responses. The endogenous P300 potential can be recorded in ways that require the listener to attend to the stimulus, which is also called the P300b (Beynon, Snik, & van den Broek, 2002; Hall, 1992; Martin et al., 2007). When the listener is not required to attend to the stimulus, a P300a will be generated.

This chapter discusses four interrelated CAEP measures: the EALR, EACC, eMMN, and P300. For each of these four measures, a basic description is provided, a brief summary of the measurement techniques (stimulus and recording) is given, and clinical uses are discussed. A summary of key points is included at the end of the chapter.

## ELECTRICALLY EVOKED AUDITORY LATE RESPONSE

### Basic Description

The EALR is composed of the P1-N1-P2 complex. The neural generators of these potentials are constantly being redefined as advances in neuroimaging methods are developed. Further, the specific neural generators vary with the paradigm used to evoke these potentials. In general, however, contributions from thalamocortical projections generate the subcomponent of the complex. N1 alone is thought to have more than three neural generators. Readers are referred to Picton (2010) for a complete review of neural generators contributing to all of the evoked potentials described here.

Figure 10–1 shows a schematic illustration of a mature EALR response. The EALR is a sensory response that can be elicited by stimulus onset, stimulus offset, or a change in a continuous stimulus (the latter of which is the acoustic change complex, described in the next section; Martin et al., 2007). As with other evoked potentials described in the earlier chapters, the morphology of the EALR is similar to that of its acoustic counterpart (ALR). Because cortical potentials are generated by central areas of the brain, there is a strong influence of sleep state and sedatives/anesthesia on the measured responses (Hall, 1992). Therefore, responses are typically obtained in the awake patient.

For both acoustic and electrical stimulation, the mature P1-N1-P2 complex occurs within 50 to 250 msec following the stimulus presentation (Brown et al., 2008; Firszt, Chambers, Kraus, & Reeder, 2002; Hall, 1992; Martin et al., 2007), although latencies may be somewhat shorter with direct electrical stimulation (Firszt, Chambers, Kraus, & Reeder, 2002; Ponton & Don, 1995; Ponton et al., 1996). For adult implant recipients, P1, N1, and P2 occur at latencies of approximately 40 to 80 msec, 75 to 150 msec, and 150 to 210 msec, respectively (Firszt, Chambers, Kraus, & Reeder, 2002; Guiraud et al., 2007; Ponton et al., 1996). EALR latencies may increase by approximately 4 to 9 ms with decreasing stimulus levels across

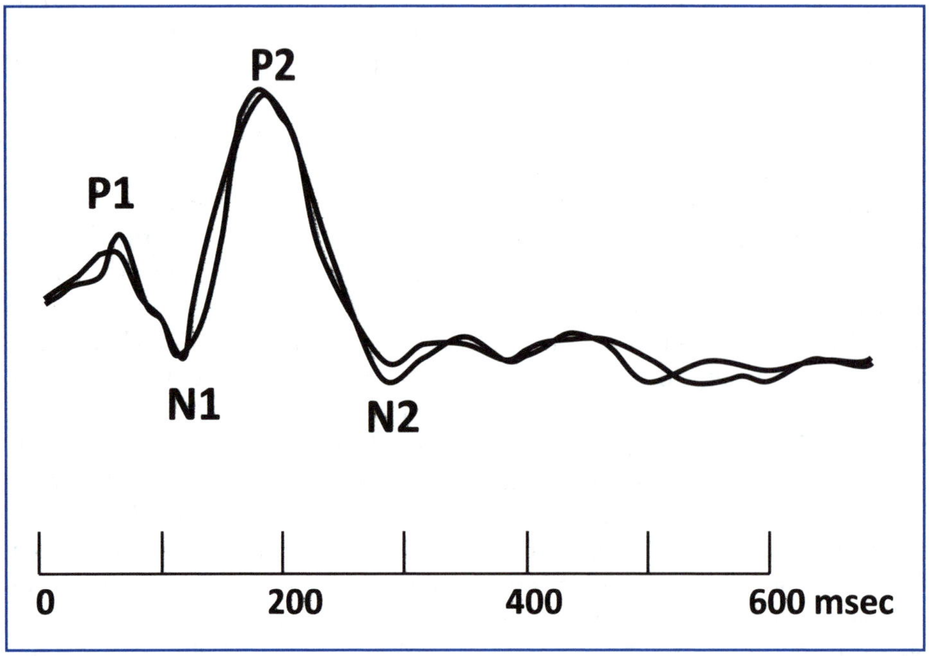


FIGURE 10–1. Example of the mature electrically evoked auditory late potential, characterized by a series of positive and negative deflections (labeled as P1, N1, P2, and N2). Time in milliseconds (msec) is given along the x-axis.

the listener's dynamic range (Firszt, Chambers, Kraus, & Reeder, 2002). For adults, EALR amplitudes are calculated from the midpoint of the N1 trough to the midpoint of the P2 peak (Firszt, Chambers, Kraus, & Reeder, 2002; Guiraud et al., 2007) because P2 is the larger response. In adults, maximum peak-to-peak amplitudes can be on the order of 3 to 12 microvolts (μV; Brown et al., 2008; Firszt, Chambers, Kraus, & Reeder, 2002), which are similar to the acoustic ALR (3 to 10 μV; Hall, 1992) and much larger than the EMLR (~2 to 3 μV; see Chapter 9). EALR response amplitudes tend to be larger for moderate rather than high-intensity stimulus levels (Firszt, Chambers, Kraus, & Reeder, 2002; Hall, 1992).

In younger children, P1 is the primary measure of interest because it is the largest component of the response, with N1 and P2 typically being absent (e.g, Gordon, Tanaka, & Papsin, 2005; Martin et al., 2007; Ponton & Eggermont, 2001; Sharma, Dorman, & Spahr, 2002a). There is some controversy over the absence of N1 responses in children: whether it reflects immaturity in the system or inadequate stimulus/recording procedures, because N1 and P2 responses have been observed when slower stimulus presentation rates are used (Wunderlich & Cone-Wesson, 2006). For individuals with normal hearing, the latency of P1 decreases as children age (Ponton et al., 1996; Ponton & Eggermont, 2001; Sharma et al., 2002a), with latencies of approximately 300 ms at birth, 125 ms at age 3 years, and 60 ms in adulthood (e.g., Dorman, Sharma, Gilley, Martin, & Roland, 2007). For children with cochlear implants, the time course of P1 maturation is affected by age at implant and duration of implant use. Children implanted at younger ages (<3.5 years) are more likely to have P1 latencies within the normal range (relative to age-matched normal-hearing peers) after approximately 6 to 8 months of implant use, and children implanted later (>7 years) are more likely to fall outside the normal range (Sharma et al., 2002a). Ponton et al. (1996) showed that the overall rate of P1 maturation for children with cochlear implants is similar to that of children with normal hearing, but is delayed by the duration of deafness prior to implant (i.e., "time in sound"). Later work by Sharma et al. (2002b) showed an initial, steeper rate of P1 maturation within the first 8 months of implant use for children who were implanted under the age of 3 years; this initial latency change occurred at a faster rate than for age-matched normal-hearing peers. Figure 10–2 shows examples of individual (thin lines) and group mean (thick lines) waveforms for a group of children with Nucleus cochlear implants (left column) and children with normal hearing (right column), matched horizontally by time in sound. As can be seen, large variability exists across individuals, particularly for the implant recipients.

In normal-hearing individuals, the P1-N1-P2 reaches a more mature stage around 10 years of age, with smaller, gradual latency decrements in the second decade of life, reaching final maturity around 18 to 21 years of age (Martin et al., 2007; Ponton & Eggermont, 2001; Sharma et al., 2002a). Over the course of maturation, the amplitude of P1 decreases while the amplitude of P2 increases. This shift is attributed to the development of the N1 component in adolescence, which partially overlays the P1, causing the P1 to appear smaller in adolescents and adults (Ponton & Eggermont, 2001). For deaf children with cochlear implants, it appears that the P1 component (from deep cortical layers) develops rather normally, but N1 (from more superficial cortical layers) does not. As a result, latency and morphology differences between children with implants and those with normal hearing emerge around the age of 10 years, when the N1 response normally begins to mature (Ponton & Eggermont, 2001).

## Measurement

### *Stimuli*

Different types of stimuli can be used to elicit electrically evoked cortical potentials. These include single pulses or pulse trains presented directly to the implant; or clicks, tones, or speech tokens (natural or synthetic) presented via a loudspeaker and processed by the recipient's sound processor. One issue with sound-field delivery of stimuli, however, is that individual differences in sound processor parameters can result in different processing of the signal across subjects, which can affect CAEP recordings in different ways. Thus,

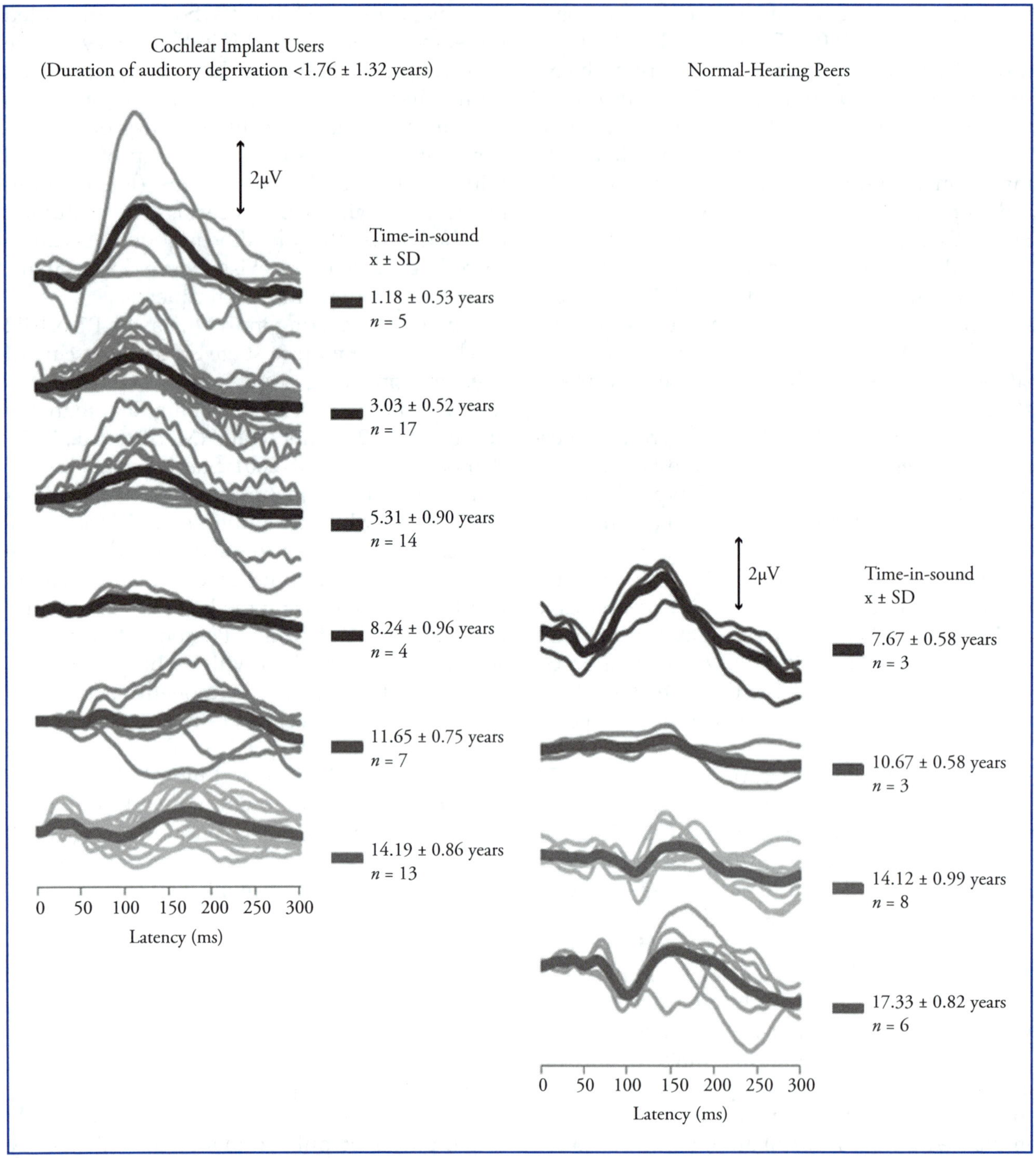


**FIGURE 10–2.** Examples of electrically evoked cortical responses from different groups of cochlear implant users (*left column*) and normal hearing peers (*right column*). In both columns, each grouping represents different durations of time in sound; this equates to duration of implant use plus any period of usable hearing prior to implantation for the left column (top to bottom: short to long duration of use) and age for the right column (top to bottom: younger to older). Roughly equivalent time-in-sound groups are aligned horizontally. In each grouping, the thinner gray lines represent individual data and the darker thick line represents the group mean. SD = standard deviation; *n* = number of subjects. Figure courtesy of Karen Gordon and Salima Jiwani, Archie's Cochlear Implant Laboratory, The Hospital for Sick Children, Toronto, Canada.

interpretation of CAEP waveforms for sound-field stimuli can be complex. It can be difficult to ascertain whether different CAEP response patterns are due to neurophysiological processes or signal processing by the implant (Tremblay & Moore, 2012).

Stimuli are typically longer in duration than what is used for more peripheral evoked potentials (such as the ECAP), and should be presented at a relatively slow repetition rate, on the order of 1 to 2 Hz (e.g., Firszt, Chambers, Kraus, & Reeder, 2002; Guiraud et al., 2007; Sharma et al., 2002a). In general, longer stimulus durations will produce more problems with stimulus artifact overlapping the measured response (Martin, 2007). The duration of the stimulus should therefore be shorter than the latency of the P1-N1-P2 to reduce this problem. Table 10–1 summarizes stimulus parameters used in selected studies evaluating the EALR P1-N1-P2 complex.

### Recording

As with the EABR and EAMLR, cortical responses are far-field measures obtained with scalp electrodes attached to a preamplifier. There are several choices for the electrode montage. The most simplistic is to place the positive (noninverting) electrode at midline either at the high forehead (Fz) or vertex (Cz), with the reference (inverting) electrode either at the nape of the neck (Firszt, Chambers, Kraus, & Reeder, 2002; Guiraud et al., 2007) or at the contralateral mastoid (Brown et al., 2008; Sharma et al., 2002a). The ground can be placed anywhere, such as at the forehead or wrist. Alternatively, electrode caps can be used, which offer multichannel recordings. An additional pair of electrodes should be placed at the lateral and superior outer canthus to monitor and reject eye-blink artifacts (e.g., Brown et al., 2008; Firszt, Chambers, Kraus, & Reeder, 2002; Kraus et al., 1993; Sharma et al., 2002a). Additional artifact rejection (±100 µV) should be employed for other myogenic responses (e.g., Gordon et al., 2005; Sharma et al., 2002a). An RF filter (low-pass, ~32 kHz) can be used to eliminate artifact from the transmitting coil (Firszt, Chambers, Kraus, & Reeder, 2002; Gordon et al., 2005).

If longer-duration stimuli are used, filtering, artifact rejection, and contralateral reference electrode placement may be insufficient, particularly when stimuli are delivered via the sound field. Alternative artifact reduction methods have been described elsewhere in detail (e.g., Gilley et al., 2006; Martin, 2007). These options include adjusting the recording electrode montage to avoid capturing stimulus artifact (zero isopotential field;

**Table 10–1.** Summary of Stimulus Parameters Used to Elicit the P1-N1-P2 Complex in Selected Studies

| Study | Stimulus | Stimulus Duration | Repetition Rate | Presentation Mode |
|---|---|---|---|---|
| Firszt et al. (2002) | Single biphasic pulse | 200 µsec | 1.1 Hz | Direct |
| Gordon et al. (2005) | 250-pps pulse train | 36 ms | 1 Hz | Direct |
| Guiraud et al. (2007) | Single biphasic pulse | 75 µsec | 1.01 Hz | Direct |
| McNeill et al. (2009) | /ba/ | 115 msec | ~1.2 Hz | Loudspeaker |
| Ponton et al. (1996, 2001) | 500-pps pulse train | 20 ms | 1.3 Hz | Direct |
| Sharma et al. (2002, 2005) | /ba/ | 90 msec | 1.4 Hz | Loudspeaker |

Gilley et al., 2006; Sharma et al., 2005), comparing across multiple recording sites for evidence of artifact polarity inversion (Martin, 2007), or employing complex offline statistical calculations, such as principal components analysis or independent components analysis (Gilley et al., 2006; Martin et al., 2007), which require a relatively large number of recording channels (16 to 64 channels). As of yet, however, there is no consensus on how to manage artifact when long duration stimuli are presented via the sound field.

The recording time window may begin approximately 100 msec prior to the stimulus and should extend approximately 300 to 600 msec beyond the stimulus onset, depending on the stimulus duration (Brown et al., 2008; Firszt, Chambers, Kraus, & Reeder, 2002; Sharma et al., 2002a). Because cortical responses are slow, broad responses, band-pass filtering should be between approximately 1 to 100 Hz (Firszt, Chambers, Kraus, & Reeder, 2002; Guiraud et al., 2007; Martin, 2007; Sharma et al., 2002a). The EALR is larger than the EMLR and EABR, so comparatively fewer sweeps are needed. Typically, 1 to 2 runs of 300 to 500 sweeps are sufficient (Firszt, Chambers, Kraus, & Reeder, 2002; Sharma et al., 2002a).

### Clinical Uses

The P1-N1-P2 of the acoustic ALR was originally used as a fairly accurate objective estimate of hearing thresholds, but lost popularity with the advent of the ABR, which is not affected by sleep state or anesthesia (see Martin et al., 2007 or Hall, 1992 for a historical perspective). At this time there do not appear to be any studies that have evaluated the relation between EALR thresholds and behavioral thresholds for electrical stimulation.

EALR morphology and latency have been studied more widely in regard to the maturation of auditory cortical pathways. In general, findings show that longer durations of deafness and later age at implant result in immature morphology and delayed EALR latencies (e.g., Gordon et al., 2005; Guiraud et al., 2007; McNeill, Sharma, & Purdy, 2009; Ponton et al., 1996; Sharma et al., 2002a). Other studies have suggested that EALR latencies (specifically P1 in children) can be used as a metric to gauge whether sufficient stimulation is being provided with hearing aids during a preimplant hearing aid trial, or to monitor auditory cortical development following cochlear implantation (Dorman et al., 2007; Sharma & Dorman, 2005, 2006; Sharma et al., 2005). These investigators described case studies of pediatric cochlear implant candidates in which no changes in P1 latency were evident over the course of 3 to 13 months of hearing aid use, but significant decreases in P1 latency occurred 3 to 6 months following cochlear implantation. It was concluded that the implant was more successful at activating the central auditory system than the hearing aid for those cases.

Finally, a few studies have examined the relation between EALR responses and speech perception. In a group of adult implant recipients, Firszt, Chambers, and Kraus (2002) found no significant relation between speech perception performance and EALR maximum amplitude, threshold, or latency. Anecdotally, however, the two subjects with no measurable N1-P2 response were also two of the poorest performers in that study. In a group of pediatric cochlear implant recipients, Gordon et al. (2005) found that children with abnormal EALR morphology tended to have poorer speech perception, and those with more typical morphology tended to have better speech perception.

## ELECTRICALLY EVOKED ACOUSTIC CHANGE COMPLEX

### Basic Description

The acoustic change complex is essentially a second N1-P2 complex that occurs in response to a change in a longer-duration continuous stimulus (i.e., a second onset response; Brown et al., 2008; Friesen & Tremblay, 2006; Martin, 2007; Martin & Boothroyd, 1999; Ostroff, Martin, & Boothroyd, 1998; Tremblay, Friesen, Martin, & Wright, 2003). The EACC (or its acoustic counterpart, the ACC) is considered a transient or exogenous auditory evoked potential because it can be recorded without the subject actively attending to the stimulus (e.g., Martin et al., 2007; Ostroff et al., 1998; Tremblay et al., 2003). A theoretical example is shown in Figure 10–3. The top panel shows a schematic of a standard P1-N1-P2 complex in response to either a 600-msec speech token /u/ (stimulus A) or a 600-msec pulse train delivered to electrode 1 (stimulus B). The bottom panel illustrates how the EACC is generated with a change in the stimulus. For stimulus C, the /u/ transitions to /i/ at the midpoint of the overall stimulus duration (300 ms). Similarly, for stimulus D, the pulse train transitions from E1 to E5 at the 300-ms point. The result is a second complex that temporally coincides with the stimulus change. Because the P1-N1-P2 nomenclature corresponds to a certain latency region and is associated with certain neural generators, the EACC in Figure 10–3 is labeled N1′-P2′ to differentiate it from the initial P1-N1-P2 complex.

## Measurement

For the EACC, stimuli can consist of speech tokens presented via a loudspeaker to the recipient's sound processor (Friesen & Tremblay, 2006; Martin, 2007) or pulse trains presented directly to the implant (i.e., bypassing the sound processor microphone; Brown et al., 2008). Stimulus artifact can be a bigger problem than for the standard

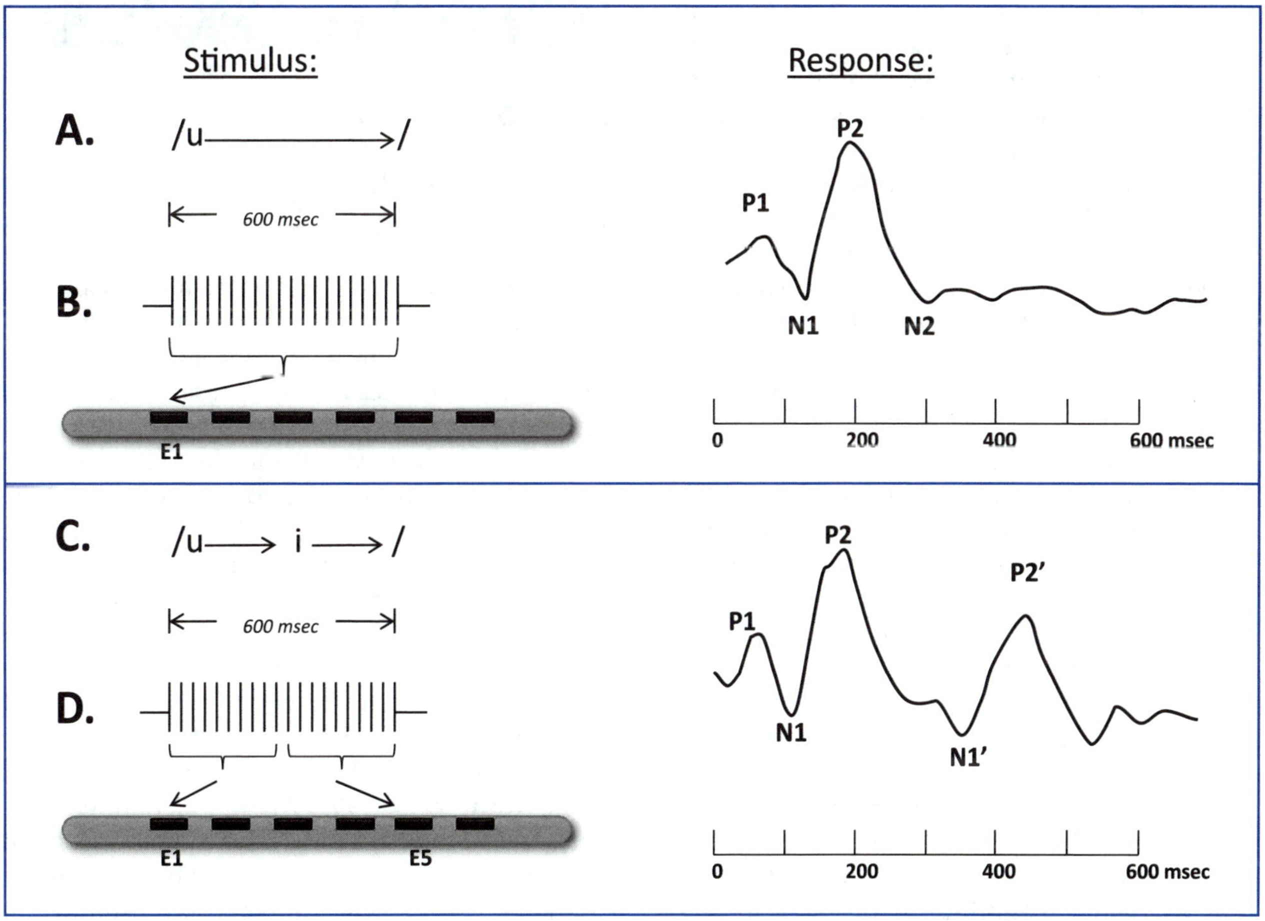


FIGURE 10–3. Schematic illustration of how the electrically evoked acoustic change complex (EACC) is generated. **Top:** Examples of two types of stimuli that can be used to elicit the standard P1-N1-P2 complex. **A.** A 600-ms vowel /u/. **B.** A 600-ms pulse train delivered to electrode 1 (E1). **Bottom:** Examples of how the stimuli in the top panel can change to produce the EACC. **C.** The vowel /u/ transitions to /i/ midway through the total stimulus duration. **D.** The pulse train delivered to electrode 1 switches to electrode 5. Either type of stimulus change will elicit an overlapping N1-P2 complex (labeled N1′ and P2′) corresponding with the temporal shift in the stimulus.

EALR because the stimulus duration for the EACC is often longer (see "Recording" under the section on EALR for suggestions regarding artifact reduction). During measurement acquisition, subjects should be instructed to ignore the stimuli; a closed-captioned video may be played during testing to keep subjects awake but distracted from the stimuli. Recording techniques are generally the same as those described above for the EALR, where either a single-channel (Brown et al., 2008) or multichannel (Friesen & Tremblay, 2006; Martin, 2007) electrode montage can be used.

### Clinical Uses

The EACC is based on cortical detection of spectral, temporal, or amplitude changes in the stimulus. Therefore, it may have clinical utility as an objective indication that a difference in the stimulus was detected by the central auditory system. It is important at this point to distinguish between detection and discrimination. The EACC represents the *detection* of a stimulus change at the level of the auditory cortex, which is a prerequisite to discrimination (e.g., Martin, 2007).

In a group of adult cochlear implant recipients, Friesen and Tremblay (2006) obtained EACC responses for sound-field presentation of two naturally produced speech tokens, /si/ ("see") and /ʃi/ ("she"). Results showed that distinct EACC responses were obtained for each of the two tokens, with latency differences between the EACC responses roughly corresponding to voice onset differences in the stimuli. In that study, the EACC test-retest reliability was strong, indicating that potential changes in response patterns across time intervals are less likely to be due to test variability.

Using direct stimulation, Brown et al. (2008) recorded the EACC using a paradigm like the one shown in Figures 10–3B and 10–3D. Results showed that the magnitude of the EACC increased with the spatial separation between the two stimulated electrodes, consistent with larger pitch differences that may have been perceived between the two electrodes. Further research is needed to determine whether EACC changes as a function of electrode separation accurately reflect the magnitude of perceptual differences in the spectral domain. Studies with acoustic stimulation have shown reasonable agreement between the ACC and perceptual detection of stimulus differences (e.g., Martin & Boothroyd, 2000); however, little work has been done to compare EACC and perceptual discrimination in cochlear implant recipients (Martin, 2007). Furthermore, it remains to be seen whether the EACC can be used to guide adjustments of sound processor settings (e.g., frequency allocations, specific electrodes activated) to optimize listening programs for individuals who cannot provide reliable perceptual feedback.

## MISMATCH NEGATIVITY

### Basic Description

The eMMN is a difference waveform derived from a change in the P1-N1-P2 complex that occurs in response to a frequent (standard) versus infrequent (deviant) stimulus presented using an "oddball" paradigm (described further in the next subsection). With this paradigm, a different (deviant) stimulus is occasionally presented in lieu of the frequent/standard stimulus. The response measured for the deviant stimulus typically presents as an enhanced N1 and/or reduced P2, as compared with the N1 and P2 waves measured in response to the standard stimulus (Martin et al., 2007). The difference between the responses to the standard and deviant stimuli is the eMMN. The eMMN presents as an enhanced negative deflection that occurs in the latency range of 140 to 300 ms with a total duration of approximately 120 ms and amplitude of approximately −2 μV to −3 μV (Kraus et al., 1993; Wable, van den Abbeele, Gallégo, & Frachet, 2000). Like the other cortical auditory evoked potentials described up to this point, the eMMN can be recorded without the subject actively attending to the stimulus. The eMMN reflects the central auditory system's ability to resolve differences in stimuli, and therefore provides an objective measure of physiological mechanisms underlying auditory discrimination (e.g., Kraus et al., 1993; Näätänen, Gaillard,

& Mäntysalo, 1978). In contrast to the acoustic change complex, which is measured in response to sustained stimuli, the eMMN is measured in response to repeated, shorter-duration stimuli and it is quantified as a difference waveform.

## Measurement

For best results, interstimulus intervals should be relatively long (~1 sec), and the deviant stimulus should only be presented in 10 to 15% of the stimulus intervals (Kraus et al., 1993; Ponton & Don, 1995). More occurrences lessen the probability that it is perceived as an infrequent/deviant stimulus. The particular characteristics of the deviant stimulus can vary in amplitude, temporal characteristics, spectral characteristics, different types of speech tokens, or even the absence of the frequent stimulus (e.g., Ponton & Don, 1995).

A common experimental paradigm that can be used to derive the eMMN is shown in Figure 10–4. In this schematic example, the same stimulus, /i/, is presented in both the standard (A) and deviant (B) conditions. In panel A, each occurrence of /i/ elicits a P1-N1-P2 complex. In panel B, the same

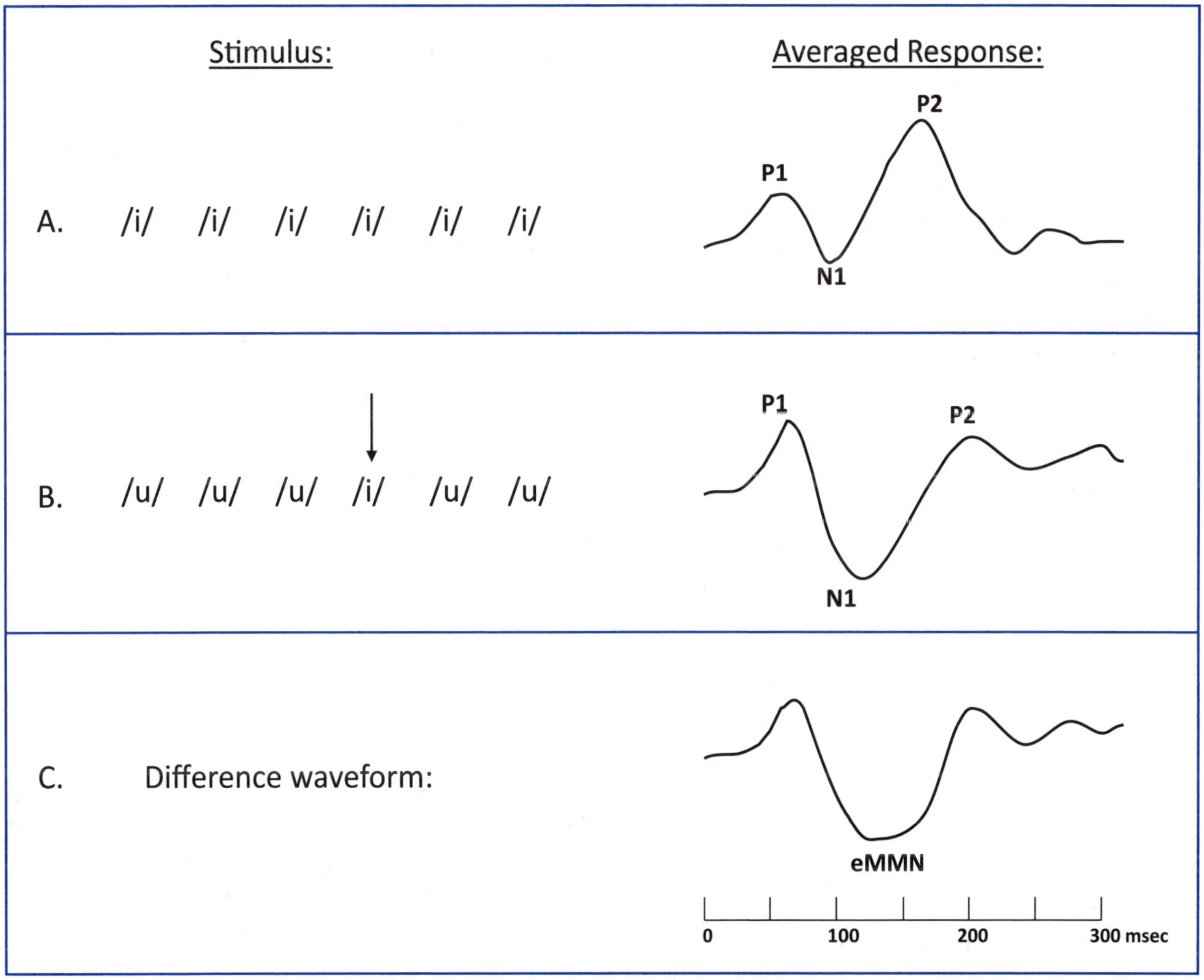


**FIGURE 10–4.** Schematic illustration of how the electrically evoked mismatch negativity (eMMN) is generated. **A.** Averaged P1-N1-P2 complex in response to the vowel /i/, presented as the standard stimulus. **B.** P1-N1-P2 complex recorded in response to the vowel /i/ presented as the deviant stimulus (standard stimulus in this case is /u/). **C.** Difference waveform between A and B is the eMMN.

vowel /i/ is presented as the deviant stimulus (among the standard stimulus /u/). The response measured for /i/ as the deviant stimulus shows an enhanced N1 and reduced P2 compared with the waveform in panel A. The eMMN (panel C) is the difference between the averaged waveforms obtained with the same stimulus presented as the standard (panel A) versus the deviant (panel B; Martin et al., 2007; Ponton & Don, 1995).

As with the EALR and EACC data collection procedures, subjects are typically given a closed-captioned video to watch to keep them engaged, and are instructed to ignore the auditory stimuli. Recording techniques are generally the same as those described above for the EALR and EACC (Kraus et al., 1993).

### Clinical Uses

Like the EACC, the eMMN may be clinically useful for providing an objective indication that a stimulus difference was detected by the central auditory system, and may have some utility in predicting speech perception ability. Kraus et al. (1993) were the first to report on measuring the eMMN in cochlear implant recipients. They successfully recorded eMMNs for a /da/-/ta/ stimulus pair in eight adult implant recipients of the Nucleus 22 who were "good users" of the device. The single "poor user" did not have a measurable eMMN for the same stimulus pair. Similar results were reported by Groenen, Snik, and van den Broek (1996), who found measurable eMMNs in a group of good performers but not for a group of "moderate performers." Finally, Kileny, Boerst, and Zwolan (1997) showed a significant negative correlation between speech perception (GASP sentences) and eMMN latency and amplitude in a group of children with cochlear implants, where better performance was found for individuals with shorter latencies and larger amplitudes. In contrast, Wable et al. (2000) found no relation between eMMN and speech perception or electrode discrimination ability. Ponton and Don (1995) showed measurable eMMNs for stimulation of different electrode pairs in a small group of cochlear implant recipients, which suggests that pitch differences between the electrodes were perceived. However, the magnitude of the eMMN was not compared with perceptual electrode discrimination ability in that study. In sum, the clinical utility of the eMMN is rather limited because responses can be difficult to define on an individual basis, and unlike the EABR, the response does not appear to be consistent enough across individuals to develop normative data.

## P300 RESPONSE

### Basic Description

A subsequent component to the EALR is the electrically evoked auditory P300 (or P3) response, which consists of the P2-N2-P3 complex (Figure 10–5). The primary difference between the P300 and the EALR, EACC, and eMMN is that the P300 is an endogenous response that requires the listener to attend to the stimulus and actively participate in the task. As such, it involves auditory detection/differentiation mechanisms as well as cognitive processes. The P300 response occurs at a latency of approximately 300 to 750 ms (Beynon et al., 2002) and can be up to twice the amplitude of the N1-P2 wave (Hall, 1992). The P300 is much larger and thus easier to resolve than the eMMN (Beynon et al., 2002). But again, there has been no movement toward using the P300 as a clinically relevant measure for the same reasons as the eMMN.

### Measurement

For the P300, stimuli are presented using an oddball paradigm as described previously for the eMMN. However, for this potential, the listener must attend to the stimuli. Typically, listeners are asked to track the number of deviant stimuli, whether by counting or pushing a button. Recording techniques are the same as those described above.

### Clinical Uses

Because the P300 reflects auditory attention and discrimination processes, it can provide some

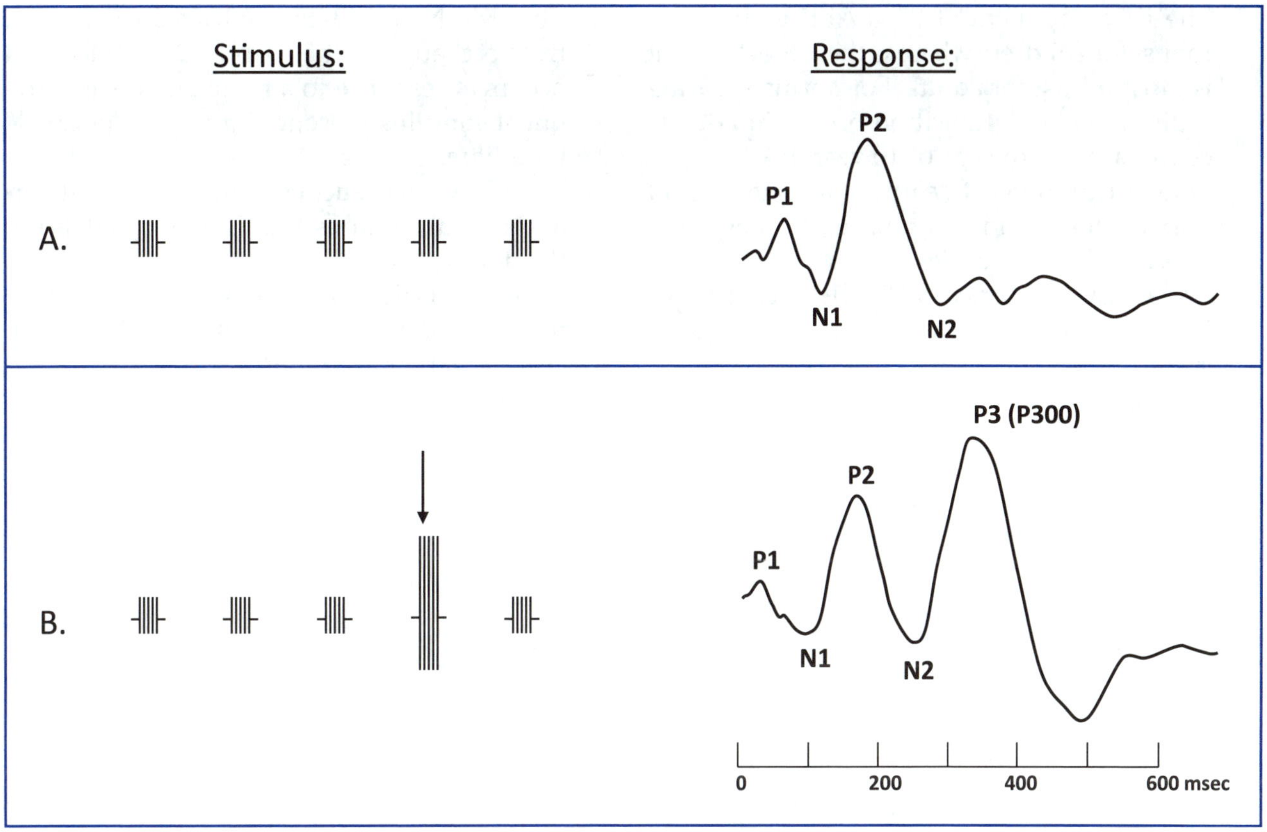


**FIGURE 10–5.** Schematic illustration of how the electrically evoked P300 is generated. **A.** Averaged P1-N1-P2 complex in response to a short pulse train of fixed amplitude. **B.** P3 (P300) waveform generated by the subject attending to intervals in which the pulse train amplitude increases (*indicated by the arrow*).

indication of how speech is differentiated at the cortical level. Several studies have shown relationships between P300 responses and speech perception with a cochlear implant. Kileny et al. (1997) showed significant correlations between speech perception and P300 latency and amplitude in a group of children with cochlear implants. Better performance was found for individuals with shorter latencies and larger amplitudes. Similar results were reported by Beynon et al. (2002), who compared P300 latencies across four different groups: (1) a group of pediatric cochlear implant recipients with open-set word recognition scores of 40% or poorer, (2) children with implants who were better performers (open-set word recognition scores of 65% or better), (3) adult cochlear implant recipients, and (4) children with normal hearing. The poorer-performing children (group 1) had significantly longer P300 latencies than the other three groups. Finally, Kubo et al. (2001) showed a significant negative correlation between P300 latency and consonant recognition for a group of 25 adult cochlear implant recipients. Individuals with better performance had shorter P300 latencies and individuals with poorer performance had longer latencies. This trend held for test intervals at 6 months and 1 to 2 years postoperatively.

## SUMMARY

Key concepts for electrically evoked CAEP measures are summarized below:

1. The EALR is composed of the P1-N1-P2 complex and represents the arrival (detection) of stimuli at the level of the auditory cortex.

2. The P1 component of the EALR is the most robust for children, whereas the P2 component is most robust for adults. For normal-hearing individuals, this transition occurs in adolescence (around the age of 10 years).
3. Longer durations of deafness and later age at implant result in immature morphology and delayed EALR latencies.
4. The EACC is a series of P1-N1-P2 complexes in response to a change in an ongoing stimulus.
5. The eMMN is a difference waveform derived from a change in the P1-N1-P2 complex that occurs in response to a frequent versus infrequent stimulus presented using an "oddball" paradigm.
6. The P300 is also elicited using an oddball paradigm, but requires the listener to attend to the deviant stimuli.
7. Several studies have shown better performance for individuals with shorter P300 latencies and larger amplitudes.

# References

Abbas, P. J., & Brown, C. J. (1988). Electrically evoked brainstem potentials in cochlear implant patients with multi-electrode stimulation. *Hearing Research, 36*, 153–162.

Abbas, P. J., & Brown, C. J. (1991a). Electrically evoked auditory brainstem response: Growth of response with current level. *Hearing Research, 51*, 123–138.

Abbas, P. J., & Brown, C. J. (1991b). Electrically evoked auditory brainstem response: Refractory properties and strength-duration functions. *Hearing Research, 51*, 139–148.

Abbas, P. J., Brown, C. J., Shallop, J. K., Firszt, J. B., Hughes, M. L., Hong, S. H., & Staller, S. J. (1999). Summary of results using the Nucleus CI24M implant to record the electrically evoked compound action potential. *Ear and Hearing, 20*, 45–59.

Abbas, P. J., Hughes, M. L., Brown, C. J., Miller, C. A., & South, H. (2004). Channel interaction in cochlear implant users evaluated using the electrically evoked compound action potential. *Audiology and Neurotology, 9*, 203–213.

Abbas, P. J., & Miller, C. A. (2004). Biophysics and physiology. In F.-G. Zeng, A. N. Popper, & R. R. Fay (Eds.), *Cochlear implants: Auditory prostheses and electric hearing* (pp. 149–212). New York, NY: Springer-Verlag.

Akin, I., Kuran, G., Saka, C., & Vural, M. (2006). Preliminary results on correlation between neural response imaging and "most comfortable levels" in cochlear implantation. *Journal of Laryngology and Otology, 120*, 261–265.

Allum, J. H. J., Greisiger, R., & Probst, R. (2002). Relationship of intraoperative electrically evoked stapedius reflex thresholds to maximum comfortable loudness levels of children with cochlear implants. *International Journal of Audiology, 41*(2), 93–99.

Battmer, R.-D., Laszig, R., & Lehnhardt, E. (1990). Electrically elicited stapedius reflex in cochlear implant patients. *Ear and Hearing, 11*(5), 370–374.

Beynon, A. J., Snik, A. F. M., & van den Broek, P. (2002). Evaluation of cochlear implant benefit with auditory cortical evoked potentials. *International Journal of Audiology, 41*, 429–435.

Bierer, J. A., & Faulkner, K. F. (2010). Identifying cochlear implant channels with poor electrode-neuron interface: Partial tripolar, single-channel thresholds and psychophysical tuning curves. *Ear and Hearing, 31*, 247–258.

Bierer, J. A., Faulkner, K. F., & Tremblay, K. L. (2011). Identifying cochlear implant channels with poor electrode-neuron interfaces: Electrically evoked auditory brain stem responses measured with the partial tripolar configuration. *Ear and Hearing, 32*, 436–444.

Bierer, J. A., & Middlebrooks, J. C. (2002). Auditory cortical images of cochlear-implant stimuli: Dependence on electrode configuration. *Journal of Neurophysiology, 87*, 478–492.

Bierer, J. A., & Middlebrooks, J. C. (2004). Cortical responses to cochlear implant stimulation: Channel interaction. *Journal of the Association for Research in Otolaryngology, 5*, 32–48.

Boëx, C., de Balthasar, C., Kós, M.-I., and Pelizzone, M. (2003). Electrical field interactions in different cochlear implant systems. *Journal of the Acoustical Society of America, 114*, 2049–2057.

Bonham, B. H., & Litvak, L. M. (2008). Current focusing and steering: Modeling, physiology, and psychophysics. *Hearing Research, 242*, 141–153.

Botros, A., & Psarros, C. (2010a). Neural Response Telemetry reconsidered: I. The relevance of ECAP threshold profiles and scaled profiles to cochlear implant fitting. *Ear and Hearing, 31*, 367–379.

Botros, A. & Psarros, C. (2010b). Neural Response Telemetry reconsidered: II. The influence of neural population on the ECAP recovery function and refractoriness. *Ear and Hearing, 31*, 380–391.

Botros, A., van Dijk, B., & Killian, M. (2007). AutoNRT™: An automated system that measures ECAP thresholds with the Nucleus Freedom™ cochlear implant via machine intelligence. *Artificial Intelligence in Medicine, 40*, 15–28.

Boymans, M., Goverts, S. T., Kramer, S. E., Festen, J. M., & Dreschler, W. A. (2008). A prospective multi-centre study of the benefits of bilateral hearing aids. *Ear and Hearing, 29*, 930–941.

Bresnihan, M., Norman, G., Scott, F., & Viani, L. (2001). Measurement of comfort levels by means of electrical stapedial reflex in children. *Archives of Otolaryngology—Head and Neck Surgery, 127*, 963–966.

Briaire, J. J., & Frijns, J. H. M. (2000). Field patterns in a 3D tapered spiral model of the electrically stimulated cochlea. *Hearing Research, 148*, 18–30.

Brown, C. J., Abbas, P. J., Fryauf-Bertschy, H., Kelsay, D., & Gantz, B. J. (1994). Intraoperative and postoperative electrically evoked auditory brain stem responses in Nucleus cochlear implant users: Implications for the fitting process. *Ear and Hearing, 15*, 168–176.

Brown, C. J., Abbas, P. J., & Gantz, B. J. (1998). Preliminary experience with Neural Response Telemetry in the Nucleus CI24M cochlear implant. *American Journal of Otology, 19*, 320–327.

Brown, C. J., Etler, C., He, S., O'Brien, S., Erenburg, S., Kim, J.-R., Dhuldhoya, A. N., & Abbas, P. J. (2008). The electrically evoked auditory change complex: Preliminary results from Nucleus cochlear implant users. *Ear and Hearing, 29*, 704–717.

Brown, C. J., Hughes, M. L., Lopez, S. M., & Abbas, P. J. (1999). Relationship between EABR thresholds and levels used to program the Clarion® speech processor. *Annals of Otology, Rhinology, and Laryngology, 108* (Suppl. 177), 50–57.

Brown, C. J., Hughes, M. L., Luk, B., Abbas, P. J., Wolaver, A., & Gervais, J. (2000). The relationship between EAP and EABR thresholds and levels used to program the Nucleus 24 speech processor: Data from adults. *Ear and Hearing, 21*, 151–163.

Brummer, S. B., & Turner, M. J. (1975). Electrical stimulation of the nervous system: The principle of safe charge injection with noble metal electrodes. *Bioelectrochemistry and Bioenergetics, 2*, 13–25.

Brummer, S. B., & Turner, M. J. (1977). Electrical stimulation with Pt electrodes: I—A method for determination of "real" electrode areas. *IEEE Transactions on Biomedical Engineering, 24*(5), 436–439.

Busby, P. A., Battmer, R.-D., & Pesch, J. (2008). Electrophysiological spread of excitation and pitch perception for dual and single electrodes using the Nucleus Freedom cochlear implant. *Ear and Hearing, 29*, 853–864.

Busby, P. A., & Plant, K. L. (2005). Dual electrode stimulation using the Nucleus CI24RE cochlear implant: Electrode impedance and pitch ranking studies. *Ear and Hearing, 26*, 504–511.

Busby, P. A., Plant, K. L., & Whitford (2002). Electrode impedance in adults and children using the Nucleus 24 cochlear implant system. *Cochlear Implants International, 3*(2), 87–103.

Cafarelli Dees, D., Dillier, N., Lai, W. K., von Wallenberg, E., van Dijk, B., Akdas, F., . . . Smoorenburg, G. F. (2005). Normative findings of electrically evoked compound action potential measurements using the Neural Response Telemetry of the Nucleus CI24M cochlear implant system. *Audiology and Neurotology, 10*, 105–116.

Caner, G., Olgun, L., Gültekin, G., & Balaban, M. (2007). Optimizing fitting in children using objective measures such as neural response imaging and electrically evoked stapedius reflex threshold. *Otology and Neurotology, 28*, 637–640.

Carlson, M. L., Archibald, D. J., Dabade, T. S., Gifford, R. H., Neff, B. A., Beatty, C. W., . . . Driscoll, C. L. W. (2010). Prevalence and timing of individual cochlear implant electrode failures. *Otology and Neurotology, 31*, 893–898.

Cartee, L. A., van den Honert, C., Finley, C. C., & Miller, R. L. (2000). Evaluation of a model of the cochlear neural membrane. I. Physiological measurement of membrane characteristics in response to intrameatal electrical stimulation. *Hearing Research, 146*, 143–152.

Carter, A. S., Noe, C. M., & Wilson, R. H. (2001). Listeners who prefer monaural to binaural hearing aids. *Journal of the American Academy of Audiology, 12*(5), 261–272.

Clark, G. M. (2003). *Cochlear implants: Fundamentals and applications*. New York, NY: Springer-Verlag.

Clark, G. M., Shute, S. A., Shepherd, R. K., & Carter, T. D. (1995). Cochlear implantation: Osteoneogenesis, electrode-tissue impedance, and residual hearing. *Annals of Otology, Rhinology, and Larnygology, 104* (Suppl. 166), 40–42.

Cohen, L. T., Richardson, L. M., Saunders, E., & Cowan, R. S. C. (2003). Spatial spread of neural excitation in cochlear implant recipients: Comparison of improved ECAP method and psychophysical forward masking. *Hearing Research, 179*, 72–87.

Cohen, L. T., Saunders, E., & Richardson, L. M. (2004). Spatial spread of neural excitation: Comparison of compound action potential and forward-masking data in cochlear implant recipients. *International Journal of Audiology, 43*, 346–355.

Cullington, H. E. (2000). Preliminary neural response telemetry results. *British Journal of Audiology, 34*, 131–140.

Cullington, H. E., & Clarke, G. P. (1997). Integrity testing of cochlear implants in the awake child. *British Journal of Audiology, 31*, 247–256.

Day, G. A., Browning, G. G., & Gatehouse, S. (1988). Benefit from binaural hearing aids in individuals with a severe hearing impairment. *British Journal of Audiology, 22*(4), 273–277.

de Balthasar, C., Boëx , C., Cosendai, G., Valentini, A., Sigrist, A., & Pelizzone, M. (2003). Channel interactions with high-rate biphasic electrical stimulation in cochlear implant subjects. *Hearing Research, 182*, 77–87.

De Ceulaer, G., Johnson, S., Yperman, M., Daemers, K., Offeciers, F. E., O'Donoghue, G. M., & Govaerts, P. J. (2003). Long-term evaluation of the effect of intracochlear steroid deposition on electrode impedance in cochlear implant patients. *Otology and Neurotology, 24*, 769–774.

Dillier, N., Lai, W. K., Almqvist, B., Frohne, C., Müller-Deile, J., Stecker, M., & von Wallenberg, E. (2002). Measurement of the electrically evoked compound action potential via a neural response telemetry system. *Annals of Otology, Rhinology, and Laryngology, 111*(5), 407–414.

Di Nardo, W., Ippolito, S., Quaranta, N., Cadoni, G., & Galli, J. (2003). Correlation between NRT measurement and behavioural levels in patients with the Nucleus 24 cochlear implant. *Acta Otorhinolaryngologica Italia, 23*, 352–355.

Donaldson, G. S., Kreft, H. A., & Litvak, L. M. (2005). Place-pitch discrimination of single- versus dual-electrode stimuli by cochlear implant users. *Journal of the Acoustical Society of America, 118*, 623–626.

Dorman, M. F., Sharma, A., Gilley, P., Martin, K., & Roland, P. (2007). Central auditory development: Evidence of CAEP measurements in children fit with cochlear implants. *Journal of Communication Disorders, 40*, 284–294.

Dorman, M. F., Smith, L. M., Dankowski, K., McCandless, G., & Parkin, J. L. (1992). Long-term measures of electrode impedance and auditory thresholds for the Ineraid cochlear implant. *Journal of Speech and Hearing Research, 35*, 1126–1130.

Dowell, R. C., Mecklenburg, D. J., & Clark G. M. (1986). Speech recognition for 40 patients receiving multichannel cochlear implants. *Archives of Otolaryngology—Head and Neck Surgery, 112*(10), 1054–1059.

Eisen, M. D., & Franck, K. H. (2004). Electrically evoked compound action potential amplitude growth functions and HiResolution programming levels in pediatric CII implant subjects. *Ear and Hearing, 25*, 528–538.

Eisen, M. D., & Franck, K. H. (2005). Electrode interaction in pediatric cochlear implant subjects. *Journal of the Association for Research in Otolaryngology, 6*, 160–170.

Fayad, J., Linthicum, F. H., Otto, S. R., Galey, F. R., & House, W. F. (1991). Cochlear implants: Histopathologic findings related to performance in 16 human temporal bones. *Annals of Otology, Rhinology, and Laryngology, 100*, 807–811.

Finley, C., Wilson, B., van den Honert, C., & Lawson, D. (1997). *Speech processors for auditory prostheses*. Sixth Quarterly Progress Report, Nov. 1, 1996–Jan. 31, 1997, NIH Project N01-DC-5-2103.

Finley, C. C., Wilson, B. S., & White, M. W. (1990). Models of neural responsiveness to electrical stimulation. In J. M. Miller & F. A. Spelman (Eds.), *Cochlear implants: Models of the electrically stimulated ear* (pp. 55–101). New York, NY: Springer-Verlag.

Firszt, J. B., Chambers, R. D., & Kraus, N. (2002). Neurophysiology of cochlear implant users II: Comparison among speech perception, dynamic range, and physiological measures. *Ear and Hearing, 23*, 516–531.

Firszt, J. B., Chambers, R. D., Kraus, N., & Reeder, R. M. (2002). Neurophysiology of cochlear implant users I: Effects of stimulus current level and electrode site on the electrical ABR, MLR, and N1-P2 response. *Ear and Hearing, 23*, 502–515.

Firszt, J. B., Holden, L. K., Skinner, M. W., Tobey, E. A., Peterson, A., Gaggl, W., . . . Wackym, P. A. (2004). Recognition of speech presented at soft to loud levels by adult cochlear implant recipients of three cochlear implant systems. *Ear and Hearing, 25*, 375–387.

Firszt, J. B., Koch, D. B., Downing, M., & Litvak, L. (2007). Current steering creates additional pitch percepts in adult cochlear implant recipients. *Otology and Neurotology, 28*, 629–636.

Firszt, J. B., Rotz, L. A., Chambers, R. D., & Novak, M. A. (1999). Electrically evoked potentials recorded in adult and pediatric CLARION® implant users. *Annals of Otology, Rhinology, and Laryngology, 108*, 58–63.

Franck, K. H. (2002). A model of a Nucleus 24 cochlear implant fitting protocol based on the electrically evoked whole nerve action potential. *Ear and Hearing, 23*, 67S–71S.

Franck, K. H., & Norton, S. J. (2001). Estimation of psychophysical levels using the electrically evoked compound action potential measured with the neural response telemetry capabilities of Cochlear Corporation's CI24M device. *Ear and Hearing, 22*, 289–299.

Friesen, L. M., & Tremblay, K. L. (2006). Acoustic change complexes recorded in adult cochlear implant listeners. *Ear and Hearing, 27*, 678–685.

Frijns, J. H. M., Briaire, J. J., de Laat, J. A. P. M., & Grote, J. J. (2002). Initial evaluation of the Clarion CII cochlear implant: Speech perception and neural response imaging. *Ear and Hearing, 23*, 184–197.

Frijns, J. H. M., de Snoo, S. L., & Schoonhoven, R. (1995). Potential distributions and neural excitation patterns in a rotationally symmetric model of the electrically stimulated cochlea. *Hearing Research, 87*, 170–186.

Frijns, J. H. M., Kalkman, R. K., Vanpouke, F. J., Snel Bongers, J., & Briaire, J. J. (2009). Simultaneous and non-simultaneous dual electrode stimulation in cochlear implants: Evidence for two neural response modalities. *Acta Oto-Laryngologica, 129*, 433–439.

Gallégo, S., Garnier, S., Micheyl, C., Truy, E., Morgon, A., & Collet, L. (1999). Loudness growth functions and EABR characteristics in Digisonic cochlear implantees. *Acta Otolaryngologica (Stockholm), 119*, 234–238.

Gantz, B. J., Tyler, R. S., Knutson, J. F., Woodworth, G., Abbas, P., McCabe, B. F., . . . Brown, C. (1988). Evaluation of five different cochlear implant designs: Audiologic assessment and predictors of performance. *Laryngoscope, 98*, 1100–1106.

Gardi, J. N. (1985). Human brainstem and middle latency responses to electrical stimulation: Preliminary observations. In R. A. Schindler & M. M. Merzenich (Eds.), *Cochlear implants* (pp. 351–363). New York. NY: Raven Press.

Gibson, W. P. R., Sanli, H., & Psarros, C. (2009). The use of insta-operative electrical auditory brainstem responses to predict the speech perception outcome after cochlear implantation. *Cochlear Implants International, 10*(Suppl. 1), 53–57.

Gilley, P. M., Sharma, A., Dorman, M., Finley, C. C., Panch, A. S., & Martin, K. (2006). Minimization of cochlear implant stimulus artifact in cortical auditory evoked potentials. *Clinical Neurophysiology, 117*, 1772–1782.

Gordin, A., Papsin, B., James, A., & Gordon, K. (2009). Evolution of cochlear implant arrays result in changes in behavioral and physiological responses in children. *Otology and Neurotology, 30*, 908–915.

Gordon, K. A., Papsin, B. C., & Harrison, R. V. (2003). Activity-dependent developmental plasticity of the auditory brain stem in children who use cochlear implants. *Ear and Hearing, 24*, 485–500.

Gordon, K. A., Papsin, B. C., & Harrison, R. V. (2004). Toward a battery of behavioral and objective measures to achieve optimal cochlear implant stimulation levels in children. *Ear and Hearing, 25*, 447–463.

Gordon, K. A., Papsin, B. C., & Harrison, R. V. (2005). Effects of cochlear implant use on the electrically evoked middle latency response in children. *Hearing Research, 204*, 78–89.

Gordon, K. A., Papsin, B. C., & Harrison, R. V. (2006). An evoked potential study of the developmental time course of the auditory nerve and brainstem in children using cochlear implants. *Audiology and Neurotology, 11*, 7–23.

Gordon, K. A., Tanaka, S., & Papsin, B. C. (2005). Atypical cortical responses underlie poor speech perception in children using cochlear implants. *NeuroReport, 16*(18), 2041–2045.

Gordon, K. A., Valero, J., & Papsin, B. C. (2007). Binaural processing in children using bilateral cochlear implants. *NeuroReport, 18*(6), 613–617.

Gordon, K. A., Valero, J., van Hoesel, R., & Papsin, B. C. (2008). Abnormal timing delays in auditory brainstem responses evoked by bilateral cochlear implant use in children. *Otology and Neurotology, 29*, 193–198.

Groenen, P., Snik, A., & van den Broek, P. (1996). On the clinical relevance of mismatch negativity: Results from subjects with normal hearing and cochlear implant users. *Audiology and Neurotology, 1*(2), 112–124.

Grolman, W., Maat, A., Verdam, F., Simis, Y., Carelsen, B., Freling, N., & Tange, R. A. (2008). Spread of excitation measurements for the detection of electrode array foldovers: A prospective study comparing 3-dimensional rotational x-ray and intraoperative spread of excitation measurements. *Otology and Neurotology, 30*, 27–33.

Guiraud, J., Gallego, S., Arnold, L., Boyle, P., Truy, E., & Collet, L. (2007). Effects of auditory pathway anatomy and deafness characteristics? Part 2: On electrically evoked late auditory responses. *Hearing Research, 228*, 44–57.

Hall III, J. W. (1992). *Handbook of auditory evoked responses*. Boston, MA: Allyn and Bacon.

Hall, R. D. (1990). Estimation of surviving spiral ganglion cells in the deaf rat using the electrically evoked auditory brainstem response. *Hearing Research, 49*, 155–168.

Han, D.-M., Chen, X.-Q., Zhao, X.-T., Kong, Y., Li, Y.-X., Liu, S., . . . Mo, L.-Y. (2005). Comparisons between Neural Response Imaging thresholds, electrically evoked auditory reflex thresholds and most comfortable loudness levels in CII Bionic Ear users with HiResolution™ sound processing strategies. *Acta Oto-Laryngologica, 125*, 732–735.

Hartmann, R., & Kral, A. (2004). Central responses to electrical stimulation. In F.-G. Zeng, A. N. Popper, & R. R. Fay (Eds.), *Cochlear implants: Auditory prostheses and electric hearing* (pp. 213–285). New York, NY: Springer-Verlag.

Hay-McCutcheon, M. J., Brown, C. J., Clay, K. S., & Seyle, K. (2002). Comparison of electrically evoked whole-nerve action potential and electrically evoked auditory brainstem response thresholds in Nucleus CI24R cochlear implant recipients. *Journal of the American Academy of Audiology, 13*, 416–427.

He, S., Brown, C. J., & Abbas, P. J. (2010). Effects of stimulation level and electrode pairing on the binaural interaction component of the electrically evoked auditory brain stem response. *Ear and Hearing, 31*, 457–470.

Henkin, Y., Kaplan-Neeman, R., Kronenberg, J., Migirov, L., Hildesheimer, M., & Muchnik, C., (2006). A longitudinal study of electrical stimulation levels and electrode impedance in children using the Clarion cochlear implant. *Acta Oto-Laryngologica, 126*, 581–586.

Henkin, Y., Kaplan-Neeman, R., Muchnik, C., Kronenberg, J., & Hildesheimer, M. (2003). Changes over time in electrical stimulation levels and electrode impedance values in children using the Nucleus 24M cochlear implant. *International Journal of Pediatric Otorhinolaryngology, 67*, 873–880.

Hochmair, I., Nopp, P., Jolly, C., Schmidt, M., Schösser, H., Garnham, C., & Anderson, I. (2006). MED-EL cochlear implants: State of the art and a glimpse into the future. *Trends in Amplification, 10*(4), 201–220.

Hodges, A. V., Balkany, T. J., Ruth, R. A., Lambert, P. R., Dolan-Ash, S., & Schloffman, J. J. (1997). Electrical middle ear muscle reflex: Use in cochlear implant programming. *Otolaryngology—Head and Neck Surgery, 117*, 255–261.

Hodges, A. V., Butts, S., Dolan-Ash, S., & Balkany, T. J. (1999). Using electrically evoked auditory reflex thresholds to fit the Clarion® cochlear implant. *Annals of Otology, Rhinology, and Laryngology, 108*, 64–68.

Holstad, B., Sonneveldt, V. G., Fears, B. T., Davidson, L. S., Aaron, R. J., Richter, M., . . . Skinner, M. W. (2009). Relation of electrically evoked compound action potential thresholds to behavioral T- and C-levels in children with cochlear implants. *Ear and Hearing, 30*, 115–127.

Hughes, M. L. (2006). Fundamentals of clinical ECAP measures in cochlear implants, Part 2: Measurement techniques and tips. *Audiology Online*, November 6, 2006, Article 1717. Retrieved November 6, 2006 from the Articles Archive on http://www.audiologyonline.com

Hughes, M. L. (2008). A re-evaluation of the relation between physiological channel interaction and electrode pitch ranking in cochlear implants. *Journal of the Acoustical Society of America, 124*(5), 2711–2714.

Hughes, M. L. (2010). Fundamentals of clinical ECAP measures in cochlear implants, Part 1: Use of the ECAP in speech processor programming (2nd ed.). *Audiology Online*, November 8, 2010, Article 2347. Retrieved November 8, 2010 from http://www.audiologyonline.com/articles/article_detail.asp?article_id=2347

Hughes, M. L., & Abbas, P. J. (2006). The relation between electrophysiologic channel interaction and electrode pitch ranking in cochlear implant recipients. *Journal of the Acoustical Society of America, 119*(3), 1527–1537.

Hughes, M. L., Abbas, P. J., Brown, C. J., Etler, C., Behrens, A., & Dunn, S. (2003). Comparison of two methods used to measure the ECAP in subjects implanted with the Clarion CII device. *Abstracts of the Third International Symposium and Workshops on Objective Measures in Cochlear Implants*, Ann Arbor, Michigan, June 26–28, 2003.

Hughes, M. L., Brown, C. J., & Abbas, P. J. (2004). Sensitivity and specificity of averaged electrode voltage measures in cochlear implant recipients. *Ear and Hearing, 25*, 431–446.

Hughes, M. L., Brown, C. J., Abbas, P. J., Wolaver, A. A., & Gervais, J. P. (2000). Comparison of EAP thresholds with MAP levels in the Nucleus 24 cochlear implant: Data from children. *Ear and Hearing, 21*, 164–174.

Hughes, M. L., & Glassman, E. K. (2011). A comparison of computer versus human methods of ECAP threshold determination. *International Journal of Pediatric Otorhinolaryngology, 75*(Suppl. 1), 94.

Hughes, M. L., Goehring, J. L., Baudhuin, J. L., & Lusk, R. P. (2012). How well do intraoperative impedance measures predict postoperative electrode function? *Abstracts of the 12th International Conference on Cochlear Implants and Other Implantable Technologies*, Baltimore, MD, May 3–5, 2012.

Hughes, M. L., & Goulson, A. M. (2011). Electrically evoked compound action potential measures for virtual channels versus physical electrodes. *Ear and Hearing, 32*, 323–330.

Hughes, M. L., & Stille, L. J. (2009). Psychophysical and physiological measures of electrical-field interaction in cochlear implants. *Journal of the Acoustical Society of America, 125*(1), 247–260.

Hughes, M. L., & Stille, L. J. (2010). Effect of stimulus and recording parameters on spatial spread of excitation and masking patterns obtained with the electrically evoked compound action potential in cochlear implants. *Ear and Hearing, 31*, 679–692.

Hughes, M. L., Vander Werff, K. R., Brown, C. J., Abbas, P. J., Kelsay, D. M. R., Teagle, H. F. B., & Lowder, M. W. (2001). A longitudinal study of electrode impedance, the electrically evoked compound action potential, and behavioral measures in Nucleus 24 cochlear implant users. *Ear and Hearing, 22*, 471–486.

Javel, E. (1989). Acoustic and electrical coding of temporal information. In J. M. Miller & F. A. Spelman (Eds.), *Cochlear implants: Models of the electrically stimulated ear* (pp. 247–296). New York, NY: Springer-Verlag.

Jeon, E. K., Brown, C. J., Etler, C. P., O'Brien, S., Chiou, L.-K., & Abbas, P. J. (2010). Comparison of electrically evoked compound action potential thresholds and loudness estimates for the stimuli used to program the Advanced Bionics cochlear implant. *Journal of the American Academy of Audiology, 21*, 16–27.

Jerger, J., Oliver, T. A., & Chmiel, R. A. (1988). Prediction of dynamic range from stapedius reflex in cochlear implant patients. *Ear and Hearing, 9*(1), 4–8.

Jyung, R. W., Miller, J. M., & Cannon, S. C. (1989). Evaluation of eighth nerve integrity by the electrically evoked middle latency response. *Otolaryngology—Head and Neck Surgery, 101*(6), 670–682.

Kiang, N. Y.-S. & Moxon, E. C. (1972). Physiological considerations in artificial stimulation of the inner ear. *Annals of Otology, Rhinology, and Laryngology, 81*, 714–730.

Kileny, P. R., Boerst, A., & Zwolan, T. (1997). Cognitive evoked potentials to speech and tonal stimuli in children with implants. *Otolaryngology—Head and Neck Surgery, 117*, 161–169.

Kileny, P. R., & Kemink, J. L. (1987). Electrically evoked middle-latency auditory potentials in cochlear implant candidates. *Archives of Otolaryngology—Head and Neck Surgery, 113*(10), 1072–1077.

Kileny, P. R., Kemink, J. L., & Miller, J. M. (1989). An intrasubject comparison of electric and acoustic middle latency responses. *American Journal of Otology, 10*, 23–27.

Kileny, P. R., Zwolan, T. A., Boerst, A., & Telian, S. A. (1997). Electrically evoked auditory potentials: Current clinical applications in children with cochlear implants. *American Journal of Otology, 18*, S90–S92.

Kileny, P. R., Zwolan, T. A., Zimmerman-Phillips, S., & Telian, S. A. (1994). Electrically evoked auditory brain-stem response in pediatric patients with cochlear implants. *Archives of Otolaryngology—Head and Neck Surgery, 120*, 1083–1090.

Kirk, K. I., Pisoni, D. B., & Osberger, M. J. (1995). Lexical effects on spoken word recognition by pediatric cochlear implant users. *Ear and Hearing, 16*(5), 470–481.

Köbler, S., & Rosenhall, U. (2002). Horizontal localization and speech intelligibility with bilateral and unilateral hearing aid amplification. *International Journal of Audiology, 41*(7), 395–400.

Kraus, N., Micco, A. G., Koch, D. B., McGee, T., Carrell, T., Sharma, A., . . . Weingarten, C. Z. (1993). The mismatch negativity cortical evoked potentials elicited by speech in cochlear-implant users. *Hearing Research, 65*, 118–124.

Krueger B., Joseph, G., Rost, U., Strau-Schier, A., Lenarz, T., & Buechner, A. (2008). Performance groups in adult cochlear implant users: Speech perception results from 1984 until today. *Otology and Neurotology, 29*, 509–512.

Kubo, T., Yamamoto, K., Iwaki, T., Matsukawa, M., Doi, K., & Tamura, M. (2001). Significance of auditory evoked responses (EABR and P300) in cochlear implant subjects. *Acta Otolaryngologica, 121*, 257–261.

Kwon, B. J., & van den Honert, C. (2006). Dual-electrode pitch discrimination with sequential interleaved stimulation by cochlear implant users. *Journal of the Acoustical Society of America, 120*, EL1–EL6.

Lai, W. K., & Dillier, N. (2007). Comparing neural response telemetry amplitude growth functions with loudness growth functions: Preliminary results. *Ear and Hearing, 28*, 42S–45S.

Landsberger, D. M., & Srinivasan, A. G. (2009). Virtual channel discrimination is improved by current focusing in cochlear implant recipients. *Hearing Research, 254*, 34–41.

Leake, P. A., & Hradek, G. T. (1988). Cochlear pathology of long term neomycin induced deafness in cats. *Hearing Research, 33*, 11–34.

Liberman, M. C., & Dodds, L. W. (1984). Single-neuron labeling and chronic cochlear pathology. III. Stereocilia damage and alternations of threshold tuning curves. *Hearing Research, 16*, 55–74.

Linthicum, F. H., Jr., Fayad, J., Otto, S. R., Galey, F. R., & House, W. F. (1991). Cochlear implant histopathology. *American Journal of Otology, 12*, 245–311.

Lo, T.-S., Chen, Y.-S., Horng, M.-J., & Hsu, C.-J. (2004). Efficacy of EABR and ECAP in programming children with Nucleus-24 cochlear implants. *Cochlear Implants International, 5*(Suppl. 1), 47–49.

Lorens, A., Walkowiak, A., Piotrowska, A., Skarzynski, H., & Anderson, I. (2004). ESRT and MCL correlations in experienced paediatric cochlear implant users. *Cochlear Implants International, 5*(1), 28–37.

Lusted, H. S., Shelton, C., & Simmons, F. B. (1984). Comparison of electrode sites in electrical stimulation of the cochlea. *Laryngoscope, 94*, 878–882.

Mahoney, M. J., & Rotz Proctor, L. A. (1994). The use of averaged electrode voltages to assess the function of Nucleus internal cochlear implant devices in children. *Ear and Hearing, 15*, 177–183.

Martin, B. A. (2007). Can the acoustic change complex be recorded in an individual with a cochlear implant? Separating neural responses from cochlear implant artifact. *Journal of the American Academy of Audiology, 18*, 126–140.

Martin, B. A., & Boothroyd, A. (1999). Cortical, auditory, event-related potentials in response to periodic and aperiodic stimuli with the same spectral envelope. *Ear and Hearing, 20*, 33–44.

Martin, B. A., & Boothroyd, A. (2000). Cortical, auditory, evoked potentials in response to changes of spectrum and amplitude. *Journal of the Acoustical Society of America, 107*, 2155–2161.

Martin, B. A., Tremblay, K. L., & Stapells, D. R. (2007). Principles and applications of cortical auditory evoked potentials. In R. F. Burkhard, M. Don, & J. J. Eggermont (Eds.), *Auditory evoked potentials: Basic principles and clinical application* (pp. 482–507). Philadelphia, PA: Lippincott Williams & Wilkins.

McDermott, H. J., & McKay, C. M. (1994). Pitch ranking with nonsimultaneous dual-electrode electrical stimulation of the cochlea. *Journal of the Acoustical Society of America, 96*, 155–162.

McKay, C. M., Fewster, L., & Dawson, P. (2005). A different approach to using neural response telemetry for automated cochlear implant processor programming. *Ear and Hearing, 26*, 38S–44S.

McKay, C. M., McDermott, H. J., & Clark, G. M. (1996). The perceptual dimensions of single-electrode and nonsimultaneous dual-electrode stimuli in cochlear implantees. *Journal of the Acoustical Society of America, 99*, 1079–1090.

McNeill, C., Sharma, M., & Purdy, S. C. (2009). Are cortical auditory evoked potentials useful in the clinical assessment of adults with cochlear implants? *Cochlear Implants International, 10*(Suppl. 1), 78–84.

Mens, L. H. M., Oostendorp, T., & van den Broek, P. (1994a). Identifying electrode failures with cochlear implant generated surface potentials. *Ear and Hearing, 15*, 330–338.

Mens, L. H. M., Oostendorp, T., & van den Broek, P. (1994b). Cochlear implant generated surface potentials: Current spread and side effects. *Ear and Hearing, 15*, 339–345.

Middlebrooks, J. C., & Bierer, J. A. (2002). Auditory cortical images of cochlear-implant stimuli: Coding of stimulus channel and current level. *Journal of Neurophysiology, 87*, 493–507.

Miller, C. A., Abbas, P. J., & Brown, C. J. (2000). An improved method of reducing stimulus artifact in the electrically evoked whole-nerve potential. *Ear and Hearing, 21*, 280–290.

Miller, C. A., Abbas, P. J., Nourski, K. V., Hu, N., & Robinson, B. K. (2003). Electrode configuration influences action potential initiation site and ensemble stochastic response properties. *Hearing Research, 175*, 200–214.

Miller, C. A., Abbas, P. J., & Robinson, B. K. (1994). The use of long-duration current pulses to assess nerve survival. *Hearing Research, 78*, 11–26.

Miller, C. A., Abbas, P. J., & Rubinstein, J. T. (1999). An empirically based model of the electrically evoked compound action potential. *Hearing Research, 135*, 1–18.

Miller, C. A., Abbas, P. J., Rubinstein, J. T., Robinson, B. K., Matsuoka, A. J., & Woodworth, G. (1998). Electrically evoked compound action potentials of guinea pig and cat: Responses to monopolar, monophasic stimulation. *Hearing Research, 119*, 142–154.

Miller, A. L., Arenberg, J. G., Middlebrooks, J. C., & Pfingst, B. E. (2001). Cochlear implant thresholds: comparison of middle latency responses with psychophysical and cortical-spike-activity thresholds. *Hearing Research, 152*, 55–66.

Miller, C. A., Brown, C. J., Abbas, P. J., & Chi, S.-L. (2008). The clinical application of potentials evoked from the peripheral auditory system. *Hearing Research, 242*, 184–197.

Miller, C. A., Robinson, B. K., Rubinstein, J. T., Abbas, P. J., & Runge-Samuelson, C. L. (2001). Auditory nerve responses to monophasic and biphasic electric stimuli. *Hearing Research, 151*, 79–94.

Miller, C. A., Woodruff, K. E., & Pfingst, B. E. (1995). Functional responses from guinea pigs with cochlear implants. I. Electrophysiological and psychophysical measures. *Hearing Research, 92*, 85–99.

Morsnowski, A., Charasse, B., Collet, L., Killian, M., & Muller-Deile, J. (2006). Measuring the refractoriness of the electrically stimulated auditory nerve. *Audiology and Neurotology, 11*, 389–402.

Näätänen, R., Gaillard, A., & Mäntysalo, S. (1978). Early selective attention effect on evoked potential reinterpreted. *Acta Psychologica, 42*, 313–329.

Neuburger, J., Lenarz, T., Lesinski-Schiedat, A., & Büchner, A. (2009). Spontaneous increases in impedance following cochlear implantation: Suspected causes and management. *International Journal of Audiology, 48*, 233–239.

Newbold, C., Richardson, R., Huang, C. Q., Milojevic, D., Cowan, R., & Shepherd, R. (2004). An in vitro model for investigating impedance changes with cell growth and electrical stimulation: implications for cochlear implants. *Journal of Neural Engineering, 1*, 218–227.

Nikolopoulos, T. P., Mason, S. M., O'Donoghue, G. M., & Gibbin, K. P. (1997). Electric auditory brain stem response in pediatric patients with cochlear implants. *American Journal of Otology, 18*, S120–S121.

Nilsson, M., Soli, S. D., & Sullivan, J. A. (1994). Development of the Hearing in Noise Test for the measurement of speech reception thresholds in quiet and in noise. *Journal of the Acoustical Society of America, 95*(2), 1085–1099.

Nilsson, M. J., Soli, S. D., & Gelnett, D. J. (1996). *Development of the Hearing in Noise Test for Children (HINT-C)*. House Ear Institute.

Opie, J. M., Allum, J. H. J., & Probst, R. (1997). Evaluation of electrically elicited stapedius reflex threshold measured through three different cochlear implant systems. *American Journal of Otology, 18*, S107–S108.

Ostroff, J. M., Martin, B. A., & Boothroyd, A. (1998). Cortical evoked response to acoustic change within a syllable. *Ear and Hearing, 19*, 290–297.

Otte, J., Schuknecht, H. F., & Kerr, A. G. (1978). Ganglion populations in normal and pathological human cochlea: Implications for cochlear implantation. *Laryngoscope, 88*, 1231–1246.

Özdamar, O., & Kraus, N. (1983). Auditory middle latency responses in humans. *Audiology, 22*, 34–49.

Paasche, G., Bockel, F., Tasche, C., Lesinski-Schiedat, A., & Lenarz, T. (2006). Changes of postoperative impedances in cochlear implant patients: The short-term effects of modified electrode surfaces and intracochlear corticosteroids. *Otology and Neurotology, 27*, 639–647.

Parkin, J. L., Eddington, D. K., Orth, J. L., & Brackmann, D. E. (1985). Speech recognition experience with multichannel cochlear implants. *Otolaryngology—Head and Neck Surgery, 93*(5), 639–645.

Pelizzone, M., Kasper, A., & Montandon, P. (1990). Binaural interaction in a cochlear implant patient. *Hearing Research, 48*, 287–290.

Pickles, J. O. (1988). *An introduction to the physiology of hearing* (2nd ed.). San Diego, CA: Academic Press.

Picton, T. W. (2010). *Human auditory evoked potentials*. San Diego, CA: Plural.

Polak, M., Hodges, A., & Balkany, T. (2005). ECAP, ESR and subjective levels for two different Nucleus 24 electrode arrays. *Otology and Neurotology, 26*, 639–645.

Ponton, C. W. & Don, M. (1995). The mismatch negativity in cochlear implant users. *Ear and Hearing, 16*, 130–146.

Ponton, C. W., Don, M., Eggermont, J. J., Waring, M. D., Kwong, B., & Masuda, A. (1995). Auditory system plasticity in children after long periods of complete deafness. *NeuroReport, 8*, 61–65.

Ponton, C. W., & Eggermont, J. J. (2001). Of kittens and kids: Altered cortical maturation following profound deafness and cochlear implant use. *Audiology and Neurotology, 6*, 363–380.

Ponton, C. W., & Eggermont, J. J. (2007). Electrophysiological measures of human auditory system maturation: Relationship with neuroanatomy and behavior. In R. F. Burkhard, M. Don, & J. J. Eggermont (Eds.), *Auditory evoked potentials: Basic principles and clinical application* (pp. 385–402). Philadelphia, PA: Lippincott Williams & Wilkins.

Potts, L. G., Skinner, M. W., Gotter, B. D., Strube, M. J., & Brenner, C. A. (2007). Relation between Neural Response Telemetry thresholds, T- and C-levels, and loudness judgments in 12 adult Nucleus 24 cochlear implant recipients. *Ear and Hearing, 28*, 495–511.

Pratt, H. (2007). Middle-latency responses. In R. F. Burkhard, M. Don, & J. J. Eggermont (Eds.), *Auditory evoked potentials: Basic principles and clinical application* (pp. 463–481). Philadelphia, PA: Lippincott Williams & Wilkins.

Robbins, A. M., Renshaw, J. J., & Berry, S. W. (1991). Evaluating meaningful auditory integration in profoundly hearing-impaired children. *American Journal of Otology, 12*(3), 144–150.

Rodenhiser, K. L., & Spelman, F. A. (1995). A method for determining the driving currents for focused stimulation in the cochlea. *IEEE Transactions on Biomedical Engineering, 42*, 337–342.

Saoji, A. A., Litvak, L. M., & Hughes, M. L. (2009). Excitation patterns in simultaneous and sequential dual-electrode stimulation in cochlear implant recipients. *Ear and Hearing, 30*, 559–567.

Saunders, E., Cohen, L., Aschendorff, A., Shapiro, W., Knight, M., Stecker, M., . . . Cowan, R. (2002). Threshold, comfortable level and impedance changes as a function of electrode-modiolar distance. *Ear and Hearing, 23*, 28S–40S.

Schulman, J. H. (1995). Using impedance telemetry to diagnose cochlear electrode history, location, and functionality. *Annals of Otology, Rhinology, and Laryngology Supplement, 166*, 85–87.

Seyle, K., & Brown, C. J. (2002). Speech perception using maps based on Neural Response Telemetry measures. *Ear and Hearing, 23*, 72S–79S.

Shallop, J. K. (1993). Objective electrophysiological measures from cochlear implant patients. *Ear and Hearing, 14*(1), 58–63.

Shallop, J. K., Beiter, A. L., Goin, D. W., & Mischke, R. E. (1990). Electrically evoked auditory brain stem responses (EABR) and middle latency responses (EMLR) obtained from patients with the Nucleus multichannel cochlear implant. *Ear and Hearing, 11*(1), 5–15.

Shallop, J. K., Carter, P., Feinman, G., & Tabor, B. (2003). Averaged electrode voltage measurements in patients with cochlear implants. In H. E. Cullington (Ed.), *Cochlear implants: Objective measures* (pp. 41–80). Philadelphia, PA: Whurr.

Shallop, J. K., Kelsall, D. C., Caleffe-Schenck, N., & Ash, K. R. (1995). Application of averaged electrode voltages in the management of cochlear implant patients. *Annals of Otology, Rhinology, and Laryngology Supplement, 166*, 228–230.

Sharma, A., & Dorman, M. F. (2005). The clinical use of P1 latency as a bio-marker for assessment of central auditory development in children with hearing impairment. *Audiology Today, 17*(3), 18–19.

Sharma, A., & Dorman, M. F. (2006). Central auditory development in children with cochlear implants: Clinical implications. In A. Møller (Ed.), *Cochlear and brainstem implants* (pp. 66–88). Basel, Switzerland: Karger.

Sharma, A., Dorman, M. F., & Spahr, A. J. (2002a). A sensitive period for the development of the central auditory system in children with cochlear implants: Implications for age of implantation. *Ear and Hearing, 23*, 532–539.

Sharma, A., Dorman, M. F., & Spahr, A. J. (2002b). Rapid development of cortical auditory evoked potentials after early cochlear implantation. *NeuroReport, 13*(10), 1365–1368.

Sharma, A., Martin, K., Roland, P., Bauer, P., Sweeney, M. H., Gilley, P., & Dorman, M. (2005). P1 latency as a biomarker for central auditory development in children with hearing impairment. *Journal of the American Academy of Audiology, 16*, 564–573.

Shepherd, R. K., Clark, G. M., & Black, R. C. (1983). Chronic electrical stimulation of the auditory nerve in cats. *Acta Otolaryngologica (Stockholm), Supplement, 399*, 19–31.

Shepherd, R. K., Hatsushika, S., & Clark, G. M. (1993). Electrical stimulation of the auditory nerve: The effect of electrode position on neural excitation. *Hearing Research, 66*, 108–120.

Smith, L., & Simmons, F. B. (1983). Estimating eighth nerve survival by electrical stimulation. *Annals of Otology, Rhinology, and Laryngology, 92*, 19–23.

Smith, Z. M., & Delgutte, B. (2007). Using evoked potentials to match interaural electrode pairs with bilateral cochlear implants. *Journal of the Association for Research in Otolaryngology, 8*, 134–151.

Smoorenburg, G. F., Willeboer, C., & van Dijk, J. E. (2002). Speech perception in Nucleus CI24M cochlear implant users with processor settings based on electrically evoked compound action potential thresholds. *Audiology and Neurotology, 7*, 335–347.

Spahr, A. J., Dorman, M. F., & Loiselle, L. (2007). Performance of patients using different cochlear implant systems: Effects of input dynamic range. *Ear and Hearing, 28*, 260–275.

Spivak, L. G., & Chute, P. M. (1994). The relationship between electrical acoustic reflex thresholds and behavioral comfort levels in children and adult cochlear implant patients. *Ear and Hearing, 15*, 184–192.

Spivak, L. G., Chute, P. M., Popp, A. L., & Parisier, S. C. (1994). Programming the cochlear implant based on electrical acoustic reflex thresholds: Patient performance. *Laryngoscope, 104*, 1225–1230.

Spoendlin, H. H. (1975). Retrograde degeneration of the cochlear nerve. *Acta Otolarygologica, 79*, 266–275.

Starr, A., & Brackmann, D. E. (1979). Brainstem potentials evoked by electrical stimulation of the cochlea in human subjects. *Annals of Otology, Rhinology, and Laryngology, 88*, 550–556.

Stephan, K., & Welzl-Müller, K. (2000). Post-operative stapedius reflex tests with simultaneous loudness scaling in patients supplied with cochlear implants. *Audiology, 39*, 13–18.

Stickney, G. S., Loizou, P. C., Mishra, L. N., Assmann, P. F., Shannon, R. V., & Opie, J. M. (2006). Effects of electrode design and configuration on channel interactions. *Hearing Research, 211*, 33–45.

Sugawara, M., Corfas, G., & Liberman, M. C. (2005). Influence of supporting cells on neuronal degeneration after hair cell loss. *Journal of the Association for Research in Otolaryngology, 6*(2), 136–147.

Thai-Van, H., Cozma, S., Boutitie, F., Disant, F., Truy, E., & Collet, L. (2007). The pattern of auditory brainstem response wave V maturation in cochlear-implanted children. *Clinical Neurophysiology, 118*, 676–689.

Tremblay, K. L., Friesen, L., Martin, B. A., & Wright, R. (2003). Test-retest reliability of cortical evoked potentials using naturally produced speech sounds. *Ear and Hearing, 24*, 225–232.

Tremblay, K. & Moore, D. (2012). Current issues in auditory plasticity and auditory training. In K. L. Tremblay & R. F. Burkhard (Eds.), *Translational perspectives in auditory neuroscience: Special topics*. San Diego, CA: Plural.

Tykocinski, M., Duan, Y., Tabor, B., & Cowan, R. S. (2001). Chronic electrical stimulation of the auditory nerve using high surface area (HiQ) platinum electrodes. *Hearing Research, 159*, 53–68.

Van Compernolle, D. (1985). *Speech processing strategies for a multi-channel cochlear prosthesis.* Ph.D. thesis, Stanford University.

van den Borne, B., Mens, L. H. M., Snik, A. F. M., Spies, T. H., & van den Broek, P. (1994). Stapedius reflex and EABR thresholds in experienced users of the Nucleus cochlear implant. *Acta Otolaryngologica (Stockholm), 114*, 141–143.

van den Honert, C., & Kelsall, D. C. (2007). Focused intracochlear electric stimulation with phased array channels. *Journal of the Acoustical Society of America, 121*(6), 3703–3716.

van den Honert, C., & Stypulkowski, P. H. (1986). Characterization of the electrically evoked auditory brainstem response (ABR) in cats and humans. *Hearing Research, 21*, 109–126.

van den Honert, C., & Stypulkowski, P. H. (1987). Single fiber mapping of spatial excitation patterns in the electrically stimulated auditory nerve. *Hearing Research, 29*, 195–206.

van Dijk, B., Botros, A. M., Battmer, R.-D., Begall, K., Dillier, N., Hey, M. . . . Offeciers, E. (2007). Clinical results of AutoNRT™, a completely automatic ECAP recording system for cochlear implants. *Ear and Hearing, 28*, 558–570.

Van Weert, S., Stokroos, R. J., Rikers, M. M. J. G., & Van Dijk, P. (2005). Effect of peri-modiolar cochlear implant positioning on auditory nerve responses: A neural response telemetry study. *Acta Oto-Laryngologica, 125*, 725–731.

Vanpoucke, F., Boermans, P.-P., & Frijns, J. (2009). Inferring the electrode trajectory from electrical spread measures. *Abstracts of the 2011 Conference on Implantable Auditory Prostheses*, 78.

Vanpoucke, F., Boermans, P.-P., & Frijns, J. (2012). Assessing the placement of a cochlear electrode array by multidimensional scaling. *IEEE Transactions on Biomedical Engineering, 59*(2), 307–310.

Vanpoucke, F., Zarowski, A., Casselman, J., Frijns, J., & Peeters, S. (2004). The facial nerve canal: An important cochlear conduction path revealed by Clarion electrical field imaging. *Otology and Neurotology, 25*, 282–289.

Vanpoucke, F. J., Zarowski, A. J., & Peeters, S. A. (2004). Identification of the impedance model of an implanted cochlear prosthesis from intracochlear potential measurements. *IEEE Transactions on Biomedical Engineering, 51*(12), 2174–2183.

Wable, J., van den Abbeele, T., Gallégo, S., & Frachet, B. (2000). Mismatch negativity: a tool for the assessment of stimuli discrimination in cochlear implant subjects. *Clinical Neurophysiology, 111*(4), 743–751.

Walden, T. C., & Walden, B. E. (2005). Unilateral versus bilateral amplification for adults with impaired hearing. *Journal of the American Academy of Audiology, 16*(8), 574–584.

White, M. W., Merzenich, M. M., & Gardi, J. N. (1984). Multichannel cochlear implants: Channel interactions and processor design. *Archives of Otolaryngology, 110*, 493–501.

Wolfe, J., & Kasulis, H. (2008). Relationships among objective measures and speech perception in adult users of the HiResolution Bionic Ear. *Cochlear Implants International, 9*(2), 70–81.

Wunderlich, J. L., & Cone-Wesson, B. K. (2006). Maturation of the CAEP in infants and children: A review. *Hearing Research, 212*, 212–223.

Xu, J., Shepherd, R. K., Millard, R. E., & Clark, G. M. (1997). Chronic electrical stimulation of the auditory nerve at high stimulus rates: A physiological and histopathological study. *Hearing Research, 105*, 1–29.

Zimmerling, M. J., & Hochmair, E. S. (2002). EAP recordings in Ineraid patients—correlations with psychophysical measures and possible implications for patient fitting. *Ear and Hearing, 23*, 81–91.

Zimmerman-Phillips, S., Osberger, M. J., & Robbins, A. M. (2000) Assessing cochlear implant benefit in very young children. *Annals of Otology, Rhinology, and Laryngology, 109*(12, Suppl. 185), 42–43.

# Index

## D



## E

## R



## S



## T



## V